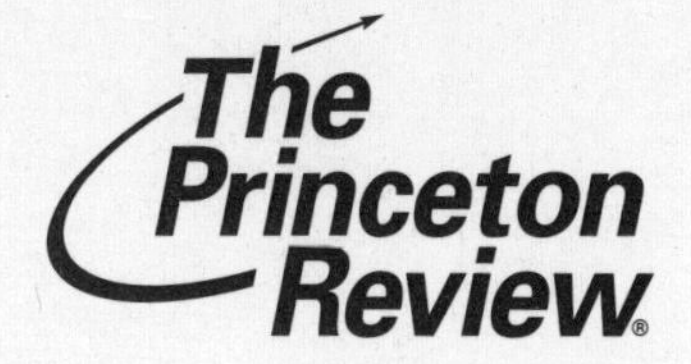

Cracking the OAT®

The Staff of The Princeton Review

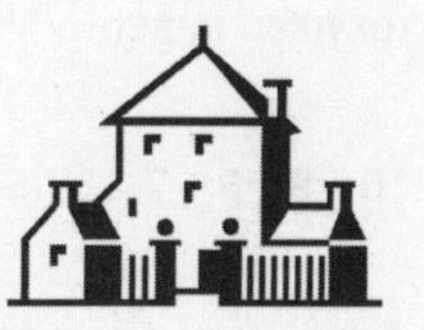

Random House, Inc. New York

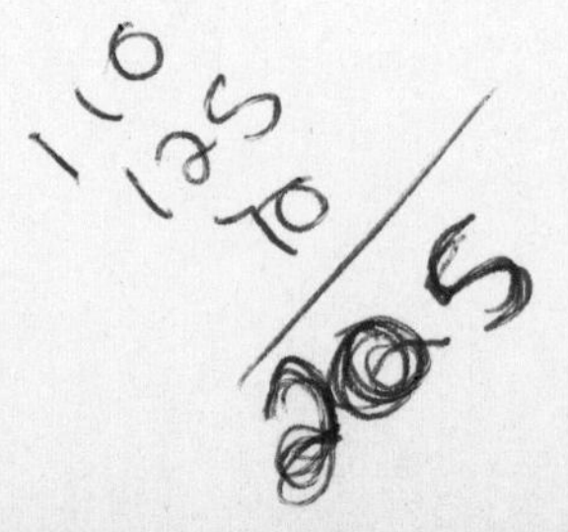

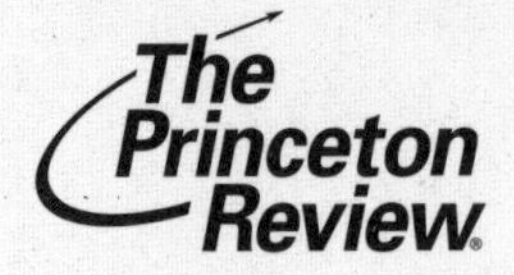

The Princeton Review, Inc.
111 Speen Street, Suite 550
Framingham, MA 01701
E-mail: editorialsupport@review.com
1-800-2-Review

ISBN: 9780375427572
ISSN: 10458725

Editor: Liz Rutzel
Production Coordinator: Deborah A. Silvestrini
Production Editor: Stephanie Tantum

Printed in the United States of America on partially recycled paper.

10 9 8 7 6 5 4 3 2 1

CONTRIBUTORS

The Princeton Review would like to thank: Jes Adams, Jeremy Belch, Laura Braswell, Liz Rutzel, Christoper Stobart, David Stradley, Stephanie Tantum, Tom Watts, and Judene Wright.

CONTENTS

Chapter 1: Introduction 1

PHYSICS **17**

Chapter 2: Vectors 19
Chapter 3: Kinematics 33
Chapter 4: Mechanics I 61
Chapter 5: Mechanics II 85
Chapter 6: Mechanics III 115
Chapter 7: Fluids and Elasticity of Solids 153
Chapter 8: Electrostatics 171
Chapter 9: Electricity and Magnetism 207
Chapter 10: Oscillations and Waves 261
Chapter 11: Light and Geometrical Optics 275
Chapter 12: Modern Physics 295
Chapter 13: Thermodynamics 311

MATH **327**

Chapter 14: Math Overview 329

READING COMPREHENSION **353**

Chapter 15: Reading Comprehension Overview 355

NATURAL SCIENCES **365**

Chapter 16: Biology 367
Chapter 17: General Chemistry 387
Chapter 18: Organic Chemistry 401

PRACTICE **409**

Physics Drill 411
Natural Sciences Drill 423

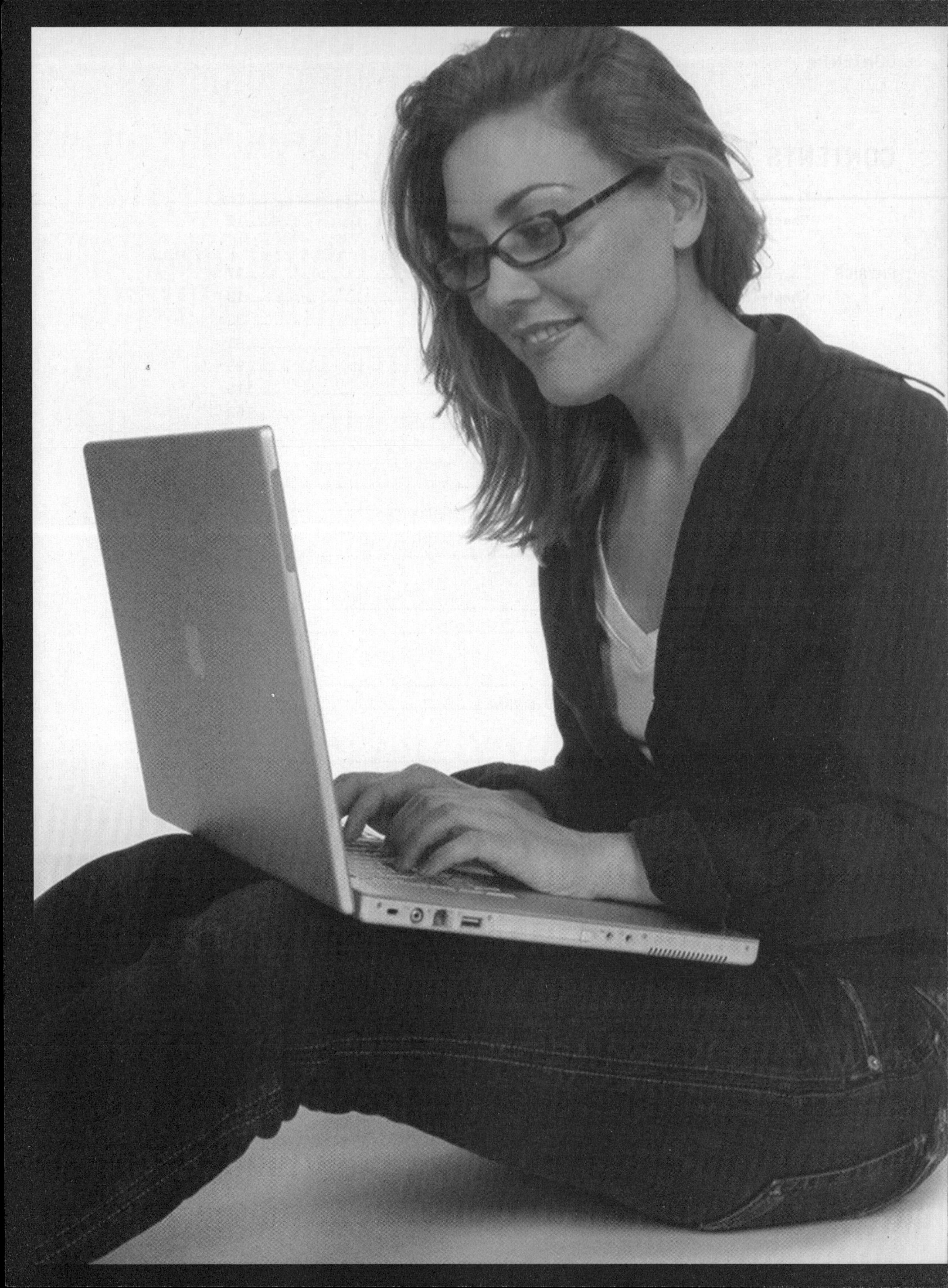

...So Much More Online!

More Practice...

- Access two full-length practice exams.
- Drills for specific strategies and content topics.
- Quick Reviews and lists of keywords to help you study.

Register Your Book Now...

- Go to PrincetonReview.com/cracking
- You'll see a welcome page where you should use the ISBN to register your book. What's an ISBN number, you ask? It's found on the back cover of your book, just above the bar code. To make your life easier, we'll write it out here too. The ISBN for *Cracking the OAT* is 9780375.
- You will then see a page where you can make an account with PrincetonReview.com so that future log-ins will be a breeze.
- Now you're good to go!

princetonreview.com/cracking

Look For This Icon Throughout The Book

Go Online

Chapter 1
Introduction

SO YOU WANT TO BE AN OPTOMETRIST

If you're reading this book, there's a pretty strong chance that you are giving serious thought to becoming an optometrist. Maybe your parents are optometrists and you always knew that you would grow up to be an optometrist. Maybe you were pre-health in college and flirted with the idea of becoming a doctor or a nurse before you decided that becoming an optometrist would suit you better. However you've come to this point, you've taken the required pre-optometry classes, and now all that remains before you can apply is to take the Optometry Admission Test (OAT).

Just the OAT.

The OAT is a long, complex, detailed exam of much of the basic biology, chemistry, and physics that you learned in your pre-optometry courses, together with math that you may not have seen since high school, and reading comprehension that only vaguely resembles any kind of reading that you've done before. And it's this monstrosity that is standing between you and optometry school.

Understandably, you may feel somewhat daunted. The path to a good OAT score is not necessarily as straightforward as the path to a good GPA or to a good letter of recommendation. While much of the OAT is about recalling facts that you learned at some point in school, much of it is not, and the test is as much about how you apply what you know as it is about what you know.

However, we would like to help. This book provides the details of the OAT that you need to know, eliminating the mystery about what is tested and how it appears. This means that we will discuss the core of the test structure and test-specific strategies. We will also review in detail the physics that you need to know, and provide a high-level overview of the other subjects.

If you want a complete review of the subjects other than physics, you should buy Cracking the DAT as well. The Dental Admission Test (DAT) is extremely similar to the OAT, and in fact the biology, organic chemistry, general chemistry, quantitative reasoning, and reading comprehension cover the same content with the same question types. This book will describe what you do and do not need to know from Cracking the DAT and what differences there are between the DAT and OAT, and it will provide the hard-to-find but necessary coverage of OAT Physics. With this book as a supplement to Cracking the DAT, you will have everything you need to do well on the OAT.

We lay it out for you here, because you want to be an optometrist. And we want to help.

WHAT IS THE OAT... REALLY?

Many students approach studying for the OAT like studying for a final exam in college. This can mean cramming lots and lots of science and math facts into your head in the few days leading up to the exam and hoping just to regurgitate what you've memorized on test day. This might have worked in college (although even then it probably wasn't the best way to go about taking a test), but it generally leads to disappointing results on the OAT.

The OAT is not a purely content-based, fact-recall test. If optometry school admission committees wanted that, they could just look at your transcript. What they want to see is both how much you know and how well you think under the intense pressure of a timed admission exam. The combination of the two is what they will try to determine from your OAT score.

The nature of the test impacts how you must study for it. Making lots of flashcards to memorize o-chem reactions (or whatever) will help you get part of the way on this exam, but it will only get you part of the way. After all, there are no facts to memorize for reading comprehension, and even on the sciences and math, you must be able to apply your knowledge to (potentially) new situations. So what else do you have to do to study for this exam, other than memorize lots of facts?

You must also practice applying the knowledge that you have to OAT-style questions. Taking the OAT is a skill in itself, and this skill, like any other, requires practice. This is much like learning to play a musical instrument or speak a foreign language; you learn to play the piano by practicing playing for an hour or two every day, not by reading about playing the piano all day before a big recital. This book contains a great many practice questions inside, and more are available online, as well. Other questions are available from the makers of the test, the American Dental Association (ADA) directly, as well. (The test is sponsored by the Association of Schools and Colleges of Optometry, ASCO, but it is actually made by ADA, which is part of why it looks so much like the DAT.) Practice as much as you can, because it is through practice that you will get better and your score will improve.

HOW TO USE THIS BOOK

Hopefully, you've picked this book up at the beginning of your OAT preparation, and you have at least two or three months to study before you take the test. If you're planning to take the test in a very short time, such as a week from now, it is unlikely that you will be able to read the whole text and do all of the practice that comes with it. Thus, how you use this book will depend on where you are in relation to your test date.

Further, how you use this book will depend on whether you also have Cracking the DAT. This book is not intended to be complete on its own. We list topics and facts for the subjects that the OAT shares with the DAT, but we do not explain them in detail. The only subject that we explain in detail is physics, which the DAT does not share with the OAT and you therefore couldn't find in Cracking the DAT.

Long-Term Prep with Cracking the OAT and Cracking the DAT

If the test is still at least a month from now, try to read the two books cover to cover, skipping only the Perceptual Ability portion of Cracking the DAT (since the OAT does not have a Perceptual Ability Test). Begin with the introduction, and progress through the sections on the different subjects in a staggered fashion (that is, read a little bit of Bio, then a bit of O-Chem, then a bit of G-Chem, and so on, until you come back to Bio). Work the chapter-end practice questions as you go, since these are important to solidify the information that you're reviewing, and read the solutions both for questions you get right and questions you get wrong, so that you can make sure you understand the proper reasoning for the questions.

Access the online practice material as soon as you can, because the most important thing you can do is take the tests that come with this book and determine your strengths and weaknesses. If you're scoring a 380 in a subject, you probably don't need to practice it much if at all, but if you're scoring a 230, it needs some serious shoring up before you take the test, and you don't know which subjects are which until you take a practice test. Thus, you should not leave the tests until the end of your practice. Take one in the middle to gauge your status, and one near the end for another assessment.

Shortly before the test, you should read the introduction again, because you'll want to remind yourself of test-day procedures, and frankly, you should read the optometry admissions information because you want to get excited for the test! You will do better if you think of this as your first step on the road to a great career in the field of optometry than if you think of this as a horrible, time-consuming, draining, boring, standardized test (which it probably is, but it's better not to think of it that way!).

Short-Term Prep with Cracking the OAT and Cracking the DAT

If the test is very soon (e.g. a week from now), then read the introduction (you could skip the admissions information if you want, although, as noted above, it might be best not to), and take one of the online practice tests. Use this to identify your areas of weakness, which could be as general as "I'm not good enough at O-Chem" or as specific as "I forget how to use sine and cosine in math," and read up on those areas. Make sure that you work some of the practice questions in those subjects.

If you don't feel comfortable with these topics even after some practice, you might consider postponing your test date to give yourself a little more time to do more detailed review and additional practice. However, don't postpone indefinitely, because then you'll never be able to go to optometry school. Choose a specific test date to move to, and prepare for that date. If you learn everything that is in this book and study the practice questions carefully, you will not be surprised by anything on the test, and you should be able to do your best. Good luck!

Prep with only Cracking the OAT

If you do not wish to purchase Cracking the DAT as well, you can use this book as an overview of most of the subjects and a detailed guide to physics. Read through the introduction and the physics portion, working through the problems. While you go, read over the lists in the other subjects, and make sure you know those topics. If you feel uncomfortable with any of them, consult some source—maybe your old class notes, maybe an online resource—to re-familiarize yourself with those topics. If there are a lot of them, though, and you feel you need a complete review, you really should purchase Cracking the DAT as well and use this book alongside that one.

OAT NUTS AND BOLTS

Sections (Sub-Tests)

There are four timed groups of questions on the OAT. These groups of questions are called "tests" by ADA, but we will usually call them "sections." Before these sections is a tutorial, in the middle is a break, and after is a survey, so the overall structure of the test is as follows.

Section	Number of Questions	Time
Tutorial		15 minutes
Survey of Natural Sciences Biology General Chemistry Organic Chemistry	100 total 40 30 30	90 minutes total
Reading Comprehension Test	40	50 minutes
Break		15 minutes
Physics Test	40	50 minutes
Quantitative Reasoning Test	40	45 minutes
Survey		15 minutes

The sections are always in this order. The test is a computer-based test (CBT), though it is fixed-form (not adaptive). You can move around within a section at your discretion, and the questions in any given test form are set before the test begins, just as on a pencil-and-paper exam.

Note that there are a few differences between the OAT and the DAT. Most obviously, the DAT has a Perceptual Ability Test that the OAT does not, and the OAT has a Physics Test that the DAT does not. Thus, you do not have to worry about Perceptual Ability when you are studying for the OAT, and you do have to worry about Physics. This is the reason that the Physics Test is covered in detail in this book.

The two other, relatively minor differences are the number of questions in the Reading Comprehension Test and the order of the sections. On the DAT, the Reading Comprehension Test has 50 questions in 60 minutes, whereas on the OAT, the Reading Comprehension Test has 40 questions in 50 minutes (10 fewer questions, 10 fewer minutes). Also, on the DAT, the second section is Perceptual Ability and the third is Reading Comprehension. On the OAT, the second section is Reading Comprehension and the third is Physics.

2.2

Scoring

You receive eight scores after taking the OAT, six for different subjects and two multi-subject scores. You receive scores ranging from 200 to 400 on the Biology, General Chemistry, Organic Chemistry, Physics Test, Reading Comprehension Test (RCT), and Quantitative Reasoning Test (QRT). Next, you receive a separate overall score for the four science subjects (Bio, G-Chem, O-Chem, and Physics). Finally, the scores for all six individual subjects are averaged, and this average is called the Academic Average.

Typically, optometry schools care most about the Academic Average. Even if the Academic Average is high, though, they will also look for any outlier scores. For example, if your four science scores are each 350, but your RCT score is 240 and your QRT score is 400, your Academic Average will be 340. However, schools may worry about your RCT score, which is 100 points lower than your Academic Average.

However, if the difference is minor, schools will generally overlook it. For example, if your Academic Average is 340 and your QRT score is 330, it is unlikely that any school will give that small difference a second thought.

There are two other important points about the OAT scoring scale. First, it is different from the DAT scoring scale (which is 1 to 30). Second, and more importantly, it was recently (in 2009) re-centered. The original scoring scale was defined in the late 1980's, and it was designed to create a bell curve centered around a 300 (the middle score). After about twenty years, though, the bell curve had shifted, and the average score on several subjects had drifted up to around 310 or 320. Thus, in 2009, ADA decided to perform what is best described as statistical voodoo on the scores to return their averages to 300.

ADA denies vigorously that this makes the test any harder, and it is true that the re-centering did not change the test questions themselves. However, obviously, if the average score on the QRT was 322 before the re-centering and is close to 300 after, they're giving lower scores for the same level of performance. Thus, while the questions aren't harder than they were before, it's harder to get (say) a 350 than it was before. This means that people will generally score lower than they did before the re-centering. Despite this, though, since you're being judged against the entire rest of the applicant pool, and everyone's scores will be lower than before the re-centering, this doesn't hurt your chances in any way. The only reason it matters is that if you talk to someone who tested before 2009, their scores won't easily compare to yours.

You might ask, "What's a good score?" This question is not as easy to answer as you might imagine. It does vary somewhat from school to school. However, a score around the mid-300's is competitive for most schools, and for any more detail, you should consult the specific schools to which you would like to apply. Because of the recent change in scoring, you should look at your percentile as well as your numerical score in order to get a sense as to where you stand with respect to other test-takers.

As a general rule, the bell curve tends to slant down dramatically away from the center. That is, a very large percentage of people score close to 300, and moving your score from a 320 to a 330 or from a 330 to a 340 will put your score past a lot of other test-takers. There is an enormous premium, therefore, on eking out every last point that you can, and we will discuss how to do this.

Non-Scored Questions

ADA says: "Each test includes equating and pretest questions. The purpose of the equating questions is to form a link among collections of items, so that examinee's standard scores can be placed on the same measurement scale. Because of these equating questions, examinee's scores have the same meaning regardless of the test they were administered. Unscored pretest questions are included on the test in order to gather information. This information is used in the test construction process to insure that these questions are appropriate before they are included among the scored items."

"Quote from the OAT Examinee Guide."

What does this mean for you? Well, certain questions will not count towards your score. There is no way to know how many or which ones. However, it does mean that you should not spend too much time on any one question, because it may not even count. As a rule of thumb, you should never spend more than three times as long on any one question as you average on the other questions. For example, if you average about 1 minute per QRT question, you should never spend more than 3 minutes on any one QRT question, unless you've already finished every other question in the section.

Registration and The Test Experience

The OAT is created by ADA, and you can register at www.ada.org/oat.aspx. It is offered by appointment at Prometric computer testing centers, which also offer many other tests, including the MCAT and the GRE (and, in fact, other test-takers in the room with you will be taking many other tests, unrelated to the one you are taking). Appointments are available for a variety of different dates and times, usually including mornings, afternoons, and evenings. Some weekend dates may be available. Convenient locations and dates often fill up well in advance, so you should sign up early (ideally at least a month or two before you are planning to take the test, just in case).

The testing center contains two parts, a waiting room and a secured computer area. In the waiting room, you are greeted by an administrator who checks your identification and signs you in. You must have two forms of identification, the primary a government issued ID with a signature and photograph (such as a driver's license), and the secondary anything with a signature (such as a credit card). Expired identification cannot be used. Test-takers are checked in as they arrive, so you may have to wait a short time before being checked in.

You will be given a small locker in which to store whatever items you brought with you (such as a small snack). Literally anything that you brought with you, other than your clothing and your IDs, must go into your locker, including books, calculators, cell phones, bags of any kind, writing implements, or food. (ADA specifically notes that, among other things, "[g]ood luck charms, statues, religious or superstitious talismans" cannot be brought into the computer room.) ADA is very explicit about the items that can and can't be brought and when they can be accessed, so make sure to read their guidelines before you go.

The security verifications during check-in can be somewhat involved and intimidating, but they are nothing to worry about (unless you are trying to cheat somehow—which you shouldn't, because you'll get caught!). Prometric testing centers are equipped with video and audio recording devices that can see and hear every part of the center, and you will be asked to sign in and out every time you enter and exit the computer room. You may also be asked to turn out your pockets, and other basic security procedures may be followed. Don't worry; they're standard.

During check-in, you will be provided with noteboards, dry-erase markers, and an eraser. These noteboards are typically two sheets of laminated, letter-sized graph paper. The two dry-erase markers are fine-tipped, usually pencil-sized but sometimes larger. The eraser works, but the noteboards often don't erase very cleanly on the first swipe without pressing fairly hard, so don't plan to erase a great deal during the middle of a section. You can, however, get a fresh set of noteboards during the break in the middle of the test, so feel free to fill up the sheets during the SNS and RCT.

Once you are checked in, you will be allowed to enter the computer room. You will be taken to a seat and asked to verify that your name is on the computer screen. At the computer will be a screen, a keyboard, a mouse, and noise-canceling headphones (which are bulky but very effective). The mouse is a two-button mouse, but the right-click is completely disabled. Once you sit down and click forward, the tutorial will begin.

During the test, other test-takers will be checking in and taking breaks sporadically. Test-takers are checked in one-by-one, so even if someone else has exactly the same appointment time as you, he or she will start the test before or after you, and most other test-takers do not have the same appointment time (and are not even taking the same test). Thus, don't worry about anyone else at the center. They are completely irrelevant to your test.

After the test, your scores pop up on the screen instantly, so steel yourself mentally when you finish the QRT. You are also given a printout of your scores. This printout is technically unofficial, since ADA must review them before they become official, though this step is usually just a formality.

TEST STRATEGIES

Strategy will be discussed at length in each the following chapters devoted to each subject, but there are a few overall test strategies that you should be familiar with at the outset.

CBT Tools

In addition to the noteboards mentioned above, you have several on-screen tools that you can use to help you on the test.

1. Mark button—This is available for each question and allows you to flag the question as one you would like to review later if time permits. When clicked, the "Mark" button turns red and says "Marked."
2. Review button—This button is found near the bottom of the screen, and when clicked, brings up a new screen showing all questions and their status (either "answered" or "unanswered," and "marked" or not). You can then choose one of three options: "review all," "review unanswered," or "review marked." You can only review questions in the section of the OAT you are currently taking.

3. Exhibit/Calculator button—Clicking this button will, on the SNS, open a periodic table. Note that the periodic table is originally large, covering most of the screen. However, this window can be resized to see the questions and a portion of the periodic table at the same time. The table text will not decrease, but scroll bars will appear on the window so you can center the section of the table of interest in the window. On the Physics Test, it will pop up a short list of physical constants: The acceleration due to gravity on the surface of the earth, the speed of light in vacuum, and the charge of an electron. On the QRT, the button says "Calculator" instead, and it pops up the on-screen calculator. This calculator will be discussed in detail later, when we discuss the QRT.

It is important to make good use of the noteboards and Mark, Review, and Exhibit/Calculator buttons as you take the test, and some recommendations for doing so follow.

Keep the noteboards organized, and use them for Process of Elimination (POE) during the test (see below for more on POE). During the tutorial, spend a minute or two using the mouse and switching from screen to screen to make sure that everything works as it should (and that the computer screen does not give you a headache).

As you work the test in the first two sections, you should use one noteboard for POE in the SNS and the other for POE in the RCT. As you work questions, on the SNS noteboard, write "1 A B C D E," then write "2 A B C D E" below it, and continue until you get to 50, which should be at the bottom of one side of the noteboard. Then put questions 51-100 on the reverse side. On the PAT noteboard, do the same thing, but number up to 90. In this way, you have answer choices on the noteboard that you can strike out as you're eliminating them, and on the side of the page, you have space for scratch work. Practice doing this with regular sheets of paper before the test; it's very useful but takes some getting used to do it properly.

For the most part, you will use the Mark and Review buttons for the Two-Pass System described below. No matter what else you do, as time runs short in the section, use the Review button to make sure that you have entered an answer for every question before time expires. You should never, ever, ever leave anything blank on the OAT, as the Guessing discussion below will explain.

Process of Elimination

Since the OAT is a multiple-choice test, knowing that one answer is right is helpful, but knowing that all of the other answers are wrong is equally helpful. You might not be sure what the primary purpose of the first paragraph of a reading passage is, but you might be able to tell what it's not, and whatever is left over after you eliminate what it cannot possibly be must be the right answer. The same is true throughout the SNS, PAT, RCT, and QRT.

As you are doing Process of Elimination (POE), use the noteboard. Strike out answers on the noteboard to indicate that you are sure that they are definitely wrong. Leave alone answers that you are not sure about. Hopefully, on the first cut through the answers, you will eliminate at least one or two, and this will leave you with only one or two answers left. If you still have more than one possible option, try to eliminate more until you only have one answer left, and then choose it. Even if you're not sure why the answer is right, if the other answers are definitely wrong, the last answer must be right, so don't waste time worrying about it and move on.

Guessing

There are no points off for wrong answers, so you should never leave blanks; a blank question is treated the same as a wrong answer, but a question with a random guess could be right. On some questions, you can eliminate answers and guess among the remaining choices. For the rest, choose your favorite guessing letter and answer that letter for anything you do not know how to answer. No letter is more often right than any other letter, but there is a slight statistical advantage to keeping a consistent guessing letter if you have no other basis for choosing among the answers. Thus, if your guessing letter is A, guess A for everything. The same goes for B, C, or D. Some questions do not have five answer choices, so if E is your guessing letter, then you have to choose E for some questions and D for the rest.

SCORING AND PACING

Introduction

Many students approach the OAT the way that they would approach tests in school: They attempt to answer every question to the best of their abilities, which in the OAT usually amounts to rushing at top speed through most sections. They expect that they will get almost all of the questions right, and that this is what they need to do to get a good score. Then they are shocked by what their actual score is.

The reason for this is that the OAT is not scored like tests in school. If you are accustomed to getting at least an A– (or possibly a B+) in most classes, and if you normally needed about 90% right on tests to achieve this score, prepare for a shock. A score around a 350 is competitive for most optometry schools, and, depending on the section, you typically need approximately 75% correct to get a 350. Combine this with the fact that there are likely to be some questions that, no matter how much time you spend on them, you just don't know how to answer, and you must come to the realization that you have to approach this test differently than other tests you've taken in your life.

Consider the following scoring grid, which converts numbers of questions answered correctly into scaled, standard scores. (This grid changes slightly from test to test, by the way, but it is often much like this one.) This grid is from before the re-centering, so the discussion that follows will be predicated on scoring as it was then; the point is essentially the same now.

RAW SCORE-STANDARD SCORE CONVERSIONS TEST PREPARATION MATERIALS							
STD SCORE	QRT	RCT*	BIO	GEN CHEM	ORG CHEM	PHY	TOTAL SCI
400	35–40	14–15	36–40	29–30	26–30	37–40	118–140
390	33–34	–	35	28	25	36	115–117
380	32	13	33–34	27	24	34–35	110–114
370	30–31	–	32	25–26	23	33	105–109
360	28–29	12	30–31	24	22	31–32	99–104
350	27	–	29	23	20–21	30	93–98
340	25–26	11	28	21–22	19	29	89–92
330	24	–	27	19–20	16–18	27–28	84–88
320	23	–	25–26	17–18	14–15	25–26	79–83
310	21–22	10	23–24	15–16	13	24	74–78
300	19–20	9	22	14	11–12	21–23	69–73
290	18	–	20–21	13	10	20	64–68
280	17	8	19	11–12	9	19	60–63
270	15–16	–	17–18	10	8	17–18	55–59
260	13–14	–	15–16	8–9	7	16	51–54
250	–	7	14	7	6	15	47–50
240	12	–	13	6	–	14	44–46
230	11	6	12	–	5	13	41–43
220	9–10	–	11	5	4	11–12	37–40
210	8	5	8–10	4	3	10	34–36
200	0–7	0–4	0–7	0–3	0–2	0–9	0–33

*The actual Reading Comprehension Test will have 40 test questions based on three reading passages.

QRT Example and Discussion

Now, let's do some calculations with the above numbers, specifically with the QRT for the sake of discussion. To get what was a competitive score around a 360 on the QRT, you could answer all 40 questions in the time allotted, at a speed of 1 minute and 7.5 seconds per question, and get roughly 70% correct. This is certainly a possibility, and it is what many test-takers try to do.

However, it is not the only way to get this score. Consider slowing down. If you completed only 30 of the 40 questions, at a speed of 1 minute and 20 seconds per question, and guessed on the rest, you would probably get about 2 or 3 questions right from random guessing (since you have a 1 in 4 or 1 in 5 chance, depending on how many answer choices there are). This means that you would only need to answer correctly about 85% of the questions that you attempted (not including the guesses) to score a 360.

Now, a difference of 12.5 seconds per question may not sound like very much. However, bear in mind that if you guess on 10 questions, you get to skip questions that you don't know how to do. This means that you get more time to answer the questions that you know how to do, instead of having to rush through both questions you know how to do and questions that you don't. Your accuracy rate has to increase, but only marginally: You must get 85% right out of the questions that you know how to do, instead of 75% right on all questions, whether you know how to do them or not. It sounds a little more reasonable, doesn't it?

This is not to say that all test-takers should skip 10 questions on the QRT. This is just to say that pacing yourself to finish all 40 questions may not be the best strategy, depending on where you are in your progress. You should make pacing goals for each test that you take. A pacing goal is a total number of questions to attempt in a given section, perhaps combined with goals for times at which to finish each group of questions (e.g. finish the first 10 in 10 minutes, then the next 10 in 15 minutes, and so on). For example, if you just scored a 270 (meaning you got about 15 questions right out of 40), it's fairly unlikely that you will immediately jump to getting all 40 questions right. On your next practice test, you should try to gain a few scaled points, perhaps 20–30, which means that your total pacing goal should be to answer about 20 questions and guess on the rest. (And remember, you'll get free points from guessing: guess on the other 20 questions, and you'll get about 4–5 right, which means you don't have to get all 20 questions right on the 20 you attempt.) This is an achievable goal, and it will improve your score. Once you score a 290 or 300, you can pace yourself to answer more questions, and more, and more, until you get to your desired final score.

Bottom line: For each test, pace yourself to gain 20–30 scaled points from your last score. Skip questions you don't need to get the score that you want.

SNS, PAT, and RCT

Similar advice applies to each of the other sections. On the old scale, a competitive 360 on the Physics could come from guessing randomly on about 8 questions and answering the rest with 90% accuracy. On the RCT, it could come from guessing randomly on about 3–4 questions and answering the rest with 90% accuracy.

On the SNS, pacing is complicated by the fact that the Biology, General Chemistry, and Organic Chemistry are scored individually as well as together. You must watch the clock to make sure that you have enough time to complete Organic Chemistry with the same level of accuracy as you complete Biology and General Chemistry. In order to manage this, you will likely want to take the section in two passes (which is often useful in QRT and PAT, too).

Two-Pass System

In the SNS, Physics, and QRT, you should move through the section in two passes. On the first pass, categorize questions as Now, Later, or Never. Now questions are those that you know how to answer quickly and accurately. Later questions are those that you can probably figure out how to answer, but they will take more time. Never questions are those that you probably don't know how to answer at all, at least not within a few minutes (and you should not spend more than a few minutes on any one question on the test).

While you are categorizing questions on the first pass, complete the Now questions as soon as you see them, and mark the Later questions in some way (either on your noteboard or with the Mark button) so that you can come back to them. Guess on the Never questions, because you don't want to spend any more time thinking about them. On your practice exams, make some indication on your simulated noteboard that you guessed on a question, so that you will know on review why you chose your answer, although this is not necessary on the real OAT.

Then, on the second pass, come back for the Later questions. At this point, you can have a good idea how much time you have left for each remaining question. For example, if you categorize 25 QRT questions as Now and 10 as Later (with 5 Never questions), and if you finish the Now questions in 25 minutes (which is fast), then you know that you have 20 minutes left for the remaining 10 Later questions and should spend about 2 minutes on each question. On the other hand, if you just tried to complete the Later questions as you came to them, you would not know whether 2 minutes was too long to spend on a single question.

Conclusion

In essence, much of this advice boils down to four simple words: accuracy first, speed second. Getting questions wrong quickly is not much better than getting questions wrong slowly; first, get them right, and then you can worry about getting them right quickly. Students who rush through questions that are easy for them to get to questions that are hard (or impossible) for them often make preventable mistakes on the easy questions that lower their score, so first you must focus on answering the questions that you know how to answer, and then you can work on answering the rest of the questions.

Of course, if you do get to the point where you are consistently scoring a 20 or higher on a section and are shooting for an extremely high score, you need to answer all of the questions and get pretty much all of them right. (To give some frame of reference, on many sections you need better than 90% right on all the questions in order to score a 25 or above.) In that case, you don't need to worry about guessing letters, but you will still probably want to take the section in two passes and follow much of the rest of the advice above. Even if you answer all of the questions, there is an advantage to having the last few questions you work be the hardest questions, so that you know exactly how much time you can allot to working them. This might, in extreme cases, mean that your first pass consists of about 35 questions, and the second pass consists of about 5 questions; just make sure that your question sequence makes sense.

OPTOMETRY OVERVIEW

PRE-OPTOMETRY CURRICULUM

Before you take the OAT, you have to take certain classes in college. These are the pre-optometry prerequisites. These may vary somewhat from school to school, but in general, you are required to take at least a year of English, general chemistry, organic chemistry, physics, and biology. Schools may also require classes in calculus, biochemistry, or other fields, such as psychology or statistics.

Most schools require you to have completed a bachelor's degree in some subject from an accredited college or university, though most do not recommend any particular major over any other, as long as you complete your prerequisite coursework. You will also find it useful in the long term to take classes that develop your interpersonal communication and business skills, as well as your core science knowledge. Thus, in addition to advanced courses in biology, chemistry, and physics, you may find it useful to take courses that require extensive reading and writing, as well as courses in statistics, accounting, or economics. Such courses are not required for admission to optometry school, but they are useful to optometrists.

As you are choosing your undergraduate courses, bear in mind that rigorous courses are viewed very positively in admissions. While GPA is important, schools also consider the context in which you earned your GPA. The strength of your overall course history is a very significant factor, perhaps as significant as your personal statement or recommendations. If you took GPA-boosting easy classes, while another student took challenging and rigorous classes, then the other student may get the benefit of the doubt even on a slightly lower GPA.

Also, sometimes students pursue graduate degrees before applying to optometry school. Such degrees are helpful, even though your undergraduate GPA will be the primary GPA considered, not your graduate GPA. Having a Master's or Ph. D. is definitely a modest advantage in admissions, in part because it shows additional academic ability.

OPTOMETRY ADMISSIONS INFORMATION

Applications for optometry school are usually processed through the Optometry's Centralized Application Service (OptomCAS), which is sort of like a Common App for optometry schools. All components of a primary application go through this service. This application usually becomes available in July each year, and you must fill it out in the year before you intend to matriculate. Admissions is rolling at most optometry schools, so applying in the summer, especially early in the summer, is advantageous.

The components of an optometry school application include several numbers (termed "hard factors") and a variety of information ("soft factors" or "softs"). The main hard factors are your undergraduate GPA, potentially with emphasis on your science or major GPA, and your OAT scores, potentially with emphasis on your Academic Average and PAT scores. The soft factors include a personal statement, letters of recommendation (often three), and a resume.

Optometry admission is typically holistic, meaning that no single factor is conclusive either way. For example, even if you have a great GPA, if your OAT is low and your personal statement is written poorly, you will likely be denied admission at most schools. Likewise, if you have an excellent overall application but one portion is a little worse than the others, that weak aspect may not hold you back. However, some optometry schools do have minimum numbers for GPA or OAT scores, so be sure to check the specific schools' admission standards to make sure that you are eligible for admission.

Despite holistic admissions, the hard factors are usually the first consideration in evaluating an applicant. If your GPA and OAT scores are above average for what the school usually accepts, you have a very good chance, but if they are both below average for the school, your chances are low. Once admission committees have examined your numbers, they will also scrutinize the rest of your application. Many also request more information through a secondary application.

If you are in serious consideration after many applications are sifted and many candidates are eliminated, you will likely be asked to interview at the school. The interview usually involves going to the school, meeting with current students and faculty, and being asked extensive personal questions about your career goals and many other topics, sometimes including specific aspects of your application. (If there are any specific weaknesses or if there is anything unusual in your application, be prepared to address it.) Being granted an interview at all is a very good sign, though it does not guarantee admission.

The interview season lasts through late fall and winter after you have submitted your application. Regular decisions (acceptance, rejection, or waitlist) are usually completed by March or April of the year in which you intend to matriculate, although some may not be given until later.

OVERVIEW OF OPTOMETRY SCHOOL

There are about 20 different optometry schools in the United States, and their educational methods are diverse, but some generalizations can be made. Optometry school programs are typically four years long, ending with a grant of the O.D. (Oculus Doctor) degree. The programs usually cover a mixture of classroom and clinical courses. Students learn about optics, visual perception, diseases of the eye, and many other topics relating to optometry. After you graduate, you can look forward to taking the national exam administered by the National Board of Examiners in Optometry.

After graduating from general optometry school, some students decide to pursue specialties. These typically involve one-year or two-year residencies. Additionally, some students pursue joint degrees. Some optometry schools offer Master of Science degrees alongside their O.D. degrees, which may be pursued concurrently or consecutively.

AFTER GRADUATION

Many optometrists work in private practice. This can be in the offices of optometrists, physicians (including ophthalmologists), or health and personal care stores (including optical goods stores). Some work in other contexts, including hospitals. Some teach and do research at universities. Roughly one-quarter of optometrists are self-employed.

In general, optometrists are extremely well compensated. The Bureau of Labor Statistics says that the median annual wages of salaries for optometrists in 2011 was approximately $95,000, and the average annual income for self-employed optometrists was $175,329 in 2007; also, job opportunities are excellent, because the employment of optometrists is expected to grow much faster than the average for all occupations.[1]

—

[1] This information is from the BLS's Occupational Outlook Handbook, 2010-2011 Edition.

Physics

Chapter 2
Vectors

TOPICS IN OAT PHYSICS

Physics on the OAT is the one topic that differentiates it from the DAT, which is why it's set out in such detail in this book. ADA describes the content of the OAT as follows[1]:

- Units and Vectors (4)
- Linear Kinematics (5)
- Statics (3)
- Dynamics (4)
- Rotational Motion (2)
- Energy and Momentum (3)
- Simple Harmonic Motion (2)
- Waves (2)
- Fluid Statics (2)
- Thermodynamics and Thermal Energy (2)
- Electrostatics (2)
- D.C. Circuits (3)
- Magnetism (1)
- Optics (4)
- Modern Physics (1)

You should pay at least some attention to the weight of the topic as you study. Magnetism is fairly complicated, but it is only worth one point out of forty. The same is true of modern physics. You can get a fairly high score on OAT Physics without studying these topics at all. On the other hand, linear kinematics is five points; if you're not solid on the concepts within that area, you're likely to miss a lot of points that you could get. Note also the relatively high weights of units and vectors, dynamics, and (not surprisingly on the OAT) optics. These three topics make up nearly a third of the test.

2.1 SCALARS AND VECTORS

Some quantities are completely described simply by a number (possibly with units). Examples include constants (like –2, 9.8, 0, and π) and physical quantities such as mass, length, time, speed, energy, power, density, volume, pressure, temperature, charge, potential, resistance, capacitance, frequency, sound level, and refractive index. All of these quantities are known as **scalars**, which you can think of as just a fancy word for *numbers*.

On the other hand, there are other quantities which are completely specified only when they're described by a number *and a direction*. Examples include displacement, velocity, acceleration, force, momentum, and electric and magnetic fields. All of these quantities are known as **vectors**. A vector is a quantity that involves *both* a number (its magnitude, which is a scalar) *and* a direction.

—

[1] Source: *OAT User Guide*

Here's an example: If I say the wind is blowing at 5 m/s, I'm giving the wind's *speed*, which is a *scalar*. However, if I say the wind is blowing at 5 m/s to the east, I'm giving the wind's *velocity*, which is a *vector*. (By the way, the distinction between speed and velocity is easy to remember: speed is a scalar, while velocity is a vector.)

Since a vector is determined by a number and a direction, we represent a vector by an arrow. The length of the arrow we draw represents the number, and the direction of the arrow represents the direction of the vector. For example, the wind velocity *5 m/s to the east* might be drawn as an arrow like this:

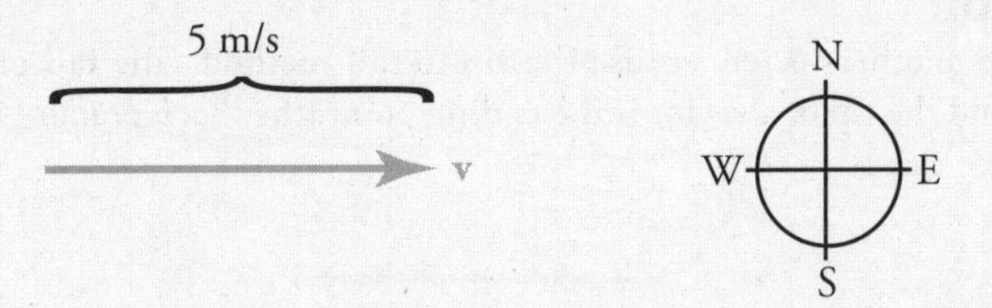

The symbol **v** is the name of this vector. In books, vector names are written as boldface letters; in handwritten work, we'd put a small arrow over the letter—like this: $\vec{v}$ or $\vec{v}$ —to signify that the quantity is a vector.

The number (or scalar) associated with a vector is its **magnitude**; it's the length of the arrow. For instance, for the vector **v** = 5 m/s to the east, the magnitude would be the scalar 5 m/s. Here's another example: If we push on something with a force of 10 N to the left,

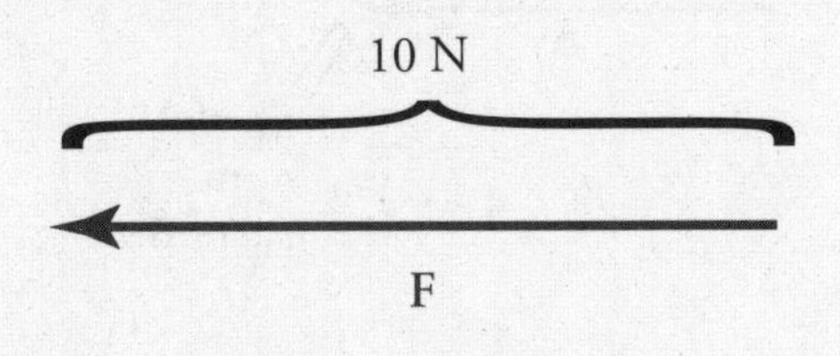

then the magnitude of the vector **F** = *10 N to the left* would be 10 N. Magnitudes are never negative.

There are two common ways to denote the magnitude of a vector. The first is to change the bold letter for the vector to an italic letter. Using this notation, the magnitude of the vector **v** would be written as *v*. As another example, the magnitude of the vector **F** would be written as *F*. The second way to denote the magnitude of a vector is to put absolute-value signs around the letter name of the vector. In this notation, the magnitude of the vector **v** would be written as $|\mathbf{v}|$ (or, in handwritten work, as $|\vec{v}|$) and the magnitude of the vector **F** would be $|\mathbf{F}|$.

2.2 OPERATIONS WITH VECTORS

For the OAT, the three most important operations we perform with vectors are (1) addition of vectors, (2) subtraction of vectors, and (3) multiplication of a vector by a scalar.

Vector Addition

To add one vector to another vector, we use the **tip-to-tail method.** The **tail** of a vector is the starting point of the arrow, and the **tip** of a vector is the ending point (the sharp point of the arrow head):

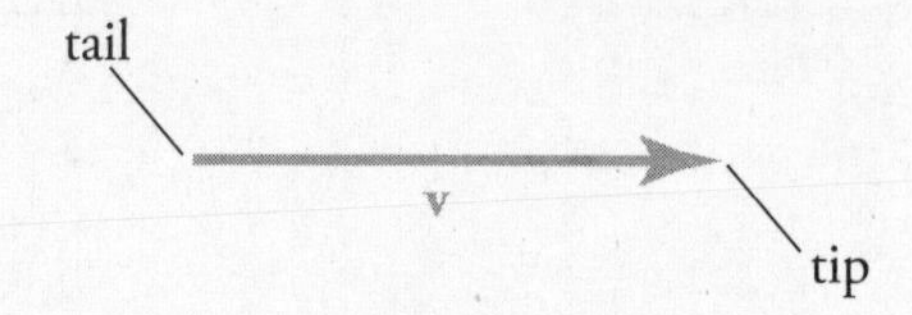

To add two vectors, we first put the tip of one of the vectors at the tail of the other one (tip-to-tail). Then we connect the exposed tail to the exposed tip; that vector is the sum of the vectors. The following figure shows this process for adding the vectors **A** and **B** to get their sum, **A** + **B**:

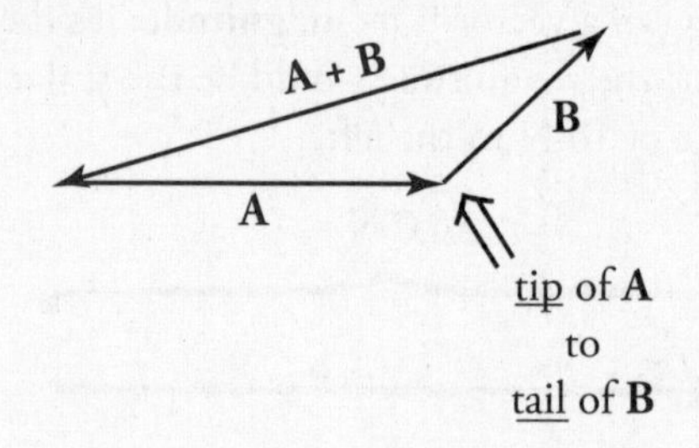

We could have put the tip of **B** at the tail of **A**, and the answer would have been the same:

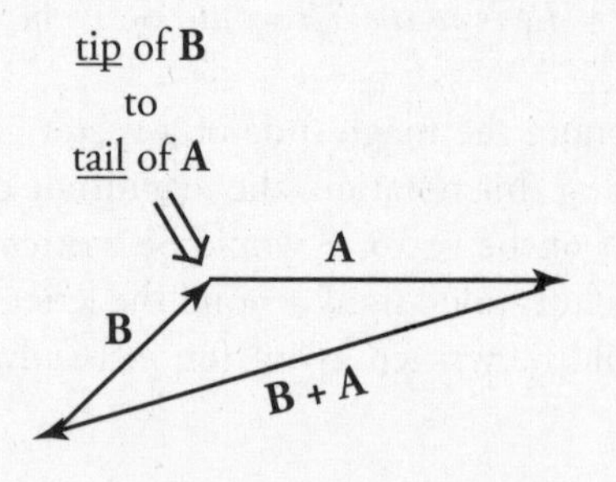

We can see from these two figures that the vector **A** + **B** has the same length *and* the same direction as the vector **B** + **A**. Therefore, the vectors are the same: **A** + **B** = **B** + **A**. We say that vectors obey the *commutative law for addition*; this means we can add them in either order, and the result is the same. (Actually, vectors *automatically* obey the commutative law for addition, by definition; that is, if **A** and **B** are vectors, then **A** + **B** will always be the same as **B** + **A**. There actually are quantities that are specified by a number and a direction but which do not obey the law **A** + **B** = **B** + **A**. Because of this failure, these quantities are not called vectors. However, you won't have to worry about such peculiar quantities for the OAT.)

Vector Subtraction

To subtract one vector from another vector, we use the familiar *scalar* equation $a - b = a + (-b)$ as motivation. That is, for any two vectors **A** and **B**, we say that **A** – **B** is equal to **A** + (–**B**). So, we first have to answer the question: Given a vector **B**, how do we form the vector –**B**? By definition, the vector –**B** has the same magnitude as **B** but the opposite direction:

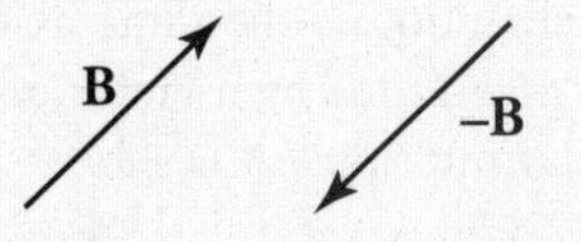

Therefore, to form the vector difference **A** – **B**, we just add –**B** to **A**:

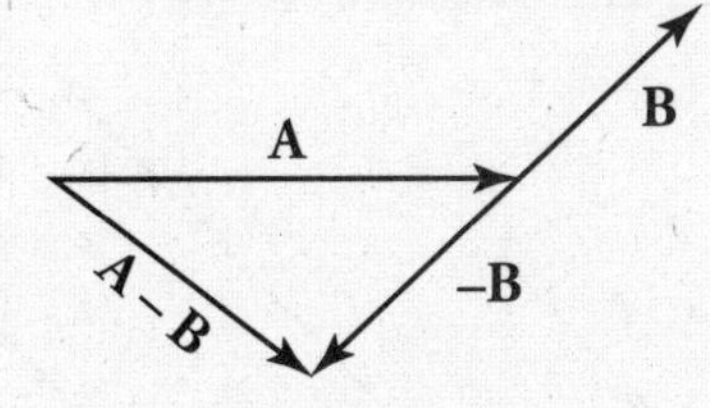

The following figure shows how to form the vector difference **B** – **A**, which is **B** + (–**A**):

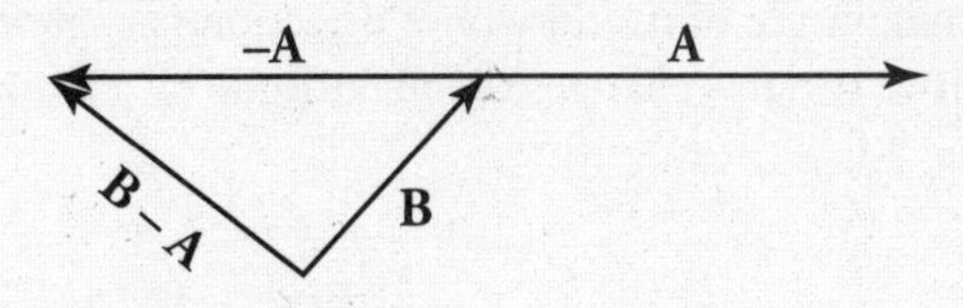

Notice that **B** – **A** is *not* the same as **A** – **B**, because their directions are not the same. That is, in general, **B** – **A** ≠ **A** – **B**; vector *subtraction* is generally *not* commutative. In fact, **B** – **A** will always be the *opposite* of **A** – **B** (same magnitude, opposite direction): **B** – **A** = –(**A** – **B**).

Another procedure you can use to subtract the vectors **A** and **B** is to put the tail of **A** at the tail of **B**, then connect the tips. (Vector *addition* uses the *tip*-to-tail method; vector *subtraction* (by this alternate procedure) uses the *tail*-to-tail method.) If you draw the resulting vector from the tip of **B** to the tip of **A**, you've constructed the vector **A** – **B**. On the other hand, if you draw the resulting vector from the tip of **A** to the tip of **B**, you've drawn the vector **B** – **A**.

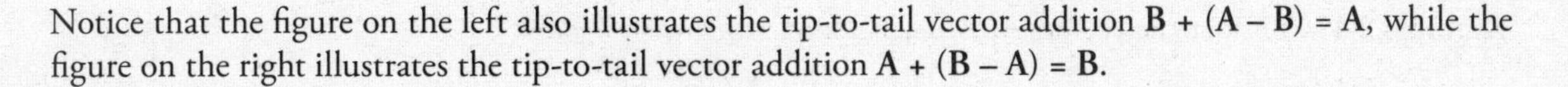

Notice that the figure on the left also illustrates the tip-to-tail vector addition **B** + (**A** – **B**) = **A**, while the figure on the right illustrates the tip-to-tail vector addition **A** + (**B** – **A**) = **B**.

2.2

Scalar Multiplication

To multiply a vector by a scalar, we consider three cases: that is, whether the scalar is positive, negative, or zero.

If k is a positive scalar, then kA, the product of k and some vector A, is a vector whose magnitude is k times the magnitude of A and whose direction is the same as that of A. In short, multiplying a vector by a positive scalar k just changes the magnitude by a factor of k (but leaves the direction of the vector unchanged). If k is less than 1, the scalar multiple kA is shorter than A; if k is greater than 1, then kA is longer than A.

If k is a negative scalar, then kA, the product of k and some vector A, is a vector whose magnitude is the *absolute value* of k times the magnitude of A and whose direction is *opposite* the direction of A. In short, multiplying a vector by a negative scalar k changes the magnitude by a factor of $|k|$ and reverses the direction of the vector.

If k is zero, then the product kA gives **0**, the **zero vector.** This unique vector has magnitude 0 and has no direction. Rather than being pictured as an arrow, the zero vector is simply pictured as a dot.

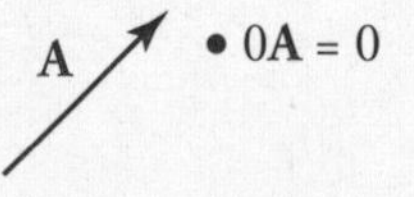

Example 2-1: Consider the vectors A, B, and C shown below:

Construct each of the following vectors:

a) $\mathbf{A} + \mathbf{B}$

b) $\mathbf{A} - 2\mathbf{C}$

c) $\frac{1}{2}\mathbf{A} - \mathbf{B} + 3\mathbf{C}$

Solution:

a) Using the tip-to-tail method for vector addition gives

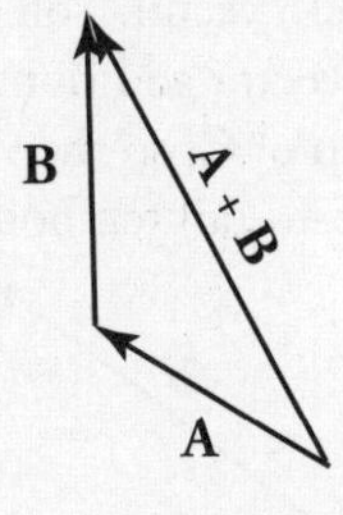

b) Since **A** – 2**C** = **A** + (–2**C**), we first multiply **C** by –2, then add the result to **A**:

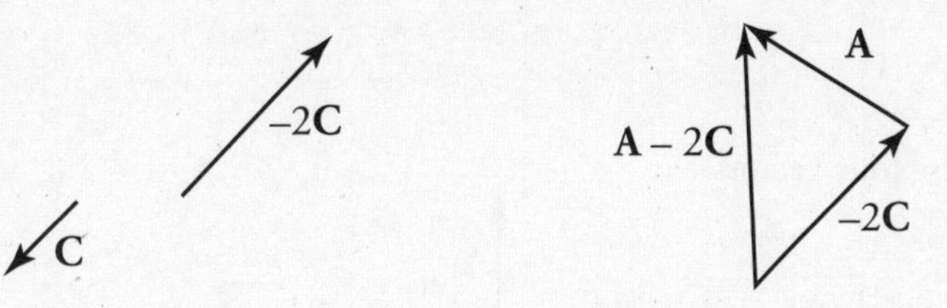

c) We multiply **A** by 1/2, then **B** by –1, then **C** by 3, and add the three results:

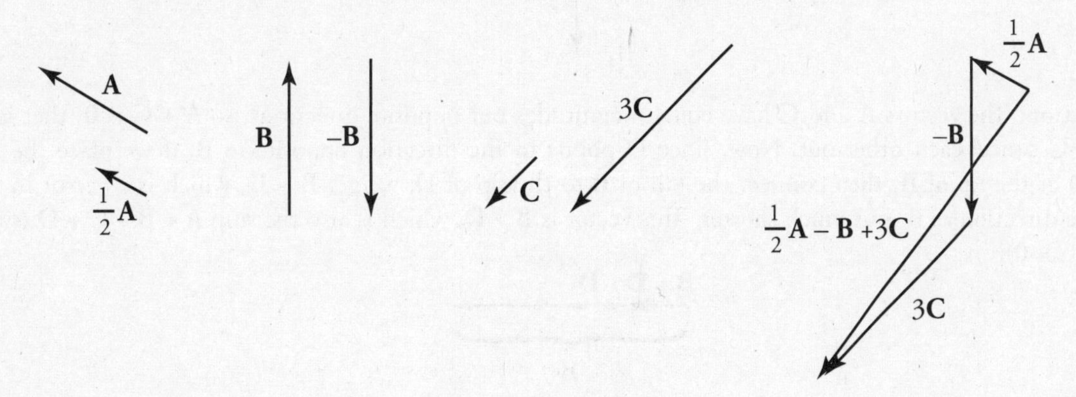

Example 2-2: Consider the vectors **A**, **B**, and **C** shown below:

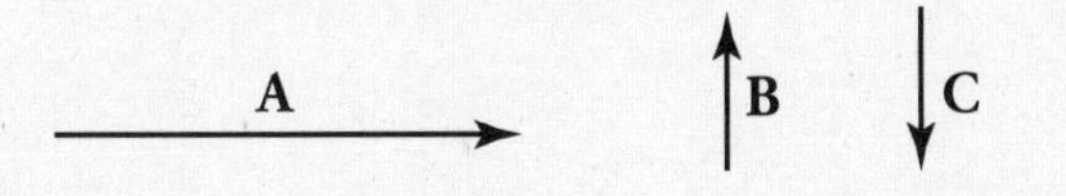

Construct each of the following vectors:

a) –**A** + **B**

b) **B** + **C**

c) **A** + 2**B**

Solution:

a) Multiplying **A** by –1 then using the tip-to-tail method to add the result to **B**, we get

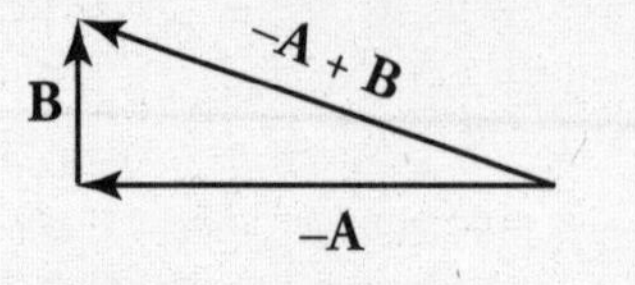

b) Since **C** has the same length as **B** but the opposite direction, **C** is equal to –**B**. So, adding **B** + **C** gives us **B** + (–**B**), which is **0**, the zero vector. You can also see that the sum of **B** and **C** will be **0** using the tip-to-tail method for vector addition: If we put the tip of **B** at the tail of **C**, then the tail of **B** *coincides* with the tip of **C**, so the vector sum is **0**.

c) Multiplying **B** by 2 then using the tip-to-tail method to add the result to **A**, we get

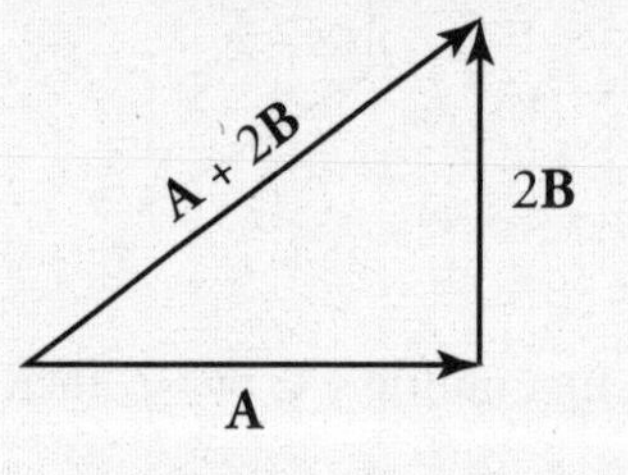

Example 2-3: Add these four vectors:

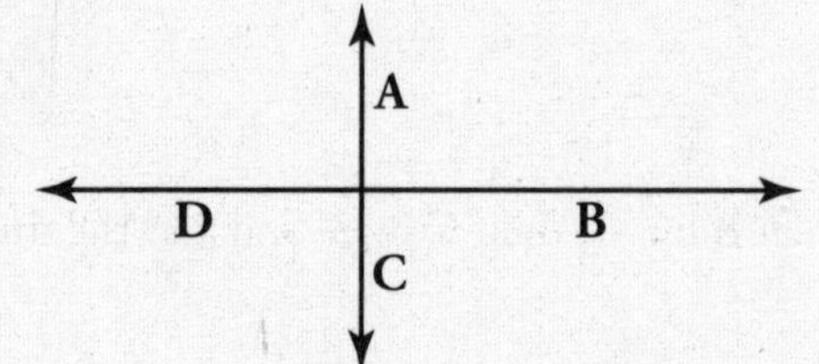

Solution: The vectors **A** and **C** have equal magnitudes but opposite directions, so **A** + **C** is **0**; that is, **A** and **C** cancel each other out. Now, since **D** points in the direction opposite to **B**, if we place the tail of **D** at the tip of **B**, then connect the tail of **B** to the tip of **D**, we get **B** + **D**, which is a vector in the same direction as **B**, but much shorter. This vector is **B** + **D**, which is also the sum **A** + **B** + **C** + **D** (since **A** + **C** = **0**):

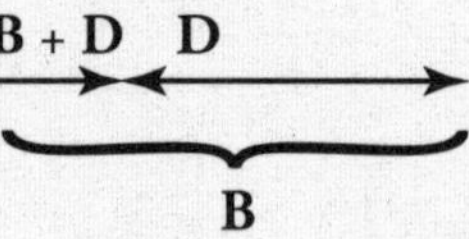

2.3 VECTOR PROJECTIONS AND COMPONENTS

In the preceding section, we performed the basic vector operations geometrically. In this section, we'll see how we can perform these operations with algebra and trig.

Let's imagine a vector **A** in a standard *x*-*y* coordinate system, with the tail of **A** at the origin. We construct perpendicular segments from the tip of **A** to the *x*-axis and to the *y*-axis. The resulting **vector projections** of **A** are denoted by $\mathbf{A}_x$ and $\mathbf{A}_y$; the vector $\mathbf{A}_x$ is the horizontal projection of **A**, and $\mathbf{A}_y$ is the vertical projection. Notice that $\mathbf{A} = \mathbf{A}_x + \mathbf{A}_y$. Therefore, *any vector* **A** *in the x-y plane can be written as the sum of a horizontal vector and a vertical vector (namely, its horizontal and vertical projections).*

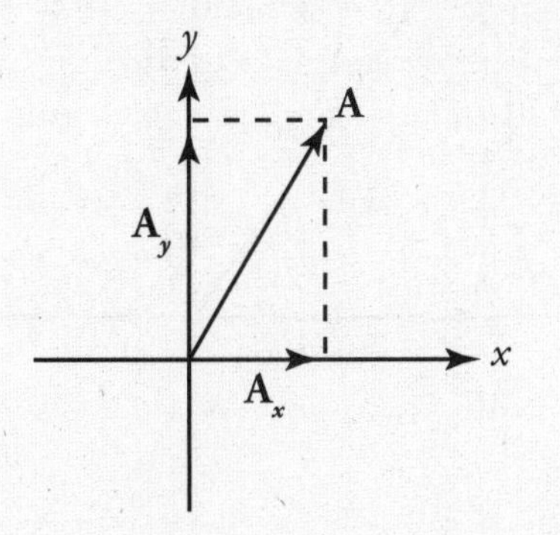

We now want to find a way to write $\mathbf{A}_x$ and $\mathbf{A}_y$ algebraically. Since any vector is specified by giving its magnitude and its direction, we need an algebraic way of describing the directions of these vectors. We do this by constructing two special vectors, one of which points in the horizontal direction, the other in the vertical direction. These two vectors are called **i** and **j**, and each has length 1:

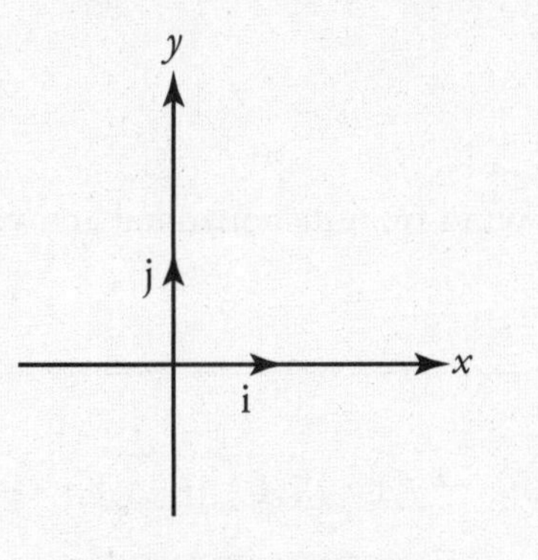

Any horizontal vector is some multiple of **i** ($\mathbf{A}_x = A_x\mathbf{i}$), and any vertical vector is some multiple of **j** ($\mathbf{A}_y = A_y\mathbf{j}$). Therefore, *any vector A in the x-y plane can be written as the sum of a multiple of* **i** *plus a multiple of* **j**:

$$\mathbf{A} = A_x\mathbf{i} + A_y\mathbf{j}$$

These multiples, A_x and A_y, are called the **components** of **A**. Notice that projections are vectors, while components are scalars.

2.3

For example, the horizontal vector of magnitude 3 that points to the right is 3**i**, and the horizontal vector of magnitude 3 that points to the left is 3(–**i**) or –3**i**. The vertical vector of magnitude 4 that points upward is 4**j**, and the vertical vector of magnitude 4 that points downward is 4(–**j**) or –4**j**. For the vector **A** = –3**i** + 4**j**, we would say that its horizontal projection is –3**i** and its horizontal component is –3; similarly, its vertical projection is 4**j** and its vertical component is 4.

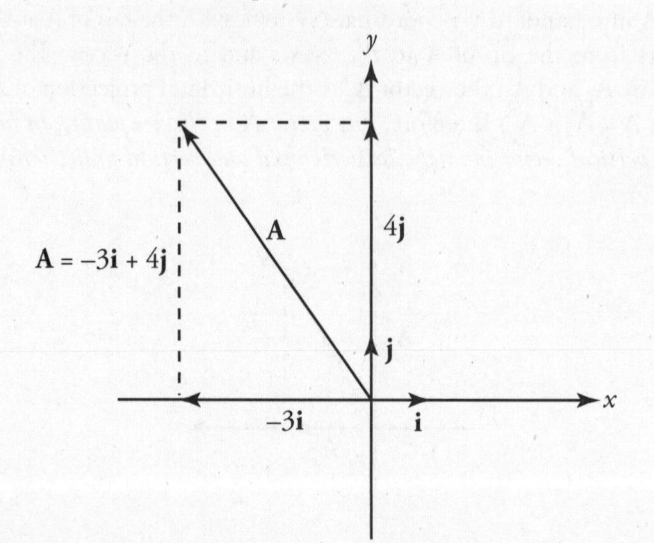

The great advantage of writing vectors algebraically is that it gives us the ability to perform vector operations quickly and precisely without having to draw the vectors (and using such procedures as the tip-to-tail method).

Magnitude

The magnitude of a vector can be found from its horizontal and vertical components using the Pythagorean theorem:

$$A = \sqrt{(A_x)^2 + (A_y)^2}$$

For example, the magnitude of the vector **A** = –3**i** + 4**j** is $A = \sqrt{(-3)^2 + 4^2} = 5$.

Direction

The direction of a vector can be described by giving the angle, θ, which the vector makes with positive x-axis. Since the components of a vector **A** are given by the formulas

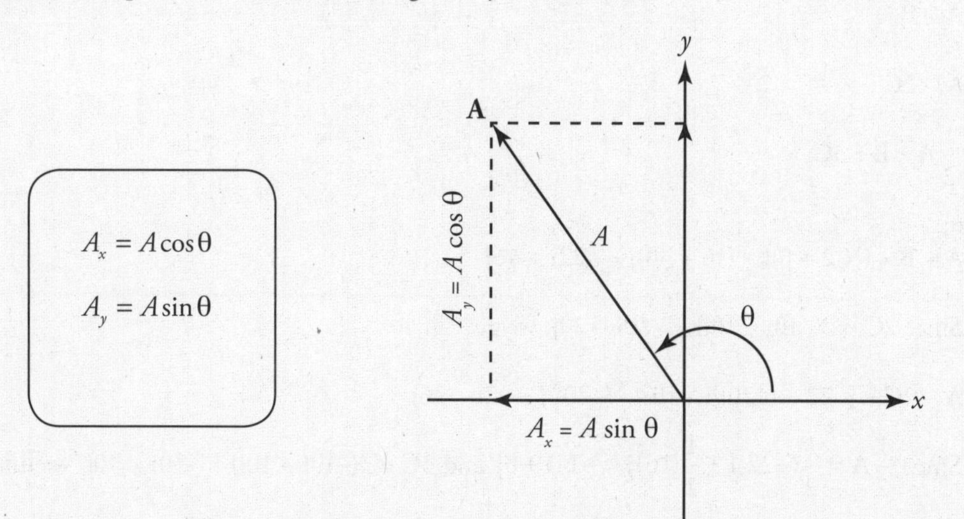

we see that

$$\frac{A_y}{A_x} = \frac{A\sin\theta}{A\cos\theta} = \tan\theta \rightarrow \quad \theta = \tan^{-1}\frac{A_y}{A_x}$$

Vector Addition and Subtraction

The operations of addition and subtraction of vectors is made especially easy by the use of components. To add the vector $\mathbf{A} = A_x\mathbf{i} + A_y\mathbf{j}$ to the vector $\mathbf{B} = B_x\mathbf{i} + B_y\mathbf{j}$, we simply add the horizontal components and add the vertical components; and to subtract the vectors, we just subtract their components:

$$\mathbf{A} + \mathbf{B} = (A_x + B_x)\mathbf{i} + (A_y + B_y)\mathbf{j}$$
$$\mathbf{A} - \mathbf{B} = (A_x - B_x)\mathbf{i} + (A_y - B_y)\mathbf{j}$$

Scalar Multiplication

To multiply a vector by a scalar, just multiply each component by the scalar:

$$k\mathbf{A} = (kA_x)\mathbf{i} + (kA_y)\mathbf{j}$$

2.3

Example 2-4: Let **A** = –22**i** + 16**j**, **B** = 30**j**, and **C** = –10**i** – 10**j**.
Find each of the following vectors:

a) **A** + **B**

b) **A** – 2**C**

c) $\frac{1}{2}\mathbf{A}-\mathbf{B}+3\mathbf{C}$

Solution:

a) **A** + **B** = (–22 + 0)**i** + (16 + 30)**j** = –22**i** + 46**j**

b) Since 2**C** = 2(–10**i** – 10**j**) = –20**i** – 20**j**, we get:

A – 2**C** = [–22 – (–20)]**i** + [16 – (–20)]**j** = –2**i** + 36**j**

c) Since $\frac{1}{2}\mathbf{A}=\frac{1}{2}(-22)\mathbf{i}+\frac{1}{2}(16)\mathbf{j}=-11\mathbf{i}+8\mathbf{j}$ and 3**C** = 3(–10**i** – 10**j**) = –30**i** – 30**j**, we find that

$$\frac{1}{2}\mathbf{A}-\mathbf{B}+3\mathbf{C}=(-11-0-30)\mathbf{i}+(8-30-30)\mathbf{j}=-41\mathbf{i}-52\mathbf{j}$$

Compare this example (and its results) with Example 3-1.

Example 2-5: What's the magnitude and direction of the vector **A** = 3**i** – 3**j**?

Solution: If we draw the vector starting at the origin, then the vector points down into Quadrant IV. Its magnitude is $A=\sqrt{3^2+(-3)^2}=3\sqrt{2}$, and its direction is given by

$$\theta=\tan^{-1}\frac{A_y}{A_x}=\tan^{-1}\left(\frac{-3}{3}\right)=\tan^{-1}(-1)=315° \text{ or } -45°$$

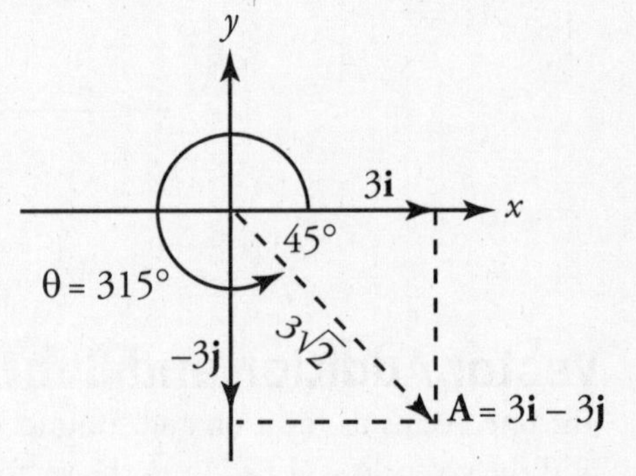

Example 2-6: Let **A** be the vector of magnitude 6 that makes an angle of 150° with the positive x-axis. Sketch this vector, determine its components, and write **A** in terms of **i** and **j**.

Solution: The figure at the right is a sketch of this vector. Its components are

$$A_x=A\cos\theta=6\cos 150°=6\left(-\frac{\sqrt{3}}{2}\right)=-3\sqrt{3}$$

$$A_y=A\sin\theta=6\sin 150°=6\left(\frac{1}{2}\right)=3$$

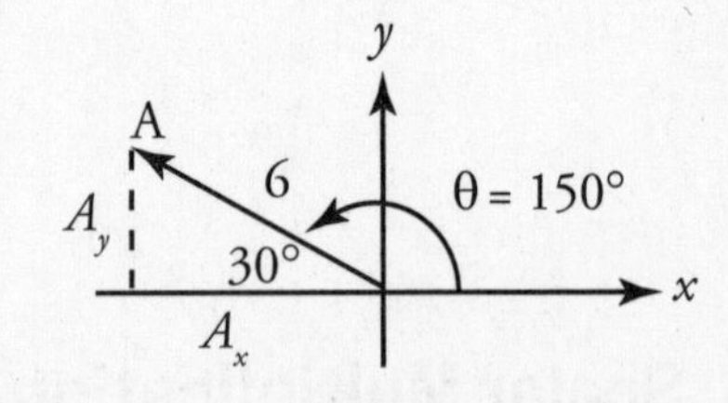

Therefore, since for any vector **A** we have $\mathbf{A} = A_x\mathbf{i} + A_y\mathbf{j}$, we can write

$$\mathbf{A} = -3\sqrt{3}\mathbf{i} + 3\mathbf{j}$$

Example 2-7: Any vector whose magnitude is 1 is called a **unit vector**. (For example, both **i** and **j** are examples of unit vectors.) Let **C** be the unit vector that makes an angle of 225° with the positive x-axis. Sketch this vector, determine its components, and write **C** in terms of **i** and **j**.
Solution: The figure at the right is a sketch of this vector. Its components are

$$C_x = C\cos\theta = 1\ \cos\ 225° = -\frac{\sqrt{2}}{2}$$

$$C_y = C\sin\theta = 1\ \sin\ 225° = -\frac{\sqrt{2}}{2}$$

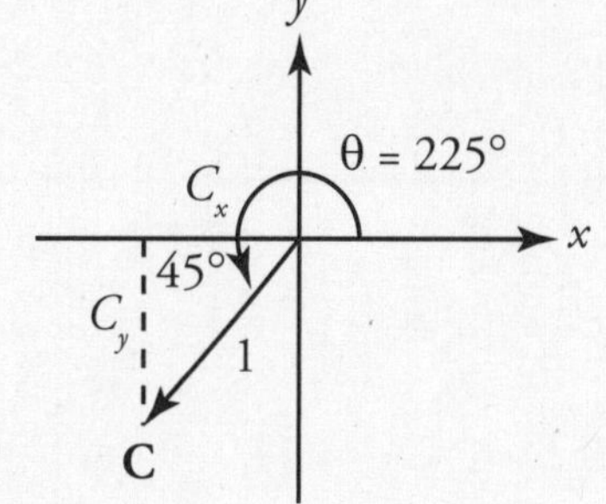

Therefore, since for any vector **C** we have $\mathbf{C} = C_x\mathbf{i} + C_y\mathbf{j}$, we can write

$$\mathbf{C} = -\frac{\sqrt{2}}{2}\mathbf{i} - \frac{\sqrt{2}}{2}\mathbf{j}$$

Example 2-8: The figure below shows a vector **W** of magnitude 100 and its projections, $\mathbf{W}_1$ and $\mathbf{W}_2$, onto two mutually perpendicular directions, such that $\mathbf{W} = \mathbf{W}_1 + \mathbf{W}_2$. Find the magnitudes of $\mathbf{W}_1$ and $\mathbf{W}_2$.

Solution: By definition of the sine and cosine, we have

$$W_1 = W\cos\theta = 100\cos 60° = 100(\frac{1}{2}) = 50$$

$$W_2 = W\sin\theta = 100\sin 60° = 100(\frac{\sqrt{3}}{2}) = 50\sqrt{3}$$

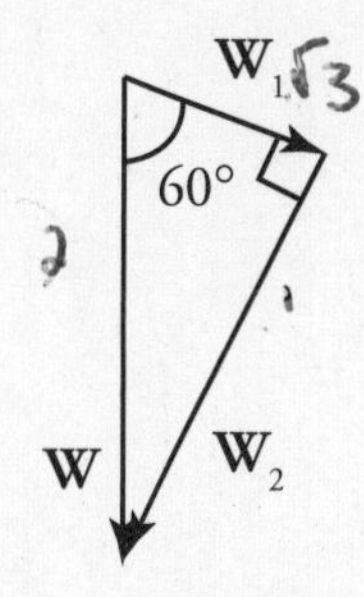

Special Triangles

SOH CAH TOA

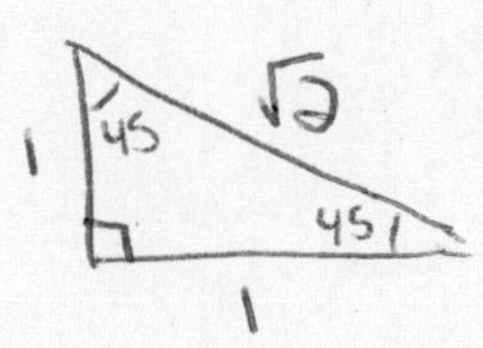

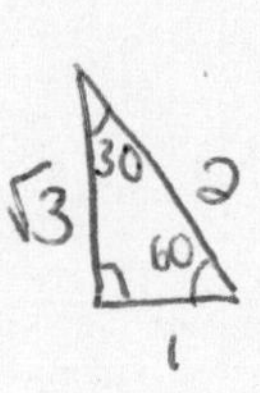

Chapter 3
Kinematics

3.1 UNITS AND DIMENSIONS

Before we begin our study of physics, we'll briefly go over metric units. Scientists —and the OAT—use the Système International d'Unités (the International System of Units), abbreviated **SI**, to express the measurements of physical quantities. The **base units** of the SI that we'll be interested in (at least for most of our study of OAT Physics) are listed below:

SI base unit	abbreviation	measures	dimension
meter	m	length	L
kilogram	kg	mass	M
second	s	time	T

This system of units is also referred to as the **mks system** (m for meters, k for kilograms, and s for seconds). Each **dimension** is simply an abbreviation for the quantity that is being measured; it does not depend on the particular unit that's used. For example, we could measure a distance in miles, meters, or furlongs—to name a few—but in all cases, we're measuring a *length*. We say that distance has the dimensions of length, L. As another example, we could measure an object's speed in miles per hour, meters per second, or furlongs per fortnight; but regardless of what units we use, we're always dividing a length by a time. Therefore, speed has dimensions of length per time (L/T).

Any physical quantity can be written in terms of the SI base units. Here are some examples:

quantity	symbol	units	dimensions
speed	v	m/s	L/T
density	ρ	kg/m^3	M/L^3
work	W	kg·m^2/s^2	ML^2/T^2

Multiples of the base units that are powers of ten are often abbreviated and precede the symbol for the unit. For example, "n" is the symbol for nano-, which means 10^{-9} (one billionth). Thus, one billionth of a second, 1 nanosecond, would be written as 1 ns. The letter "M" is the symbol for mega-, which means 10^6 (one million), so a distance of one million meters, 1 megameter, would be abbreviated as 1 Mm.

Some of the most common power-of-ten prefixes are given in the following list:

prefix	symbol	multiple
pico	p	10^{-12}
nano-	n	10^{-9}
micro-	μ	10^{-6}
milli-	m	10^{-3}
centi-	c	10^{-2}
kilo-	k	10^{3}
mega-	M	10^{6}
giga-	G	10^{9}

You should memorize this list.

On the OAT, you won't need to convert between the American system of units (which uses things like inches, feet, yards, and pounds) and the metric system, so don't bother memorizing conversions like 2.54 cm = 1 inch or 39.37 inches = 1 meter, etc. You will need to be able to convert within the metric system using the powers-of-ten prefixes.

Example 3-1: Express a density of 5500 kg/m^3 in g/cm^3.

Solution: All we want to do with this physical measurement is to change the units in which it's expressed. For that, we need conversion factors. A **conversion factor** is simply a fraction whose value is 1, that multiplies a measurement in one set of units to give the equivalent measurement in a different set of units. In this case, we'd write

$$\rho = 5.5 \times 10^3 \frac{\text{kg}}{\text{m}^3} \times \left(\frac{10^3 \text{ g}}{1 \text{ kg}}\right) \times \left(\frac{1 \text{ m}}{10^2 \text{ cm}}\right)^3 = 5.5 \frac{\text{g}}{\text{cm}^3}$$

Notice that each of these conversion factors is written so that the unit we want to change (that is, the unit we want to eliminate) cancels out. The fraction

$$\frac{1 \text{ kg}}{10^3 \text{ g}}$$

is also a conversion factor for mass, but writing it like this would not have been helpful in this particular problem because then the "kg" would not have canceled.

Example 3-2: If a ball is dropped from a great height, then the force of air resistance it feels at any point during its descent is given by the equation $F = KD^2v^2$, where D is the diameter of the ball and v is its speed. If the units of F are kg·m/s^2, what are the units of K?

Solution: If the equation $F = KD^2v^2$ is to be valid, then the units of the left-hand side must be the same as the units of the right-hand side. To specify the unit of a quantity, we put brackets around it; for example, $[F]$ denotes the units of F; that is, $[F]$ = kg·m/s^2. So we need to make sure that $[F] = [KD^2v^2]$, which means

$$\begin{aligned}
[F] &= [K][D]^2[v]^2 \\
\frac{\text{kg} \cdot \text{m}}{\text{s}^2} &= [K] \cdot \text{m}^2 \cdot \left(\frac{\text{m}}{\text{s}}\right)^2 \\
&= [K] \cdot \frac{\text{m}^4}{\text{s}^2} \\
\text{kg} \cdot \text{m} &= [K] \cdot \text{m}^4 \\
\therefore [K] &= \frac{\text{kg}}{\text{m}^3}
\end{aligned}$$

3.2 KINEMATICS

Kinematics is the description of motion in terms of an object's position, velocity, and acceleration. The OAT will expect not only that you can answer mathematical questions about these quantities but also that you know the definitions of these quantities.

Displacement

The **displacement** of an object is its change in position. For example, let's say we were measuring an object moving along a straight line by laying a meter stick along the object's line of motion. If the object starts at, say, the *10 cm* mark on the meter stick and moves to the *70 cm* mark, then its position changed by 70 cm – 10 cm = 60 cm, so we'd say its displacement is 60 cm.

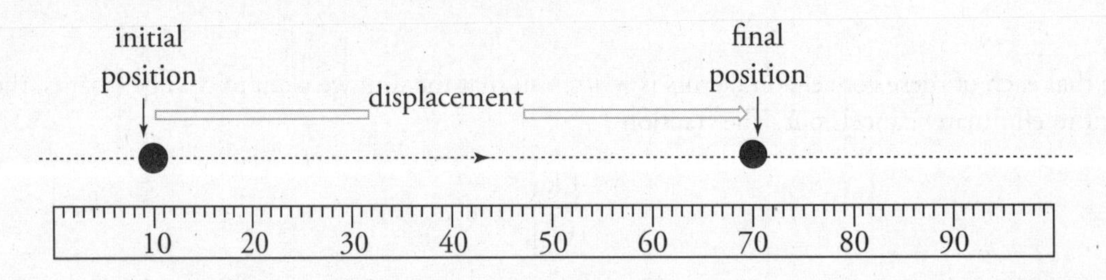

We find the displacement by subtracting the object's initial position from its final position:

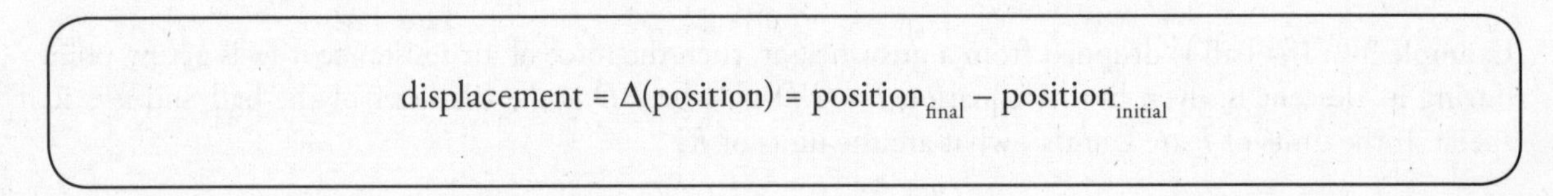

$$\text{displacement} = \Delta(\text{position}) = \text{position}_{\text{final}} - \text{position}_{\text{initial}}$$

Now, what if the object moved from the *70 cm* mark on the meter stick to the *10 cm* mark? Then its displacement would be 10 cm – 70 cm = –60 cm.

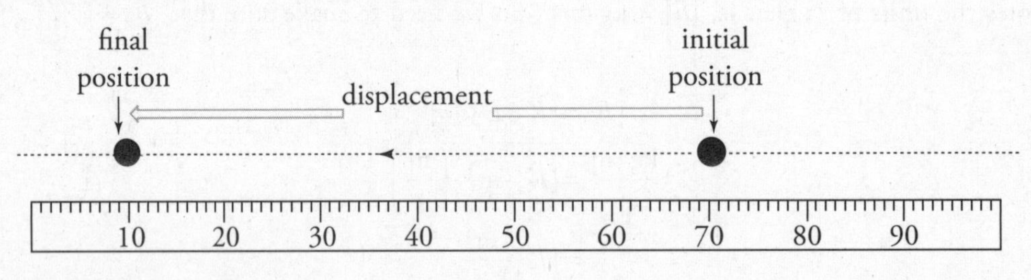

In both cases, the object moved a distance of 60 cm, but in the first case it moved to the right, and in the second case, it moved to the left. Displacement is a vector, so it takes direction into account. If we call *to the right* the positive direction (so *to the left* automatically becomes the negative direction) then in the first case, we'd say the displacement is +60 cm, and in the second case, it's –60 cm.

The motion of the object can be more complicated. For example, what if the object started at the *10 cm* mark, moved to the *50 cm* mark, back to the *40 cm* mark, and then over to the *70 cm* mark?

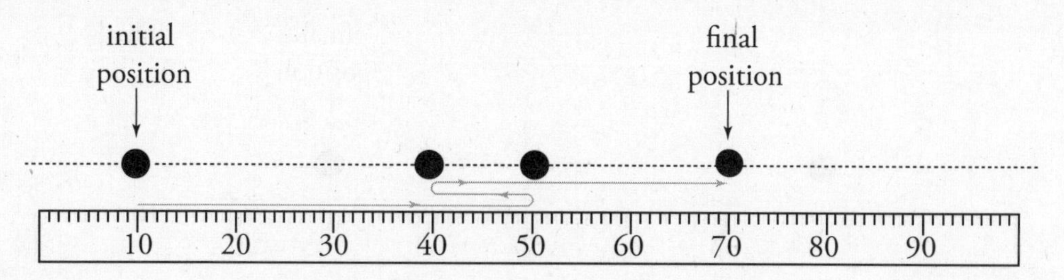

This example brings up a crucial point about displacement. The *total* distance that the object travels is (40 cm) + (10 cm) + (30 cm) = 80 cm, but the object's displacement is still

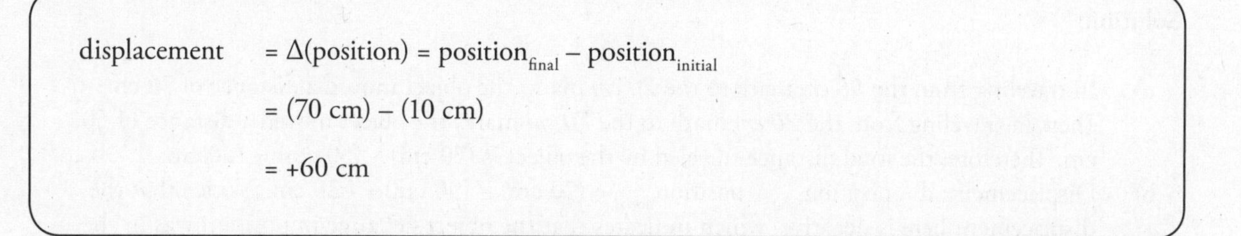

$$\text{displacement} = \Delta(\text{position}) = \text{position}_{\text{final}} - \text{position}_{\text{initial}}$$
$$= (70 \text{ cm}) - (10 \text{ cm})$$
$$= +60 \text{ cm}$$

Displacement gives us the *net* distance traveled by the object, which may very well be less than the total distance. So, the displacement is a vector that always points from the object's initial position to its final position, *regardless of the path the object took*, and whose magnitude is the *net* distance traveled by the object. There are multiple different symbols that are used to represent the displacement vector, but the most common one is the single letter **d**. Sometimes, we use $\Delta\mathbf{x}$ if we know the displacement is horizontal, or $\Delta\mathbf{y}$ if we know the displacement is vertical. Be aware that the OAT also uses the word *displacement* to mean just the magnitude of the displacement vector (that is, just the net distance traveled by the object without regard for direction); the question will make it clear which meaning is intended.

Displacement

$$\mathbf{d} = \text{position}_{\text{final}} - \text{position}_{\text{initial}} = \text{net distance plus direction}$$

For example, if a sprinter runs 400 meters around a circular track and returns to her starting point, she has covered a *total* distance of 400 meters, but her *displacement* is zero. If a sprinter runs 300 meters north, then 400 meters east, he's covered a total distance of 700 m, but his displacement is only 500 meters.

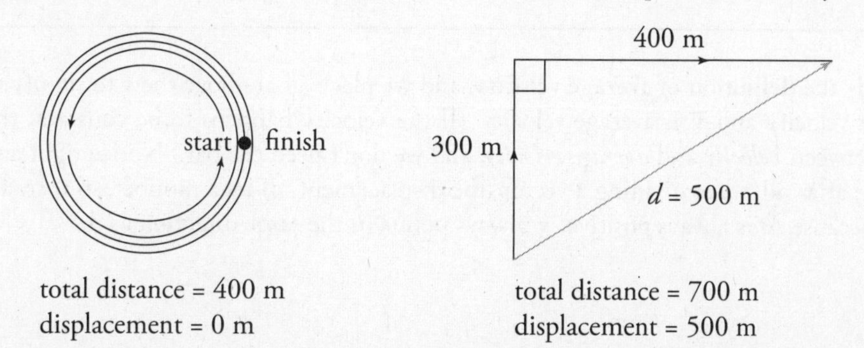

Example 3-3: The object shown below begins at the *90 cm* mark on the meter stick, moves to the *20 cm* mark, then to the *70 cm* mark.

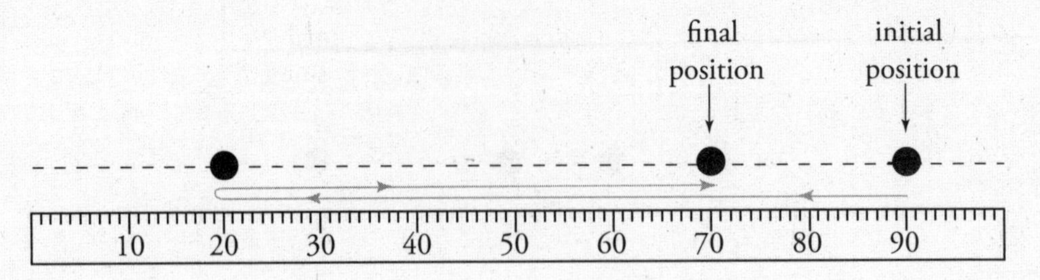

a) What's the total distance traveled by this object?
b) What's the object's displacement?

Solution:

a) In traveling from the *90 cm* mark to the *20 cm* mark, the object moved a distance of 70 cm. Then, in traveling from the *20 cm* mark to the *70 cm* mark, the object moved a distance of 50 cm. Therefore, the total distance traveled by the object is (70 cm) + (50 cm) = 120 cm.
b) Displacement: $\mathbf{d} = \text{position}_{\text{final}} - \text{position}_{\text{initial}} = (70\text{ cm}) - (90\text{ cm}) = -20\text{ cm}$. Notice that the displacement here is negative, which indicates that the object's change in position was in the negative direction (it ended up to the *left* of where it started).

Velocity

Displacement tells us how much an object's position changes. **Velocity** tells us how *fast* an object's position changes. If you're in a car traveling at 60 miles per hour along a long, straight highway, then this means your position changes by 60 miles every hour. To calculate velocity, simply divide how much the position has changed by how much time it took for it to change; in other words, divide displacement by time.

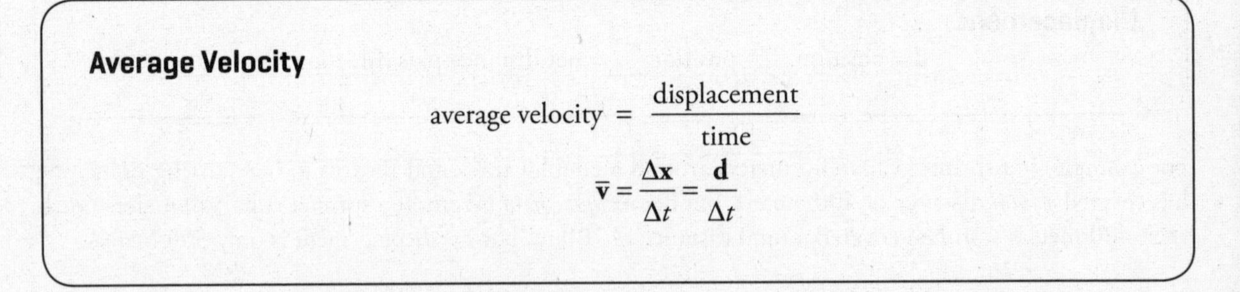

This is actually the definition of **average velocity**, and we place a bar above the **v** to signify that it's an *average*. So, **v** is velocity and $\bar{\mathbf{v}}$ is average velocity. (If the velocity happens to be constant, then there's no distinction between *velocity* and *average velocity*, and we don't need the bar.) Notice right away that velocity is a vector; after all, we're dividing a vector (the displacement, **d**) by a number, so we're left with a vector. In fact, because Δt is always positive, $\bar{\mathbf{v}}$ always points in the same direction as **d**.

The magnitude of the velocity vector is called the **speed.** Speed is a scalar; it has no direction and can never be negative. (Notice that the speedometer in your car is well-named; it only tells you how fast the car is moving, not the direction of motion. It's not a "velocity-o-meter.") Velocity is a vector that specifies both speed and direction.

Velocity

v = speed & direction

In the figure below, each vector represents the car's velocity. Both cars have the same speed (let's say 20 m/s), so the magnitudes of their velocity vectors are the same. Nevertheless, they have different velocities, because the directions are different. (By the way, if the car on the right looks bigger than the car on the left, it's an optical illusion. Grab a ruler and check it for yourself. They're the same size!)

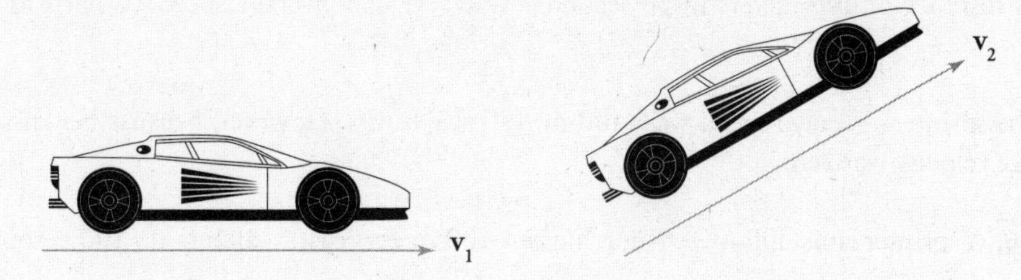

These two cars have the same speed but different velocities. Is it possible for two cars to have the same velocity but different speeds? No. Velocity is speed plus direction, so if the velocities are the same, then the speeds (and the directions) are the same.

Example 3-4: The object shown below begins (time t = 0) at the *90 cm* mark on the meter stick. At time t = 3 sec, it has moved to the *20 cm* mark, and at time t = 5 sec, it's at the *70 cm* mark.

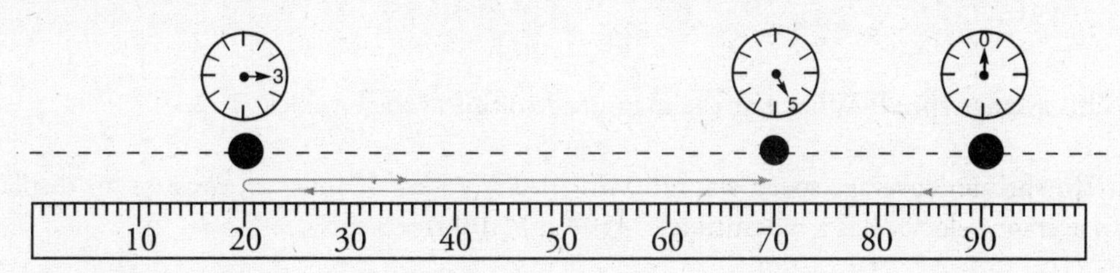

a) What was the average velocity of this object?
b) What was the object's average speed?

Solution:

a) We figured out in Example 3-3(b) that the object's displacement was –20 cm. Therefore,

$$\mathbf{v} = \frac{\mathbf{d}}{\Delta t} = \frac{-20 \text{ cm}}{5 \text{ s}} = -4 \text{ cm/s or } -0.04 \text{ m/s}$$

The minus sign indicates the direction of $\overline{\mathbf{v}}$ the object's displacement was to the left, so its average velocity is also to the left.

b) *Average speed* is not the magnitude of the average velocity. (Confusing, but true.) By definition, **average speed** is the *total* distance traveled divided by the time. We figured out in Example 3-3(a) that the total distance traveled by this object was 120 cm, so the object's average speed is (120 cm)/(5 s) = 24 cm/s = 0.24 m/s.

Example 3-5: A sprinter runs 400 meters around a circular track and returns to her starting point, covering a total distance of 400 meters in 50 seconds. What was her average speed? What was her average velocity?

Solution: The sprinter's average speed was (400 m)/(50 s) = 8 m/s. However, because her displacement is 0, her average velocity was zero.

Example 3-6: A sprinter runs 300 meters north, then 400 meters east, which takes 100 seconds.

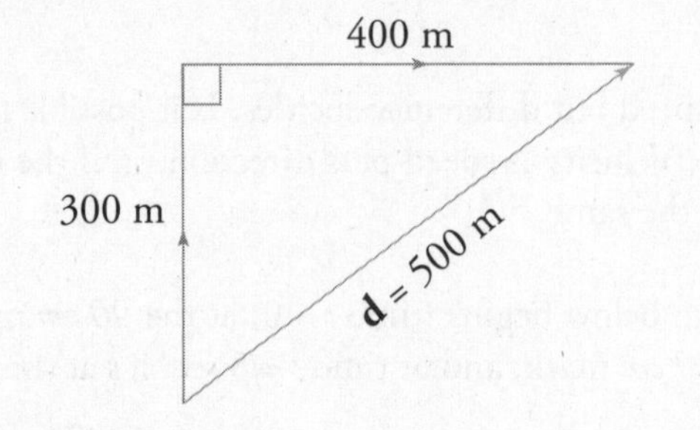

What was his average speed? What was the magnitude of his average velocity?

Solution: The sprinter's average speed was (700 m)/(100 s) = 7 m/s. However, because his displacement is 500 m, his average velocity has a magnitude of (500 m)/(100 s) = 5 m/s.

Example 3-7: An object moves from Point A to Point B in 4 seconds.

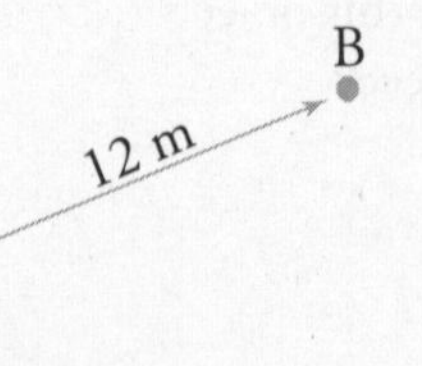

What was the object's velocity?

A. 3 m/s
B. 8 m/s
C. 6 m/s
D. 48 m/s

Solution: Notice that the question is asking for velocity (which is a vector) but all the choices are scalars. Strictly speaking, the answer should include the correct direction as well as the magnitude. However, the OAT (as well as textbook authors and teachers) will often use the word *velocity* when they mean *speed*; usually, it won't cause confusion. From the choices given, we know it's the magnitude of the velocity that is the desired quantity, and this is

$$v = \frac{d}{\Delta t} = \frac{12\text{ m}}{4\text{ s}} = 3\text{ m/s}$$

Choice A is the answer we'd choose.

Acceleration

Velocity tells us how fast an object's position changes. **Acceleration** tells us how fast an object's *velocity* changes.

Average Acceleration

$$\text{average acceleration} = \frac{\text{change in velocity}}{\text{time}}$$

$$\bar{\mathbf{a}} = \frac{\Delta \mathbf{v}}{\Delta t}$$

Acceleration is a little trickier than velocity. Even though both involve how fast something changes, acceleration is how fast velocity changes, and an object's velocity changes if the speed *or* the direction changes. So, for example, an object can be accelerating even if its speed is constant. This is a very important point and a potential OAT trap.

In everyday language, we use the word *acceleration* to describe what happens when we step on the gas pedal and go faster. Well, that's certainly an example of acceleration even from the "proper" physics perspective, but it isn't the only example of acceleration.

What happens when you step on the brake? You slow down. Is that acceleration? Yes, although we might also call it a *deceleration*, because our speed changes.

Now, imagine that you set the car on cruise control at, say, 60 miles per hour. Up ahead you see a curve in the road, so as you approach it, you slowly turn the wheel to stay on the road. Even though your speed remains constant, your direction of motion changes, which means your velocity vector changes. Thus, you experience an acceleration.

Let's try this one. Throw a baseball straight up into the air. It rises, gets to the top of its path, then falls back down. At the moment it's at the top of its path, its velocity is zero. What is the ball's acceleration at this point?

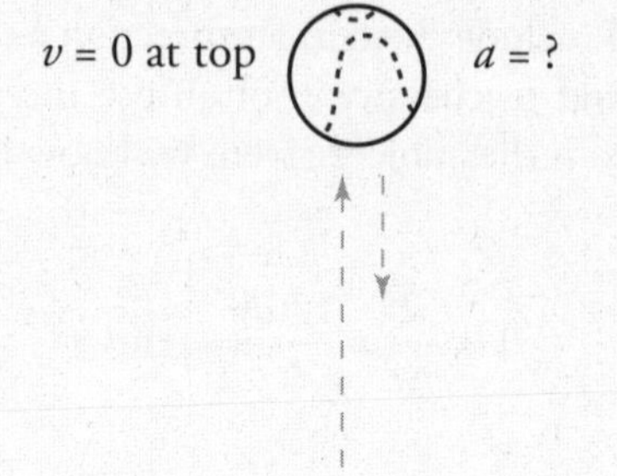

A common answer is, "If the velocity is 0, then the acceleration is 0, too." Let's see why this isn't the case here. What's happening to the baseball's velocity at the top of the path? Its direction is changing from up to *down*. The fact that the velocity is changing means there's an acceleration, so the acceleration can't be zero at the top of the path. Here's another way of looking at it: What if the acceleration *were* zero at the top? Zero acceleration means no change in velocity, so if $a = 0$ at a certain point, then whatever velocity there is at that point will stay constant. Does the velocity of the baseball remain zero? No, because the ball immediately starts to fall toward the ground.

Example 3-8: The velocity of an object moving along a straight line changes from $\mathbf{v}_i = 4$ m/s at time $t_i = 0$ to $\mathbf{v}_f = 10$ m/s at time $t_f = 2$ sec.

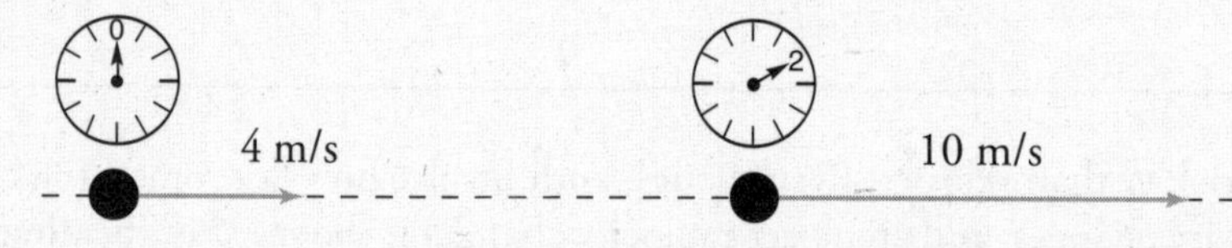

What was the object's average acceleration during this time interval?

Solution: By definition of average acceleration, we have

$$\bar{\mathbf{a}} = \frac{\Delta \mathbf{v}}{\Delta t} = \frac{\mathbf{v}_f - \mathbf{v}_i}{t_f - t_i} = \frac{10\,\text{m/s} - 4\,\text{m/s}}{(2\text{ s}) - 0\text{ s}} = 3\,\text{m/s}^2$$

Notice that $\bar{\mathbf{a}}$ is positive, which means that it points to the right, just like $\mathbf{v}_i$. If the acceleration points in the *same* direction as the initial velocity, then the object's speed is *increasing*.

Example 3-9: The velocity of an object moving along a straight line changes from $\mathbf{v}_i = 7$ m/s at time $t_i = 0$ to $\mathbf{v}_f = 1$ m/s at time $t_f = 3$ sec.

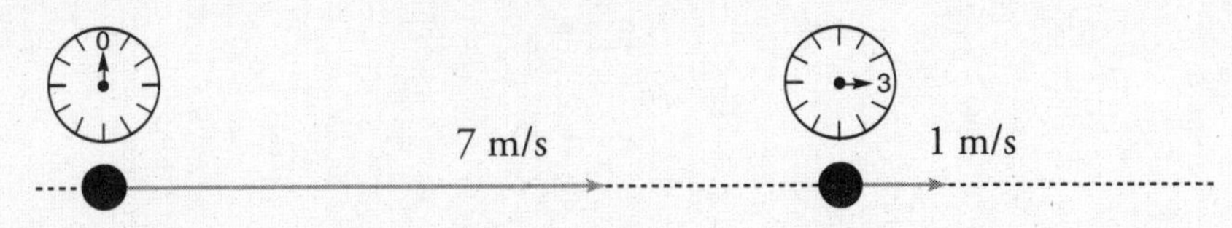

What was the object's average acceleration during this time interval?

Solution: By definition of average acceleration, we have

$$\bar{\mathbf{a}} = \frac{\Delta \mathbf{v}}{\Delta t} = \frac{\mathbf{v}_f - \mathbf{v}_i}{t_f - t_i} = \frac{1\text{ m/s} - 7\text{ m/s}}{(3\text{ s}) - 0\text{ s}} = -2\text{ m/s}^2$$

Notice that $\bar{\mathbf{a}}$ is negative, which means that it points to the left, in the direction opposite to $\mathbf{v}_i$. If the acceleration points in the direction *opposite* to the initial velocity, then the object's speed is *decreasing.*

Example 3-10: The velocity of an object moving along a straight line changes from $\mathbf{v}_i = -2$ m/s at time $t_i = 0$ to $\mathbf{v}_f = -5$ m/s at time $t_f = 2$ sec.

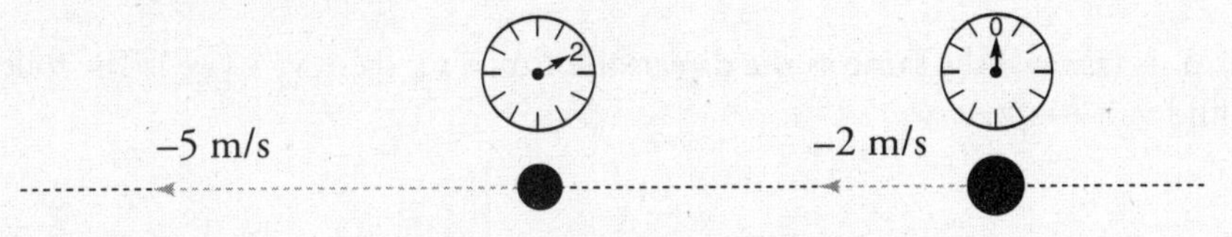

What was the object's average acceleration during this time interval?

Solution: By definition of average acceleration, we have

$$\bar{\mathbf{a}} = \frac{\Delta \mathbf{v}}{\Delta t} = \frac{\mathbf{v}_f - \mathbf{v}_i}{t_f - t_i} = \frac{-5\text{ m/s} - (-2\text{ m/s})}{(2\text{ s}) - 0\text{ s}} = -1.5\text{ m/s}^2$$

Notice that $\bar{\mathbf{a}}$ is negative, which means that it points to the left, just like $\mathbf{v}_i$. If the acceleration points in the *same* direction as the initial velocity, then the object's speed is *increasing.*

Example 3-11: The velocity of an object changes from $\mathbf{v}_1$ at time $t_i = 0$ to $\mathbf{v}_2$ at time $t_f = 2$ sec.

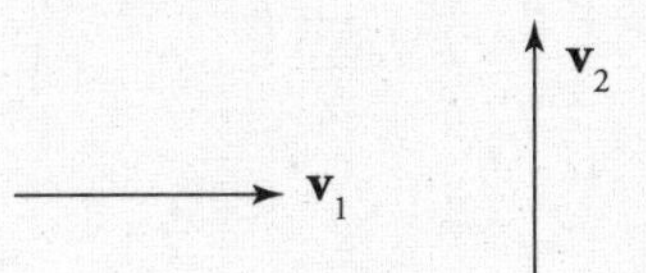

Which of the following best illustrates the object's average acceleration during this time interval?

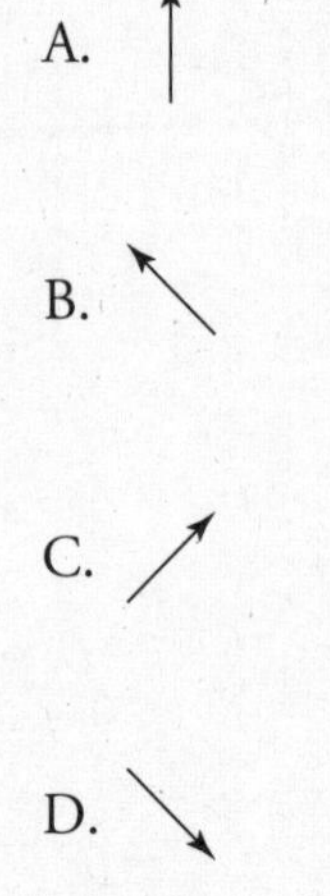

Solution: By definition of average acceleration, we have

$$\bar{\mathbf{a}} = \frac{\Delta \mathbf{v}}{\Delta t} = \frac{\mathbf{v}_2 - \mathbf{v}_1}{t_f - t_i} = \frac{\mathbf{v}_2 - \mathbf{v}_1}{2\text{ s}}$$

The direction of $\bar{\mathbf{a}}$ is (always) the same as the direction of $\Delta\mathbf{v} = \mathbf{v}_2 - \mathbf{v}_1 = \mathbf{v}_2 + (-\mathbf{v}_1)$. The following diagram shows how we find $\mathbf{v}_2 + (-\mathbf{v}_1)$:

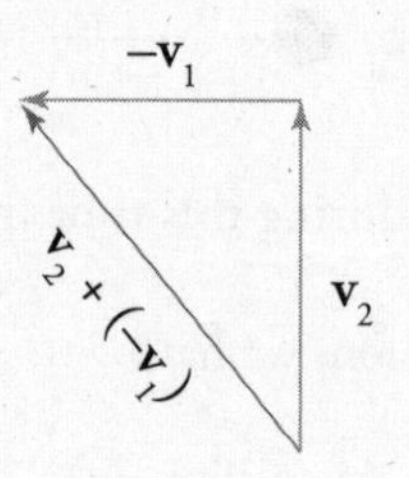

Therefore, choice B is the best answer.

The direction of **a** tells **v** how to change; the following diagrams summarize the possibilities:

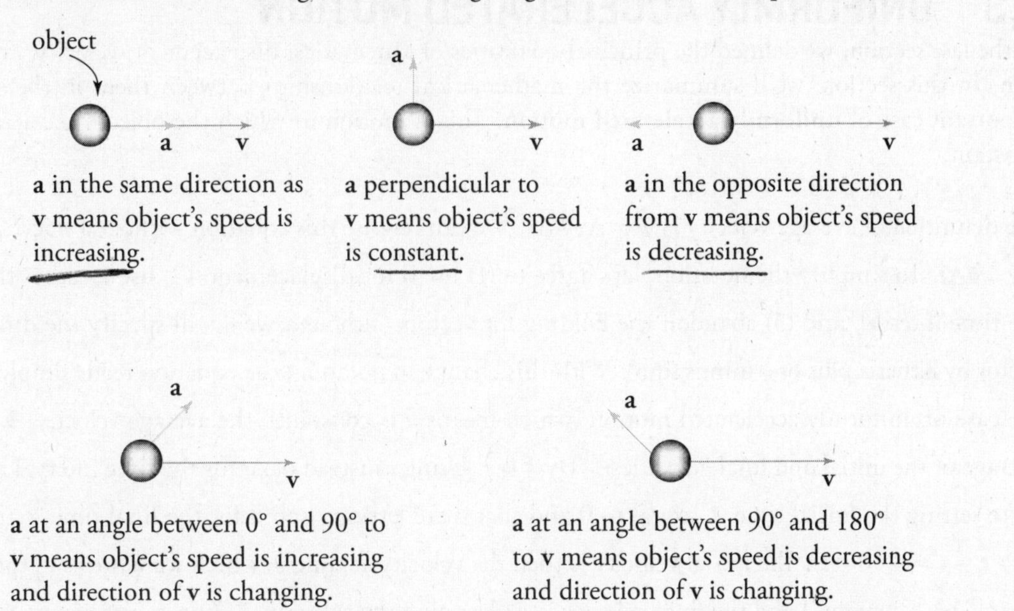

Example 3-12: The velocity and acceleration of an object at a certain point are shown in the diagram below.

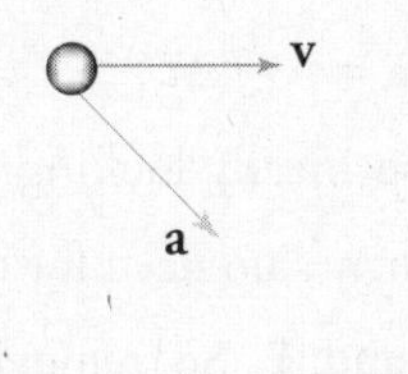

Describe the object's velocity a short time later.

Solution: We split the acceleration vector into components, one along the direction of **v** and one perpendicular to the direction of **v**:

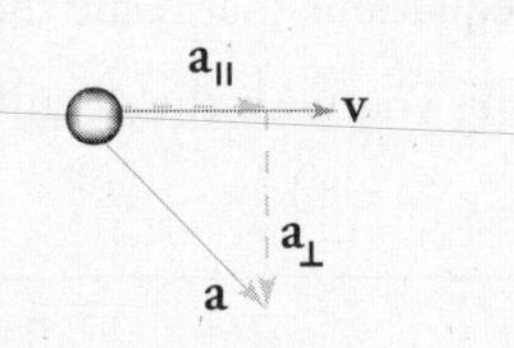

The component $\mathbf{a}_{\parallel}$ points along the line of the object's motion, so the *speed* of the object will change; in particular, the speed will *increase*, since $\mathbf{a}_{\parallel}$ points in the *same* direction as **v**. The component of **a** that's perpendicular to **v**, $\mathbf{a}_{\perp}$, will make the *direction* of **v** change; in particular, it will turn downward (since $\mathbf{a}_{\perp}$ points downward). Therefore, we'd expect the object to increase in speed as it turns downward.

3.3 UNIFORMLY ACCELERATED MOTION

In the last section, we defined the principal quantities of kinematics: displacement, velocity, and acceleration. In this section, we'll summarize the mathematical relationships between them in the special but important case of **uniformly accelerated motion.** This is motion in which the object's acceleration, **a**, is constant.

The definition of average velocity is $\bar{\mathbf{v}} = \Delta x / \Delta t$. We can rewrite this equation without a fraction like this: $\Delta x = \bar{\mathbf{v}}\Delta t$. To simplify the notation, let's agree to (1) use **d** for displacement, (2) use t, rather than Δt, for the time interval, and (3) abandon the bolding for vectors (although we'll still specify the direction of a vector by either a plus or a minus sign). With this change in notation, the equation reads simply $d = \bar{v}t$. In the case of uniformly accelerated motion (which means a is constant), the average velocity, $\bar{v}$ is just the average of the initial and final velocities: $\frac{1}{2}(v_i + v_f)$. Using t instead of Δt for the time interval means that we're setting the initial time, t_i, equal to 0 and that we're letting t stand for the final time, t_f (notice that $\Delta t = t_f - t_i = t - 0 = t$). The initial velocity is then the velocity at time 0, which we write as v_0 (pronounced "v zero" or "v naught") and the final velocity is v (dropping the subscript "f" on v_f just like we're dropping the subscript "f" on t_f). Therefore, the average velocity can be written as $\bar{v} = \frac{1}{2}(v_0 + v)$, and the equation for d becomes $d = \frac{1}{2}(v_0 + v)t$.

The definition of average acceleration is $\bar{\mathbf{a}} = \Delta\mathbf{v} / \Delta t$. We can rewrite this equation without a fraction like this: $\Delta\mathbf{v} = \bar{\mathbf{a}}\Delta t$. Now, since we are specifically looking at uniformly accelerated motion (motion in which the acceleration is constant), then there's no need for the bar on the **a**. After all, if **acceleration** is a constant, there's no distinction between **a** and $\bar{\mathbf{a}}$. So, removing the bar and using the simplified notation described in the last paragraph, the equation becomes $\Delta v = at$, or $v = v_0 + at$.

The two equations $d = \frac{1}{2}(v_0 + v)t$ and $v = v_0 + at$ follow directly from the definitions of average velocity and acceleration. There are three other equations that relate these quantities, but they would require more algebra to derive them. Instead of boring you with the details, we'll just state them. Since there are five equations, we call them **The Big Five:**

The Big Five

1. $d = \frac{1}{2}(v_0 + v)t$ missing a
2. $v = v_0 + at$ missing d
3. $d = v_0 t + \frac{1}{2}at^2$ missing v
4. $d = vt - \frac{1}{2}at^2$ missing v_0
5. $v^2 = v_0^2 + 2ad$ missing t

Notice that these equations involve *five* quantities, d, v_0, v, a, and t, and there are *five* equations. Each equation has exactly one of those quantities missing, and this is how you decide which equation to use in a particular problem. A quantity is *missing* from the problem if it's *not given and not asked for*. For example, if a question does not give or ask for v, then use Big Five #3; if a question does not give or ask for t, then use Big Five #5. On the OAT, the Big Five equations that are used most frequently are #2, #3, and #5.

Example 3-13: An object has an initial velocity of 3 m/s and a constant acceleration of 2 m/s² in the same direction. What will the object's velocity be at $t = 6$ s?

Solution: We're given v_0, a; and t, and asked for v. Since the displacement, d, is neither given nor asked for, we use Big Five #2:

$$v = v_0 + at = 3\text{ m/s} + (2\text{ m/s}^2)(6\text{ s}) = 15\text{ m/s}$$

Example 3-14: A particle has an initial velocity of 10 m/s and a constant acceleration of 3 m/s² in the same direction. How far will the particle travel in 4 seconds?

Solution: We're given v_0, a, and t, and asked for d. Since the final velocity, v, is missing, we use Big Five #3:

$$d = v_0 t + \tfrac{1}{2}at^2 = (10\text{ m/s})(4\text{ s}) + \tfrac{1}{2}(3\text{ m/s}^2)(4\text{ s})^2 = 64\text{ m}$$

Example 3-15: An object starts from rest and travels in a straight line with a constant acceleration of 4 m/s² in the same direction until its final velocity is 20 m/s. How far does it travel during this time?

Solution: We're given v_0, a, and v, and asked for d. Since the time, t, is neither given nor asked for, we use Big Five #5. Because the object starts from rest, we know that $v_0 = 0$, so we get

$$v^2 = v_0^2 + 2ad \rightarrow v^2 = 2ad \rightarrow d = \frac{v^2}{2a} = \frac{(20\text{ m/s})^2}{2(4\text{ m/s}^2)} = 50\text{ m}$$

Example 3-16: A particle has an initial velocity of 6 m/s and moves with constant acceleration in the same direction for 5 seconds until its final velocity is 16 m/s. How far does it travel during this time?

Solution: We're given v_0, t, and v, and asked for d. Since the acceleration, a, is missing, we use Big Five #1:

$$d = \tfrac{1}{2}(v_0 + v)t = \tfrac{1}{2}(6\text{ m/s} + 16\text{ m/s})(5\text{ s}) = 55\text{ m}$$

Example 3-17: An object whose final velocity is 24 m/s traveled for 4 seconds at a constant acceleration of 2 m/s² in the same direction. How far did it travel?

Solution: We're given v, t, and a, and asked for d. Since the initial velocity, v_0, is neither given nor asked for, we use Big Five #4:

$$d = vt - \tfrac{1}{2}at^2 = (24\text{ m/s})(4\text{ s}) - \tfrac{1}{2}(2\text{ m/s}^2)(4\text{ s})^2 = 80\text{ m}$$

3.4 KINEMATICS WITH GRAPHS

The OAT will expect you to not only handle kinematics problems algebraically (as we did in the last five examples) but also *graphically.* There are two types of graphs that we'll look at: the **position vs. time** graph and the **velocity vs. time** graph.

Consider the following graph, which gives an object's position, x, as a function of time, t:

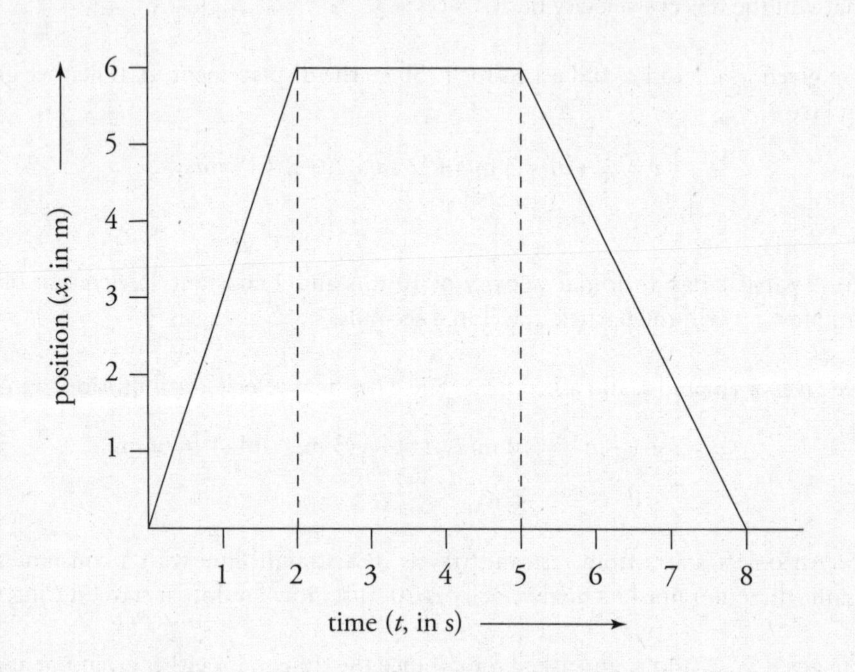

The object starts at $x = 0$, then moves to $x = 6$ m at $t = 2$ s. From $t = 2$ s to $t = 5$ s, it remains at position $x = 6$ m. Then, from $t = 5$ s to $t = 8$ s, the object moves from $x = 6$ m back to $x = 0$.

Let's figure out its velocity during these time intervals. From $t = 0$ to $t = 2$ s, its velocity is

$$v = \frac{\Delta x}{\Delta t} = \frac{x - x_0}{t_f - t_i} = \frac{(6\text{ m}) - (0\text{ m})}{2\text{ s}} = 3\text{ m/s}$$

Note that Δx is the vertical change in this graph and Δt is the horizontal change, from $t = 0$ to $t = 2$ s. Dividing a vertical change by the corresponding horizontal change gives the *slope* of a graph. So, we have this rule:

> The slope of a position vs. time graph gives the velocity.

From $t = 2$ s to $t = 5$ s, the object remained at position $x = 6$ m. Since the object didn't move, we expect its velocity during this time interval to be zero. But notice that the graph is flat here, and the slope of a flat line is 0.

Finally, from $t = 5$ s to $t = 8$ s, the velocity is

$$v = \frac{\Delta x}{\Delta t} = \frac{x - x_0}{t_f - t_i} = \frac{(0 \text{ m}) - (6 \text{ m})}{(8 \text{ s}) - (5 \text{ s})} = -2 \text{ m/s}$$

This is the slope of the graph from $t = 5$ s to $t = 8$ s.

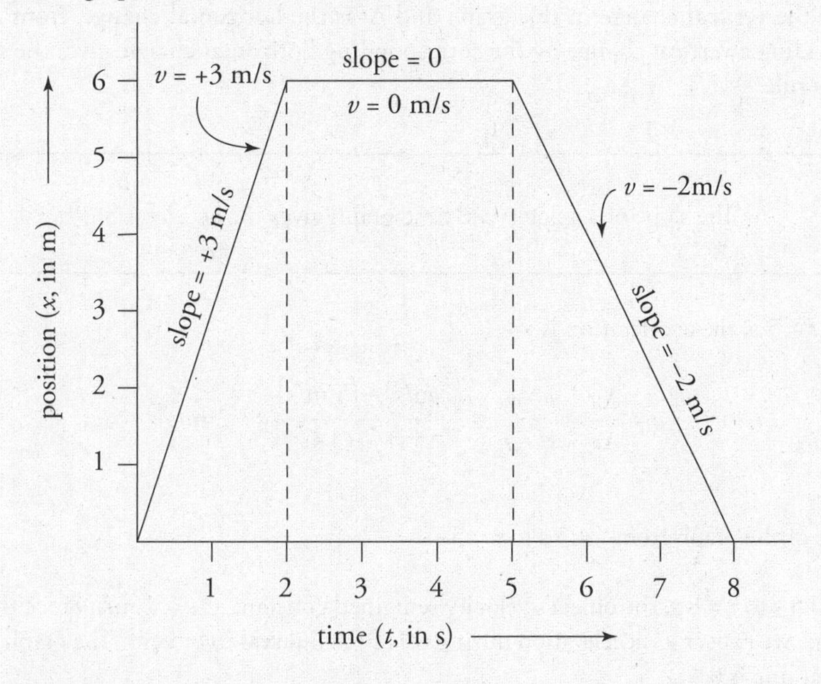

Now consider the following graph, which gives an object's velocity, v, as a function of time, t:

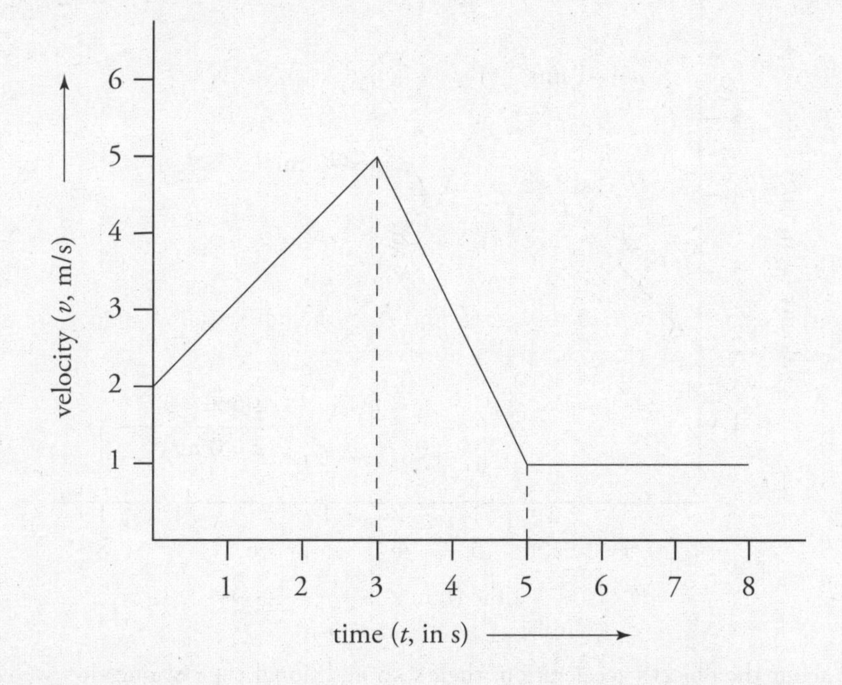

The object's velocity at $t = 0$ is $v = 2$ m/s, and steadily increases to $v = 5$ m/s at time $t = 3$ s. From $t = 3$ s to $t = 5$ s, the velocity decreases to $v = 1$ m/s. Then, from $t = 5$ s to $t = 8$ s, the object's velocity remains constant at $v = 1$ m/s.

Let's figure out the object's acceleration during these time intervals. From $t = 0$ to $t = 3$ s, its acceleration is

$$a = \frac{\Delta v}{\Delta t} = \frac{v - v_0}{t} = \frac{(5 \text{ m/s}) - (2 \text{ m/s})}{3 \text{s}} = 1 \text{ m/s}^2$$

Note that Δv is the vertical change in this graph and Δt is the horizontal change, from $t = 0$ to $t = 3$ s. Once again, dividing a vertical change by the corresponding horizontal change gives the slope of a graph. So, we have this rule:

The slope of a velocity vs. time graph gives the acceleration.

From $t = 3$ s to $t = 5$ s, the acceleration is

$$a = \frac{\Delta v}{\Delta t} = \frac{v - v_0}{t_f - t_i} = \frac{(1 \text{ m/s}) - (5 \text{ m/s})}{(5 \text{ s}) - (3 \text{ s})} = -2 \text{ m/s}^2$$

This is the slope of the graph from $t = 3$ s to $t = 5$ s.

Finally, from $t = 5$ s to $t = 8$ s, the object's velocity remained constant at $v = 1$ m/s. Since the object's velocity didn't change, we expect its acceleration during this time interval to be zero. The graph is flat here, and the slope of a flat line is 0.

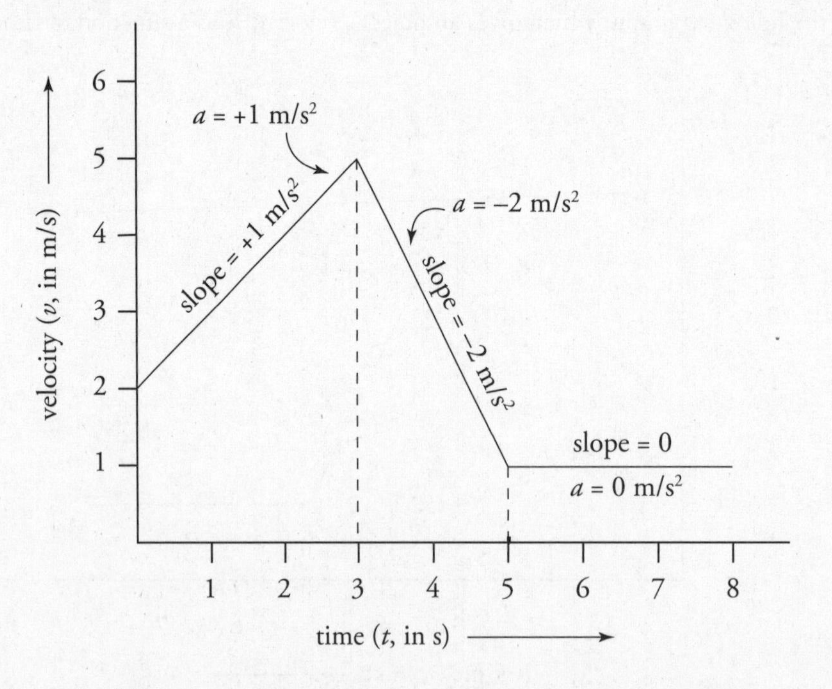

Besides asking about the object's acceleration, there's an additional type of question we could be asked given an object's velocity vs. time graph. For example, what was the object's *displacement* from $t = 5$ s to

$t = 7$ s? Since the object's velocity was a constant $v = 1$ m/s, we just use the basic equation *distance* = *rate* × *time* (which is really just Big Five #1 in the case where v is constant) to find that $d = (1 \text{ m/s})(2 \text{ s}) = 2$ m. But if we look at the graph, we realize that what we've just found is the *area* under the graph from $t = 5$ s to $t = 7$ s. After all, the area under the graph is just a bunch of squares whose height is a velocity and whose base is a time. The area of a square is *base* × *height* (*bh*), so we're multiplying velocity × time, and that gives us displacement. The same rule applies even if the graph isn't flat:

> The area under a velocity vs. time graph gives the displacement.

What is the object's displacement from $t = 0$ to $t = 3$ s? It will be the area under the velocity vs. time graph from $t = 0$ to $t = 3$ s. The figure below shows that we can split this area into two pieces: a triangle whose area is $\frac{1}{2}bh = \frac{1}{2}(3\text{s})(3 \text{ m/s}) = \frac{9}{2}$ m, and a rectangle whose area is $bh = (3\text{s})(2 \text{ m/s}) = 6\text{m}$. Therefore, the object's displacement from $t = 0$ to $t = 3$ s, which is the *total* area under the graph between $t = 0$ and $t = 3$ s, is $\left(\frac{9}{2}\text{ m}\right) + (6\text{m}) = 10.5\text{m}$.

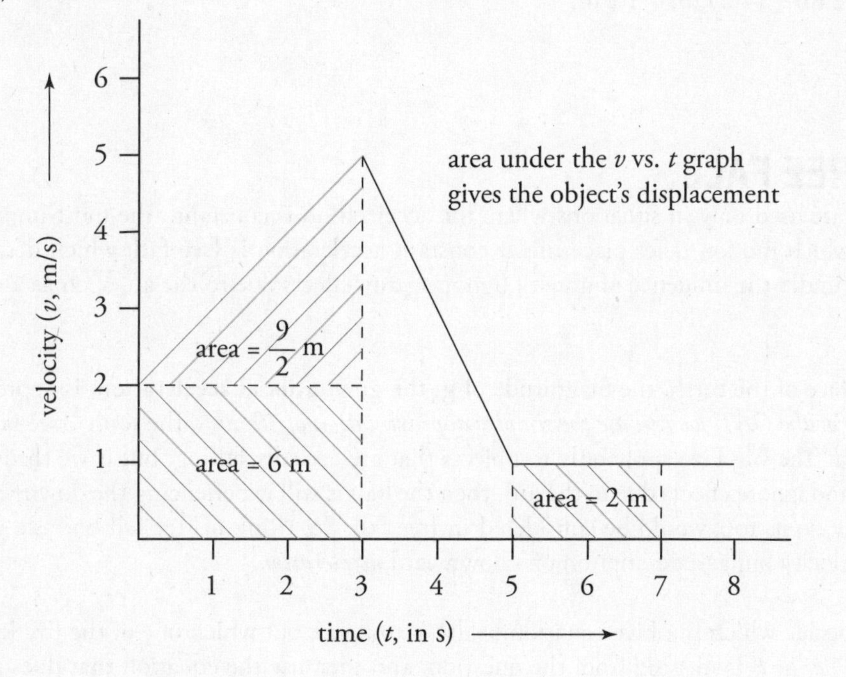

We can check this result using Big Five #1:

$$d = \frac{1}{2}(v_0 + v)t = \frac{1}{2}(2 \text{ m/s} + 5 \text{ m/s})(3\text{s}) = 10.5\text{m}$$

Example 3-18: For the object whose velocity vs. time graph is shown below, what is its displacement from $t = 2$ s to $t = 5$ s?

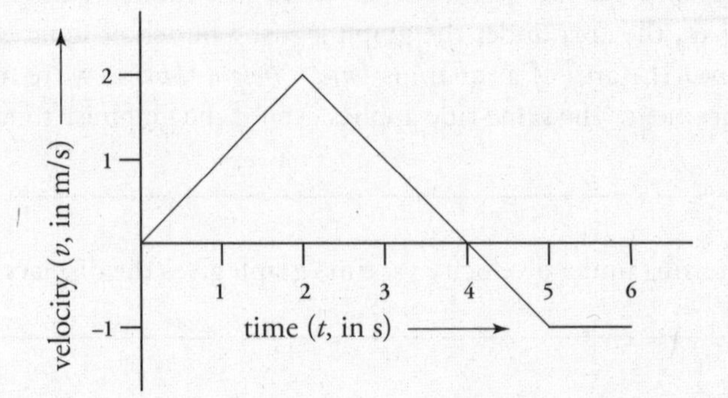

Solution: The area under the graph (or, more precisely, the area between the graph and the t axis) gives the object's displacement. The area under the graph from $t = 2$ s to $t = 4$ s is $\frac{1}{2}bh = \frac{1}{2}(2\text{ s})(2\text{ m/s}) = 2\text{ m}$. After $t = 4$ s, the graph is *below* the t axis, so any area here counts *negative*. From $t = 4$ s to $t = 5$ s, the area is $\frac{1}{2}bh = \frac{1}{2}(1\text{ s})(-1\text{ m/s}) = -0.5\text{ m}$. Therefore, the total area between the graph and the t axis, from $t = 2$ s to $t = 5$ s, is (2 m) + (–0.5 m) = 1.5 m.

3.5 FREE FALL

The Big Five are used only in situations where the acceleration is constant. The most important "real life" situation in which motion takes place under constant acceleration is **free fall**, which describes an object moving only under the influence of gravity (ignoring any effects due to the air, such as air resistance and buoyancy).

Near the surface of the earth, the magnitude of **g**, the **gravitational acceleration**, is approximately equal to 9.8 m/s^2. *For the OAT, we can use the simpler approximation of 10 m/s^2*. The term "free fall" might make you think that The Big Five apply only to objects that are actually falling, but if we throw a baseball up into the air (and ignore effects due to the air), then the ball is still experiencing the downward acceleration due to gravity, so it, too, would be considered in free fall. So, think of free fall not as a description of a downward velocity but as a description of a downward *acceleration*.

The way we decide which Big Five equation to use is to figure out which one of the five kinematics quantities (d, v_0, v, a, or t) is missing from the question, and then use the equation that does not involve this missing quantity. Often, in questions asking about objects in free fall, the acceleration will not be given because it's known implicitly. As soon as you realize the question involves an object moving under the influence of gravity, then you know that a is automatically known; on Earth, the magnitude of this a is about 10 m/s^2.

However, there is one thing you will have to decide on once you've selected which Big Five equation to use. Gravitational acceleration, like any acceleration, is a vector, so it has magnitude and direction. We know the magnitude is 10 m/s^2 and the direction is downward, but is it *down* the positive direction or the negative direction? The answer is: it's up to you. I suggest letting the direction of the object's displacement be the positive direction in every problem (this is almost always the simplest, most intuitive, decision). If the object's displacement is *down*, then call *down* the positive direction, and use $a = +g = +10\ \text{m/s}^2$ in whichever Big Five equation you've selected. If the object's displacement is *up*, call *up* the positive direction (and thus *down* is automatically the negative direction) and use $a = -g = -10\ \text{m/s}^2$.

It's important to remember that once you make your decision about which direction, up or down, is the positive direction, your decision applies to all other vectors in that problem: namely, v_0, v, and d. Therefore, if *down* is positive, for example, then in addition to the downward acceleration being positive, a downward initial velocity is positive, a downward final velocity is positive, and a downward displacement is positive. (This would mean that an upward initial velocity is negative, an upward final velocity is negative, and an upward displacement is negative.) Of course, if you follow the suggestion of always calling the direction of the displacement positive, then d will always be positive.

Example 3-19: An object is dropped from a height of 80 m. How long will it take to strike the ground?

Solution: We're given v_0, a, and d, and asked for t. Since the final velocity, v, is neither given nor asked for, we use Big Five #3. Because the object is falling, its displacement is downward, so let's call *down* the positive direction; this means that $a = +g = +10\ \text{m/s}^2$. Since the term *dropped* means that the object's initial velocity is 0 m/s, we find that

$$d = v_0 t + \tfrac{1}{2}at^2 \rightarrow d = \tfrac{1}{2}at^2 \rightarrow t = \sqrt{\frac{2d}{a}} = \sqrt{\frac{2d}{+g}} = \sqrt{\frac{2(80\ \text{m})}{+10\ \text{m/s}^2}} = 4\ \text{s}$$

Example 3-20: An object is dropped from a height of 80 m. What is its velocity as it strikes the ground?

Solution: (Don't make the common mistake of thinking that the answer is 0 because once the object hits the ground, it stops. The question is really asking for the velocity of the object *as* it slams into the ground, and this won't be zero.) We're given v_0, a, and d, and asked for v. Since the time, t, is neither given nor asked for, we use Big Five #5. Because the object is falling, its displacement is downward, so let's call *down* the positive direction. This means that $a = +g = +10\ \text{m/s}^2$. Since the term *dropped* means that the object's initial velocity is 0, we find that

$$v^2 = v_0^2 + 2ad \rightarrow v^2 = 2ad \rightarrow v = \sqrt{2ad} = \sqrt{2(+g)d} = \sqrt{2(+10\ \text{m/s}^2)(80\ \text{m})} = 40\ \text{m/s}$$

Example 3-21: A ball is thrown straight upward with an initial speed of 30 m/s. How high will it go?

Solution: We're given v_0, a, and v, and asked for d. (We know v because the question is asking how high the ball will go; at the top of the ball's path, its velocity at this point is 0.) Since the time, t, is missing, we use Big Five #5. Since we're interested only in the object's upward motion, let's call *up* the positive direction. This means that $v_0 = +30\ \text{m/s}$ and $a = -g = -10\ \text{m/s}^2$. Because the velocity of the ball is 0 at its highest point, we find that

$$v^2 = v_0^2 + 2ad \rightarrow 0 = v_0^2 + 2ad \rightarrow d = -\frac{v_0^2}{2a} = -\frac{v_0^2}{2(-g)} = -\frac{(+30\ \text{m/s})^2}{2(-10\ \text{m/s}^2)} = 45\,\text{m}$$

Notice that the displacement *d* turned out to be positive; that's because we chose *up* to be our positive direction, and the ball moves *up* to its highest position.

Example 3-22: A ball of mass 10 kg and a ball of mass 1 kg are dropped simultaneously from a tower of height 45 m. If air resistance could be ignored, which ball will hit the ground first and how long does it take?

Solution: We're given v_0, a, and d, and asked for t. Since the final velocity, v, is missing, we use Big Five #3. Because each object is falling, its displacement is downward, so let's call *down* the positive direction. This means that $a = +g = +10 \text{ m/s}^2$. Remembering that the term *dropped* means that $v_0 = 0$, Big Five #3 becomes $d = \frac{1}{2}at^2$, so

$$t = \sqrt{\frac{2d}{a}} = \sqrt{\frac{2d}{+g}} = \sqrt{\frac{2(45 \text{ m})}{+10 \text{ m/s}^2}} = 3 \text{ s}$$

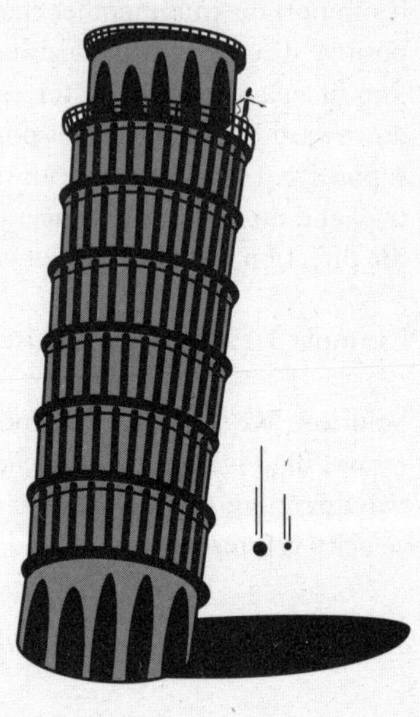

Because none of the Big Five equations involves the *mass* of the object, this is how long it takes *each* ball to strike the ground. The free-fall acceleration of an object does not depend on its mass (or size or shape), so in the absence of effects due to the air, both objects will hit the ground *at the same time.*

3.6 PROJECTILE MOTION

The examples we've worked through so far have involved objects that move along a straight line, either horizontal or vertical. However, if we were to throw a baseball up at an angle to the ground, the path the ball would follow (its **trajectory**) would not be a straight line. If we neglect effects due to the air, the path will be a *parabola.*

In this case, the motion of an object, experiencing only the constant, downward acceleration due to gravity (free fall), is called **projectile motion.** This is also a case of uniformly accelerated motion.

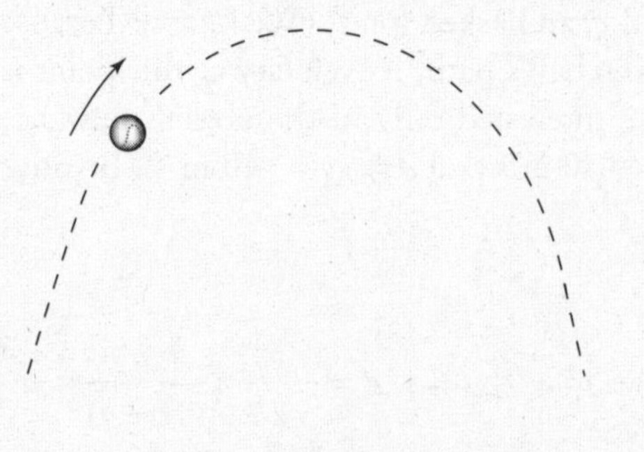

Because the projectile is experiencing both horizontal and vertical motion, we'll need to analyze both. But the trick is to analyze them *separately*. We'll use The Big Five to look at the horizontal motion, simply specializing the variables to horizontal motion; for example, we'll use x instead of d, we'll use v_{0x} and v_x instead of v_0 and v, and we'll use a_x instead of a. We'll use The Big Five to look at the vertical motion, too, and simply specialize the variables to vertical motion; we'll use y instead of d, v_{0y} and v_y instead of v_0 and v, and a_y instead of a. In this case, a_y will be equal to the gravitational acceleration.

In order to make an object follow a parabolic path, we'll need to launch the object at an angle to the horizontal. Therefore, the initial velocity vector $\mathbf{v}_0$ will have a nonzero horizontal component (v_{0x}) *and* a nonzero vertical component (v_{0y}). In terms of the **launch angle**, θ_0, which is the angle the initial velocity vector makes with the horizontal, we have $v_{0x} = v_0 \cos \theta_0$ and $v_{0y} = v_0 \sin \theta_0$.

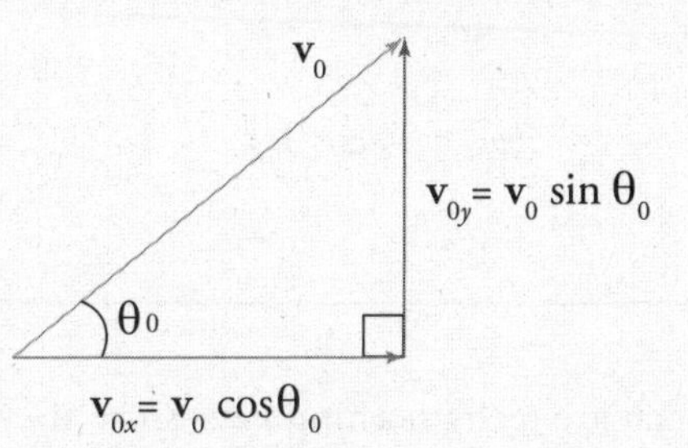

Let's first take care of the horizontal motion. This is the easier of the two for one important reason: once the projectile is launched, it no longer experiences a horizontal acceleration. That is, a_x will be zero throughout the projectile's flight. If the horizontal acceleration is zero throughout the projectile's flight, then *the horizontal velocity will be constant throughout the flight.* (This is a very important point and something the OAT loves to ask about.) If the horizontal velocity does not change, then whatever it was initially is all it'll ever be; that is, the horizontal velocity of the projectile at any point during its flight will be equal to the initial horizontal velocity, v_{0x}. Finally, if v_x is always equal to v_{0x}, then by using Big Five #1, we have $x = v_{0x}t$ (this is just *distance* = *rate* × *time* in the case where the rate is constant).

For the vertical motion, we realize that there *is* an acceleration; after all, the gravitational acceleration is vertical. In order to write down the equations for the vertical motion, we need to make a decision about which direction is positive. Let's call *up* the positive direction, so that *down* is the negative direction; this will mean that $a_y = -g$. Big Five #2 now tells us that the vertical component of the velocity, v_y, will be $v_{0y} + a_y t = v_{0y} + (-g)t$ at time t. Big Five #3 tells us that the vertical displacement of the projectile, y, will be $v_{0y}t + \frac{1}{2}a_y t^2 = v_{0y}t + \frac{1}{2}(-g)t^2$.

3.6

Projectile Motion

	Horizontal Motion	Vertical Motion
displacement:	$x = v_{0x}t$	$y = v_{0y}t + \frac{1}{2}(-g)t^2$
velocity:	$v_x = v_{0x}$ (constant!)	$v_y = v_{0y} + (-g)t$
acceleration:	$a_x = 0$	$a_y = -g$
	$(v_{0x} = v_0 \cos\theta_0)$	$(v_{0y} = v_0 \sin\theta_0)$

In addition to these formulas (which are really nothing new, since they're just a few of the Big Five equations), there are a couple of other facts worth knowing. The first involves the projectile's velocity at the top of its trajectory. Since the top of the parabola is the parabola's turning point, and an object's velocity is always tangent to its path (whatever the shape of the trajectory), the projectile's velocity will be horizontal at the top of the parabola. This means that the vertical velocity is zero. (*Be careful* not to say that the velocity is zero at the top. For a projectile moving in a parabolic path, it's only the *vertical* velocity that's zero at the top; the horizontal velocity is still there!)

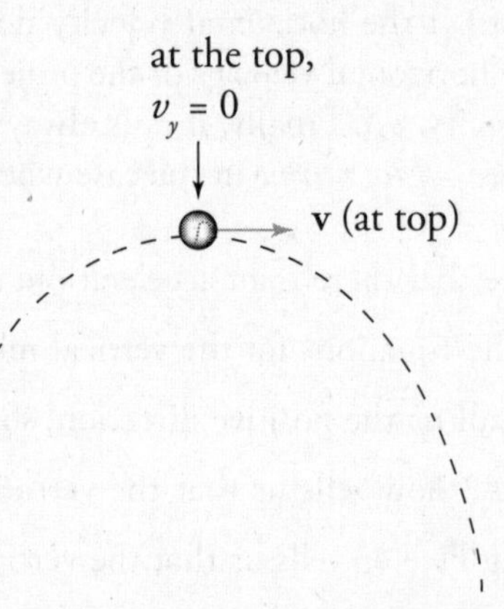

The second fact reflects the symmetry of the parabolic shape of the path. If we were to draw a vertical line up from the ground through the top point on the parabola, we'd notice that the left and right sides are just mirror images of each other. One of the consequences of this observation is that the time the projectile takes to reach the top will be the same as the time it takes to drop back down (to the same height from which it was launched). Therefore, *the projectile's total flight time will be twice the time required to reach the top*. So, for example, if the time it takes the projectile to reach the top of the parabola is 3 seconds, then the total flight time will be 6 seconds, because it'll take another 3 seconds to come back down.

Example 3-23: A cannonball is shot from ground level with an initial velocity of 100 m/s at an angle of 30° to the ground.

a) How high will the cannonball go?
b) What is the cannonball's velocity at the top of its path?
c) What will be the cannonball's total flight time?
d) How far will the cannonball travel horizontally?

Solution:

a) The maximum height reached by the projectile is the displacement y at the moment the cannonball is at the top of the parabola. What does it mean for the projectile to be at the top of the parabola? It means the vertical velocity is zero. So, we'll set the vertical velocity equal to zero:

$$v_y = v_{0y} + (-g)t \text{ with } v_y = 0 \rightarrow v_{0y} + (-g)t = 0 \rightarrow t = \frac{v_{0y}}{g} = \frac{v_0 \sin\theta_0}{g}$$

This is how long it'll take the projectile to reach the top. If we plug in $v_0 = 100$ m/s, $\theta_0 = 30°$, and $g = 10$ m/s^2, we find that

$$t = \frac{v_0 \sin\theta_0}{g} = \frac{(100 \text{ m/s})\sin 30°}{10 \text{ m/s}^2} = 5 \text{ s}$$

So now the question is, "What is y when $t = 5$ s?" All we need to do is take the equation for the vertical displacement of the projectile and plug in $t = 5$ s:

$$\begin{aligned} y &= v_{0y}t + \tfrac{1}{2}(-g)t^2 \\ &= (v_0 \sin\theta_0)t + \tfrac{1}{2}(-g)t^2 \end{aligned}$$

$$\therefore y \text{ (at } t = 5 \text{ s)} = (100 \text{ m/s} \cdot \sin 30°)(5 \text{ s}) + \tfrac{1}{2}(-10 \text{ m/s}^2)(5 \text{ s})^2 = 125 \text{ m}$$

b) At the top of its path, the cannonball's velocity is horizontal, and the horizontal velocity is the same throughout the flight, equal to the initial horizontal velocity:

$$v_x = v_{0x} = v_0 \cos\theta_0 = (100 \text{ m/s})\cos 30° \approx (100 \text{ m/s})(0.85) = 85 \text{ m/s}$$

c) The projectile's total flight time is just equal to twice the time required for it to reach the top. Since we found in part (a) that it takes 5 seconds for the cannonball to reach the top, its total flight time will be 2 × (5 s) = 10 s.

d) The question is asking for the horizontal displacement at the time when the cannonball strikes the ground. We found in part (b) that the cannonball's horizontal velocity is a constant 85 m/s, and we found in part (c) that the cannonball's total flight time is 10 seconds. Therefore, the total horizontal displacement is

$$x = v_{0x}t = (85 \text{ m/s})(10 \text{ s}) = 850 \text{ m}$$

(The total horizontal displacement is called the **range** of the projectile.)

Example 3-24: A projectile is launched from a height of 5 m with an initial velocity of 80 m/s at an angle of 40° to the horizontal. If v_{x1} is the horizontal velocity of the projectile 1 second after launch, and v_{x2} is the horizontal velocity 2 seconds after launch, what is the value of $v_{x2} - v_{x1}$?

Solution: Sounds complicated, doesn't it? The OAT would love this question, because although it seems like solving it would be messy, the solution actually requires only applying one simple fact. You remember that once a projectile is launched, its horizontal velocity remains constant during the entire flight. Therefore, $v_{x2} = v_{x1}$, and the value of $v_{x2} - v_{x1}$ is zero.

Example 3-25: A rock is thrown horizontally, with an initial speed of 10 m/s, from the edge of a vertical cliff. It strikes the ground 5 s later.

a) How high is the cliff?
b) How far from the foot of the cliff does the rock land?

Solution:

a) The height of the cliff will be the vertical distance the rock falls. Because the rock is thrown horizontally, it has no initial vertical velocity: $v_{0y} = 0$. Therefore, the equation for the projectile's vertical displacement becomes $y = \frac{1}{2}(-g)t^2$. Considering the time it takes the rock to fall is $t = 5$ s, we have $y = \frac{1}{2}(-10\text{ m/s}^2)(5\text{s})^2 = -125\text{m}$. This tells us that the rock falls 125 m in 5 s, so the height of the cliff is 125 m.

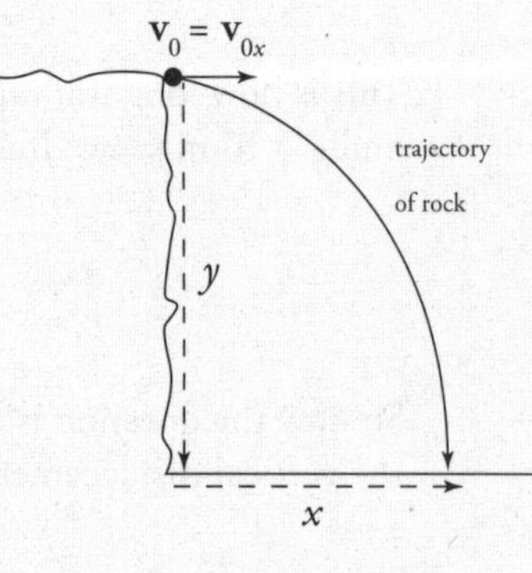

b) The horizontal displacement of the rock is given by the equation $x = v_{0x}t$. Since $v_{0x} = 10$ m/s and $t = 5$ s, we get $x = (10\text{ m/s})(5\text{s}) = 50\text{m}$.

Example 3-26: A ball is kicked from ground level, travels as an ideal projectile in a parabolic path, and hits the ground 4 seconds after it was kicked. If its initial vertical speed was 20 m/s, how high did the ball go?

Solution: If the total flight time was 4 seconds, that means it took half that time, 2 seconds, to reach the top of the parabola (its highest point). Therefore, since we're given that $v_{0y} = 20$ m/s, the vertical displacement of the ball at $t = 2$ s was

$$\begin{aligned} y &= v_{0y}t + \tfrac{1}{2}(-g)t^2 \\ &= (20\text{ m/s})(2\text{ s}) + \tfrac{1}{2}(-10\text{ m/s}^2)(2\text{ s})^2 \\ &= 20\text{ m} \end{aligned}$$

Summary of Formulas

displacement $\mathbf{d} = \Delta x =$ (final position) – (initial position) = *net* distance [plus direction]

average velocity: $\bar{\mathbf{v}} = \frac{\Delta x}{\Delta t} = \frac{\mathbf{d}}{\Delta t}$

average acceleration: $\bar{\mathbf{a}} = \frac{\Delta \mathbf{v}}{\Delta t}$

The **BIG FIVE** (for Uniformly Accelerated Motion: a = constant):

1. $d = \frac{1}{2}(v_0 + v)t$
2. $v = v_0 + at$
3. $d = v_0 t + \frac{1}{2}at^2$
4. $d = vt - \frac{1}{2}at^2$
5. $v^2 = v_0^2 + 2ad$

Position (x) vs. time (t) graph: slope = velocity (v)

Velocity (v) vs. time (t) graph: slope = acceleration (a)

area under graph = displacement (d)

Projectile Motion :

(Downward = Negative Direction)

	Horizontal Motion	**Vertical Motion**
displacement:	$x = v_{0x}t$	$y = v_{0y}t + \frac{1}{2}(-g)t^2$
velocity:	$v_{0x} = v_x$ (constant!)	$v_y = v_{0y} + (-g)t$
acceleration:	$a_x = 0$	$a_y = -g$
acceleration:	$(v_{0x} = v_0 \cos\theta_0)$	$(v_{0y} = v_0 \sin\theta_0)$

$v_y = 0$ at the top of the trajectory

$v_x \neq 0$ at the top of the trajectory

Total flight time = (time from launch to top) + (time from top to landing)

Chapter 4
Mechanics I

4.1 MASS, FORCE, AND NEWTON'S LAWS

In the preceding chapter, we studied kinematics, which is the description of motion in terms of an object's position, velocity, and acceleration. In this chapter, we'll begin our study of **dynamics**, which is the *explanation* of motion in terms of the forces that act on an object.

Simply put, a **force** is a push or pull exerted by one object on another. If you pull on a rope attached to a crate, you create a *tension* in the rope that pulls the crate. When a sky diver is falling through the air, the earth exerts a downward pull called the *gravitational force*, and the air exerts an upward force called *air resistance*. When you stand on the floor, the floor provides an upward, supporting force called the *normal force*. If you slide a book across a table, the table exerts a *frictional force* against the book, so the book slows down and eventually stops. Static cling provides a simple example of the *electrostatic force*. (In fact, all of the forces mentioned above, with the exception of gravity, are due ultimately to the electromagnetic force.)

Newton's First Law

An object's state of motion—its *velocity*—will not change unless a net force acts on the object.

That is, if no net force acts on an object, then:

if the object is at rest, it will remain at rest;

and

if the object is moving, then it will continue to move with constant velocity

(constant speed in a straight line).

Or, more simply: **no net force = no acceleration.**

How forces affect motion is described by three physical laws, known as **Newton's laws**. They form the foundation of mechanics, and you should memorize them.

The first law says that objects naturally resist changing their velocity. In other words, objects at rest don't just suddenly start moving all on their own. Some external source must exert a force to make them move. Also, an object that's already moving doesn't change its velocity. It doesn't go faster, or slower, or change direction all by itself; something must exert some force on it to make any of these changes happen. This property of objects, their natural resistance to change in their state of motion, is called **inertia**. In fact, the first law is often referred to as the *law of inertia*.

It's important to note that the first law applies when there is no *net* force on an object. This could mean there are no forces at all, though that couldn't happen in our universe; more commonly, it means the forces on an object balance out, in other words, the total of all the forces, in each dimension, is zero. We'll work examples of computing net force when we get to Newton's second law.

The **mass** of an object is the quantitative measure of its inertia; intuitively, mass measures how much matter is contained in an object. Mass is measured in *kilograms*, abbreviated kg. (Note: An object whose mass is 1 kg weighs a little more than 2 pounds on Earth, but be careful not to confuse mass with weight; they're different things.) Compared to an object whose mass is just 1 kg, an object whose mass is 100 kg has 100 times the inertia. Intuitively, we'd find it 100 times more difficult to cause the same change in its motion than we would with the 1 kg object. This point will be clearer after we state the second of Newton's laws.

Newton's Second Law

If $\mathbf{F}_{net}$ is the net—or total—force acting on an object of mass m, then the resulting acceleration of the object, $\mathbf{a}$, satisfies this simple equation:

$$\mathbf{F}_{net} = m\mathbf{a}$$

Notice that the first law is really just a special case of the second law: the case in which $\mathbf{F}_{net} = 0$.

Forces are represented by vectors, because a force has a magnitude and a direction. If two different forces (let's call them $\mathbf{F}_1$ and $\mathbf{F}_2$) act on an object, then the total—or *net*—force on the object is the sum of these individual forces: $\mathbf{F}_{net} = \mathbf{F}_1 + \mathbf{F}_2$. Since forces are vectors, they must be added as vectors; that is, their directions must be taken into account. The following figures show some examples of obtaining $\mathbf{F}_{net}$ from the individual forces that act on an object:

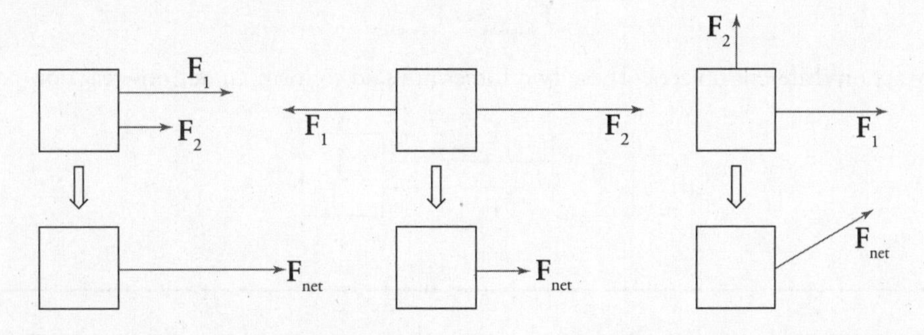

Note the following facts about the equation $\mathbf{F}_{net} = m\mathbf{a}$:

1. $\mathbf{F}_{net}$ is the sum of all the forces that act *on* the object; namely, the object whose mass, m, is on the other side of the equation. Any force exerted *by* the object is *not* included in $\mathbf{F}_{net}$.
2. Because m is a *positive* number, the direction of $\mathbf{a}$ is always the same as the direction of $\mathbf{F}_{net}$. Therefore, an object will accelerate in the direction of the net force it feels. This does not mean that an object will always *move* in the direction of $\mathbf{F}_{net}$. Be sure that this distinction makes sense because it can be a source of confusion, and therefore a potential OAT trap. Newton's second law tells us about the direction of an object's *acceleration* but does not define the direction of an object's velocity.
3. What if $\mathbf{F}_{net} = 0$? Then $\mathbf{a} = 0$. What does $\mathbf{a} = 0$ mean? It means that the object's velocity does not change, which is also what Newton's *first* law says. But how about this question: Does $\mathbf{F}_{net} = 0$ mean that $\mathbf{v} = 0$? Not necessarily! $\mathbf{F}_{net} = 0$ means that an object won't *accelerate*, not that it won't move. This is a key point and another potential OAT trap. If the object is already moving at, say, 100 m/s toward the north, then it will continue to move at 100 m/s toward the north as long as the net force on the object remains zero.

4. Because $\mathbf{F}_{net} = m\mathbf{a}$ is a vector equation, it automatically means that the components of both sides must be the same. In other words, $\mathbf{F}_{net}$ could be written as the sum of a force in the horizontal direction, ($\mathbf{F}_{net,x}$) plus a force in the vertical direction ($\mathbf{F}_{net,y}$); these would be the horizontal and vertical components of $\mathbf{F}_{net}$. The equation $\mathbf{F}_{net} = m\mathbf{a}$ would then tell us that $\mathbf{F}_{net,x} = m\mathbf{a}_x$ and $\mathbf{F}_{net,y} = m\mathbf{a}_y$. So, dividing the horizontal component of the net force by m gives us the horizontal component of the object's acceleration, and dividing the vertical component of the net force by m gives us the vertical component of the object's acceleration.
5. The unit of force is equal to the unit of mass times the unit of acceleration:

$$[F] = [m][a] = \text{kg} \cdot \text{m/s}^2$$

A force of 1 kg·m/s² is called 1 **newton** (abbreviated N). A force of 1 N is about equal to a quarter of a pound, or about the weight of a medium-sized apple (on Earth).

Newton's Third Law

If Object 1 exerts a force, $\mathbf{F}_{1\text{-on-}2}$, on Object 2, then Object 2 exerts a force, $\mathbf{F}_{2\text{-on-}1}$, on Object 1. These forces, $\mathbf{F}_{1\text{-on-}2}$ and $\mathbf{F}_{2\text{-on-}1}$, have the same magnitude but act in opposite directions, so

$$\mathbf{F}_{1\text{-on-}2} = -\mathbf{F}_{2\text{-on-}1}$$

and they act on different objects. These two forces are said to form an **action–reaction pair.**

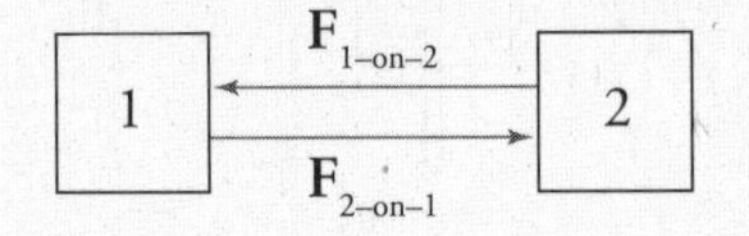

This is the law commonly stated as, "For every action, there is an equal but opposite reaction." Unfortunately, this popular version of Newton's third law can lead to confusion. Essentially, Newton's third law says that the *forces* in an action–reaction pair have the same magnitude and act in opposite directions (and on "opposite" objects). It does *not* say that the *effects* of these forces will be the same. For example, suppose that two skaters are next to and facing each other on a skating rink. Let's say that Skater 1 has a mass of 50 kg and Skater 2 has a mass of 100 kg. Now, what if Skater 1 pushes on Skater 2 with a force of 50 N? Then $\mathbf{F}_{1\text{-on-}2} = 50$ N and $\mathbf{F}_{2\text{-on-}1} = -50$ N, by Newton's third law.

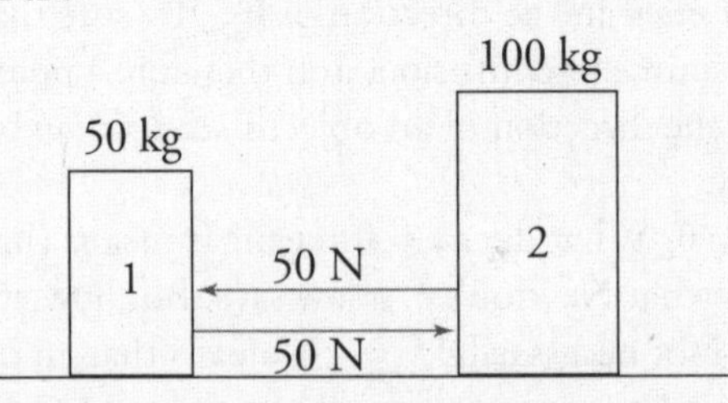

But will the *effects* of these equal-strength forces be the same? No, because the masses of the objects are different. The accelerations of the skaters will be

$$\mathbf{a}_1 = \frac{\mathbf{F}_{2\text{-on-}1}}{m_1} = \frac{-50\text{ N}}{50\text{ kg}} = -1\text{ m/s}^2 \text{ and } \mathbf{a}_2 = \frac{\mathbf{F}_{1\text{-on-}2}}{m_2} = \frac{+50\text{ N}}{100\text{ kg}} = +0.5\text{ m/s}^2$$

So, Skater 2 will move away with an acceleration of 0.5 m/s^2, while Skater 1 moves away, in the opposite direction, with an acceleration of twice that magnitude, 1 m/s^2.

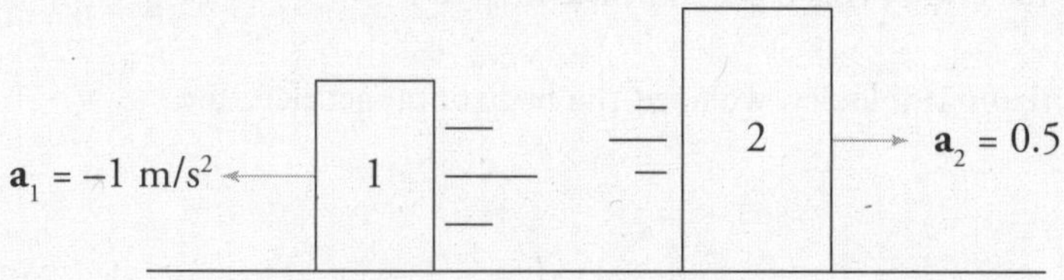

$\mathbf{a}_1 = -1$ m/s^2 ← 1 2 → $\mathbf{a}_2 = 0.5$ m/s^2

Therefore, while the forces are the same (in magnitude), the effects of these forces —that is, the resulting accelerations (and velocities)—are not the same, because the masses of the objects are different. Newton's third law says nothing about mass; it only tells us that the action and reaction forces will have the same magnitude. So, the point is not to interpret "equal but opposite reaction" as meaning "equal but opposite effect," because if the masses of the interacting objects are not the same, then the resulting accelerations (and velocities) of the objects will not be the same.

The key to distinguishing Newton's first law from Newton's third law is to focus on the description of the forces. In Newton's first law, all of the forces must be acting on a *single* object; thus, the net force on a single object is calculated by adding those vectors. However, in Newton's third law, each force must be acting on a *different* object in an action-reaction pair.

There are two aspects of Newton's third law that frequently give students trouble. First, just because two forces are equal and opposite does *not* mean they form an action-reaction pair; the forces also have to be from two objects acting on each other, not two objects acting on a third object. Second, the third law applies even when the objects are accelerating; even if one object is accelerating, the second object pushes or pulls just as hard on the first as the first pushes or pulls on the second.

Example 4-1: An object of mass 50 kg moves with a constant velocity of magnitude 1000 m/s. What is the net force on this object?

Solution: If the object moves with constant velocity, then the net force it feels must be zero, regardless of the object's mass or speed.

Example 4-2: The net force on an object of mass 10 kg is zero. What can you say about the speed of this object?

Solution: If the net force on an object is zero, all we can say is that it will not accelerate; its velocity may be zero, or it may not. Without more information, we cannot determine the object's speed; all we know is that whatever the speed is, it will remain constant.

Example 4-3: For 6 seconds, you push a 120 kg crate along a frictionless horizontal surface with a constant force of 60 N parallel to the surface. If the crate was initially at rest, what will its velocity be at the end of this 6-second time interval?

Solution: Using Newton's second law, we find that the acceleration of the crate is $a = F/m$ = (60 N)/(120 kg) = 0.5 m/s^2. Using Big Five #2, we now find that $v = v_0 + at = 0 + (0.5 \text{ m/s}^2)(6 \text{ s}) = 3$ m/s.

Example 4-4: For 6 seconds, you pull a 120 kg crate along a frictionless horizontal surface with a constant force of 60 N directed at an angle of 60° to the surface. If the crate was initially at rest, what will its horizontal velocity be at the end of this 6-second time interval?

Solution: To find the horizontal velocity, we need the horizontal acceleration.

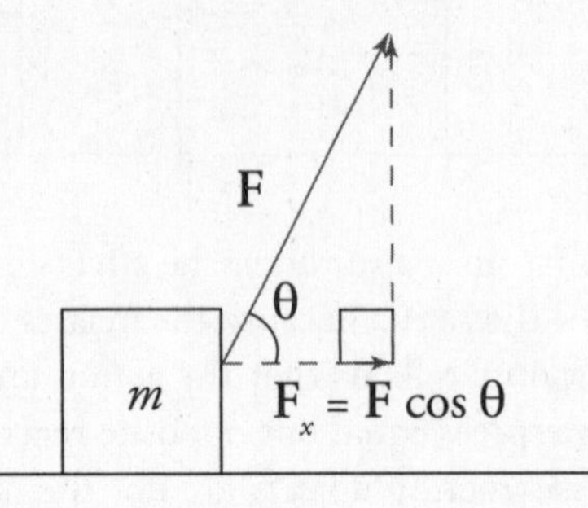

Using Newton's second law, we find that the horizontal acceleration of the crate is $a_x = F_x/m = (F \cos \theta)/m = (60 \text{ N} \cos 60°)/(120 \text{ kg}) = (30 \text{ N})/(120 \text{ kg}) = 0.25 \text{ m/s}^2$. Using Big Five #2, we now find that $v_x = v_{0x} + a_x t = 0 + (0.25 \text{ m/s}^2)(6 \text{ s}) = 1.5 \text{ m/s}$.

Example 4-5: Two crates are moving along a frictionless horizontal surface. The first crate, of mass $M = 100$ kg, is being pushed by a force of 300 N. The first crate is in contact with a second crate, of mass $m = 50$ kg.

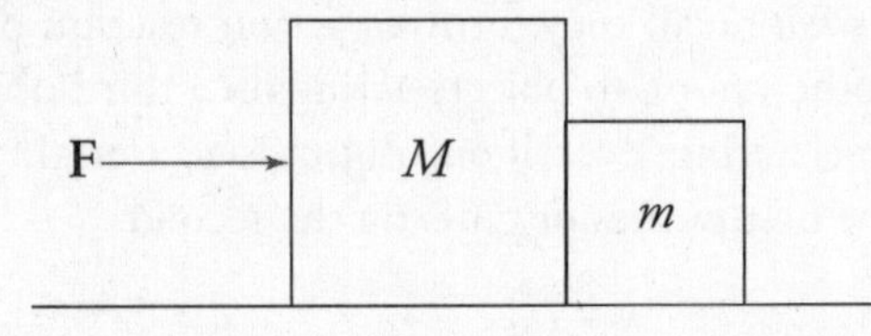

a) What's the acceleration of the crates?
b) What's the force exerted by the larger crate on the smaller one?
c) What's the force exerted by the smaller crate on the larger one?

Solution:

a) The force **F** is pushing on a combined mass of 100 kg + 50 kg = 150 kg, so by Newton's second law, the acceleration of both crates will be $a = (300 \text{ N})/(150 \text{ kg}) = 2 \text{ m/s}^2$.
b) Because M and m are in direct contact, each is pushing on the other with a certain force. Let $\mathbf{F}_2$ be the force that M exerts on m. Then we must have $F_2 = ma$, so $F_2 = (50 \text{ kg})(2 \text{ m/s}^2) = 100$ N.
c) By Newton's third law, if the force that M exerts on m is $\mathbf{F}_2$, then the force that m exerts on M must be $-\mathbf{F}_2$. So, if we call "to the right" our positive direction, then the force that m exerts on M is –100 N. We can check that this is correct by looking at all the forces acting on M. We have **F** pushing to the right and $-\mathbf{F}_2$ pushing to the left. The net force on M is therefore $\mathbf{F}_{\text{net on } M} = \mathbf{F} + (-\mathbf{F}_2) = (300 \text{ N}) + (-100 \text{ N}) = 200$ N. If this is correct, then $F_{\text{net on } M}$ should equal Ma. Since $M = 100$ kg and $a = 2 \text{ m/s}^2$, we get $Ma = 200$ N, which does match what we found for $F_{\text{net on } M}$. (In effect, what's happening here is that M is using 200 N of the 300 N force from **F** for its own motion and passing the remaining 100 N along to m, so that both move together with the same acceleration.)

Example 4-6: Two forces act on an object of mass $m = 5$ kg. One of the forces has a magnitude of 6 N, and the other force, perpendicular to the first, has a magnitude of 8 N. What's the acceleration of the object?

Solution: Forces are vectors, and when we find the net force on this object, we see that it's the hypotenuse of a 6-8-10 right triangle.

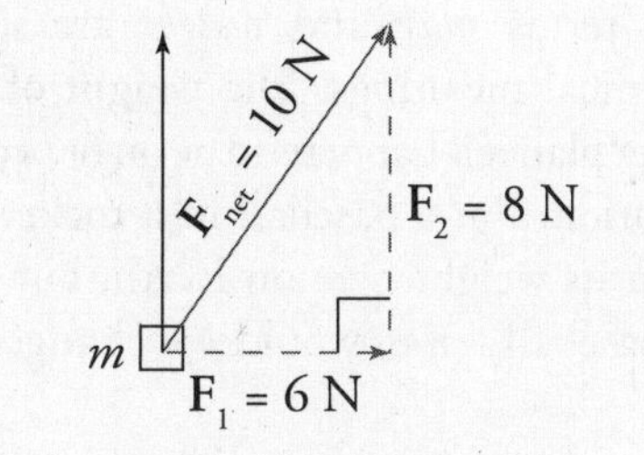

Since $F_{net} = 10$ N, the acceleration of the object will be $a = F_{net}/m = (10 \text{ N})/(5 \text{ kg}) = 2 \text{ m/s}^2$.

Example 4-7: The figure below shows all the forces acting on a 5 kg object. The magnitude of $\mathbf{F}_1$ is 50 N. If the acceleration of the object is 8 m/s², what's the magnitude of $\mathbf{F}_2$?

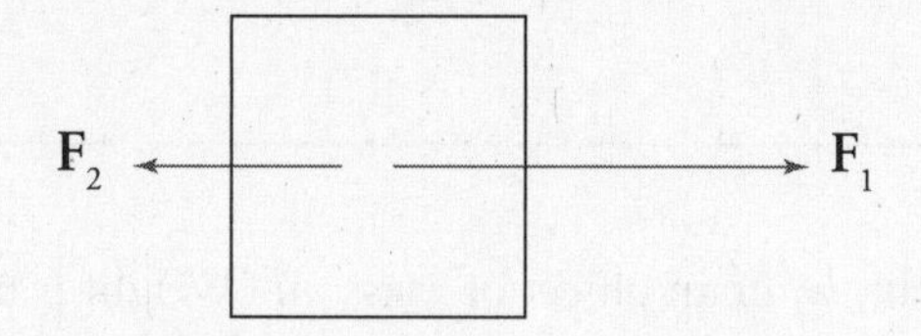

Solution: The net force on the block is just the sum of $\mathbf{F}_1$ and $\mathbf{F}_2$, so $\mathbf{F}_{net} = \mathbf{F}_1 + \mathbf{F}_2 = (+50 \text{ N}) + \mathbf{F}_2$, if we call "to the right" our positive direction. The net force must be $ma = (5 \text{ kg})(8 \text{ m/s}^2) = 40$ N. Since (+50 N) + $\mathbf{F}_2$ must be 40 N, we know that $\mathbf{F}_2 = -10$ N; that is, $\mathbf{F}_2$ has magnitude 10 N (and points to the left).

Example 4-8: According to Newton's third law, every force is "accompanied by" an equal but opposite force. If this is true, shouldn't these forces cancel out to zero? How could we ever accelerate an object?

Solution: The answer does not involve the masses of the objects; Newton's third law says nothing about mass. The key is to remember what $\mathbf{F}_{net}$ means; it's the sum of all the forces that act *on* an object, not *by* the object. Let's say we have a pair of objects, 1 and 2, and an action–reaction pair of forces between them, and we wanted to find the acceleration of Object 2. We'd find all the forces that act on Object 2. One of these forces is $\mathbf{F}_{1\text{-on-}2}$. The reaction force, $\mathbf{F}_{2\text{-on-}1}$, is *not* included in $\mathbf{F}_{net\text{-on-}2}$ because it doesn't act on Object 2; it's a force *by* Object 2. So, the reason why the two forces in an action–reaction pair don't cancel each other is that we'd never add them in the first place because they don't act on the same object.

4.2 NEWTON'S LAW OF GRAVITATION

The mass of an object is a measure of its inertia, its resistance to acceleration. We'll now look at the related concept of an object's weight.

Although in everyday language the terms *mass* and *weight* are sometimes used interchangeably, in physics they have very different technical meanings. The **weight** of an object is the gravitational force exerted on it by the earth (or by whatever planet it happens to be on or near). **Mass** is an intrinsic property of an object and does not change with location. Put a baseball in a rocket and send it to the moon. The baseball's *weight* on the moon is less than its weight here on Earth, but you'd have as much "baseball stuff" there as you would here; that is, the baseball's *mass* would *not* change.

Since weight is a force, we can use $\mathbf{F} = m\mathbf{a}$ to compute it. What acceleration would the gravitational force (which is what *weight* means) impose on an object? The gravitational acceleration, of course! Therefore, setting $\mathbf{a} = \mathbf{g}$, the equation $\mathbf{F} = m\mathbf{a}$ becomes

$$\mathbf{w} = m\mathbf{g}$$

This is the equation for the weight, $\mathbf{w}$, of an object of mass m. (Weight is often symbolized by $\mathbf{F}_{grav}$, rather than $\mathbf{w}$; we'll use both notations.) Note that mass and weight are proportional but not identical. Furthermore, mass is measured in kilograms, while weight is measured in newtons.

Example 4-9:

a) Find the weight of an object whose mass is 50 kg.
b) Find the mass of an object whose weight is 50 N.

Solution:

a) To find an object's weight, we multiply its mass by g. Using $g = 10$ m/s^2 (or, equivalently, $g = 10$ N/kg), we find that $w = mg = (50 \text{ kg})(10 \text{ N/kg}) = 500$ N.
b) To find an object's mass, we divide its weight by g. With $g = 10$ N/kg, we find that $m = w/g = (50 \text{ N})/(10 \text{ N/kg}) = 5$ kg.

Most of the time, we'll use the formula $w = mg$ to find the weight of an object whose mass is m. However, the value of g can change, and if we're not near the surface of the earth (where we know that g is approximately 10 m/s^2) we may not know the value of g. In that case, we'll invoke another law discovered by Newton:

Newton's Law of Gravitation

Every object in the universe exerts a gravitational pull on every other object. The magnitude of this gravitational force is proportional to the product of the objects' masses and inversely proportional to the square of the distance between them. The constant of proportionality is denoted by G and known as Newton's universal gravitational constant.

$$F_{grav} = G\frac{Mm}{r^2}$$

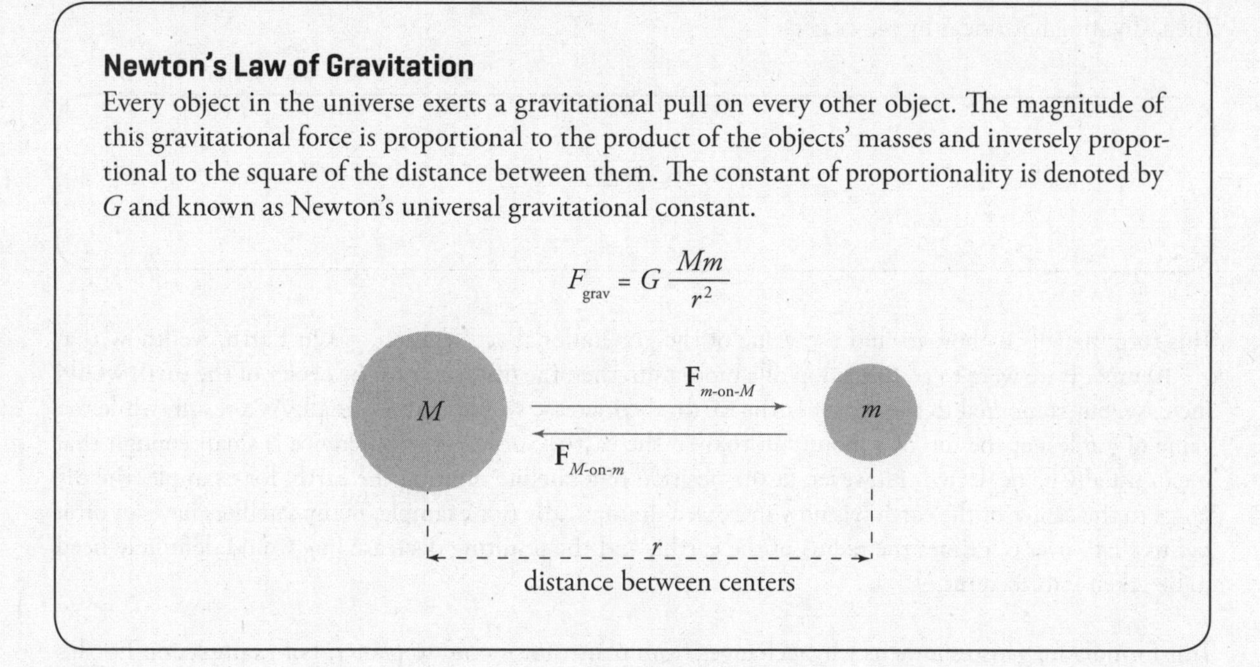

The value of G is roughly 6.7×10^{-11} N·m²/kg², but don't bother memorizing this constant. If you actually need the value on the OAT (which is unlikely), it will be provided. Unfortunately, sometimes it will be provided even when you don't need it.

One of the most important features of Newton's law of gravitation is that it's an **inverse-square law.** This means that the magnitude of the gravitational force is *inversely* proportional to the *square* of the distance between the centers of the objects. (Another important physical law, Coulomb's law [for the electrostatic force between two charges], which we'll see later, is also an inverse-square law.)

Also notice that the forces illustrated in the box above form an action–reaction pair. Even if M and m are different, the gravitational force that M exerts on m has the same magnitude as the gravitational force that m exerts on M. (If the directions of the force vectors in the box above seem backward, remember that gravity is always a *pulling* force; therefore, in the figure above, $\mathbf{F}_{M\text{-on-}m}$ pulls to the left, toward M, while $\mathbf{F}_{m\text{-on-}M}$ pulls to the right, toward m.) Of course, the accelerations of the objects will have different magnitudes if the masses are different, as we discussed earlier when we studied Newton's third law.

Example 4-10: What will happen to the gravitational force between two objects if the distance between them is doubled? What if the distance is cut in half?

Solution: Since the gravitational force obeys an inverse-square law, if r increases by a factor of 2, then F_{grav} will *decrease* by a factor of $2^2 = 4$. On the other hand, if r decreases by a factor of 2, then F_{grav} will *increase* by a factor of $2^2 = 4$.

Notice that the two formulas given in this section, $w = mg$ and $F_{grav} = GMm/r^2$, are really formulas for the same thing. After all, weight *is* gravitational force. Therefore, we could set these expressions equal to each other:

$$mg = G\frac{Mm}{r^2}$$

Then, dividing both sides by m, we get

$$g = G\frac{M}{r^2}$$

This formula tells us how to find the value of the gravitational acceleration, g. On Earth, we know that $g \approx 10$ m/s^2. If we were to go to the top of a mountain, then the distance r to the center of the earth would increase, but compared to the radius of the earth, the increase would be very small. As a result, while the value of g *is* less at the top of a mountain than at the earth's surface, the difference is small enough that it can usually be neglected. However, at the position of a satellite orbiting the earth, for example, the distance to the center of the earth has now increased dramatically (for example, many satellites have an orbit radius that's over 6.5 times the radius of the earth), and the resulting decrease in g would definitely need to be taken into account.

This formula for g also shows us why g changes from planet (or moon) to planet. For example, on Earth's moon, the value of g is only about 1.6 m/s^2 (about a sixth of what it is on Earth) because the mass of the moon is so much smaller than the mass of the earth. It's true that the radius of the moon is smaller than the radius of the earth, which would, by itself, make g bigger, but M is *much* smaller, and this is why the value of g on the surface of the moon is smaller than its value on the surface of the earth. So, while big G is a universal gravitational constant, the value of little g depends on where you are.

Example 4-11: The radius of the Earth is approximately 6.4×10^6 m. What's the mass of the Earth?

Solution: We can use the formula $g = GM/r^2$ to solve for M:

$$M = \frac{gr^2}{G} = \frac{(10 \text{ m/s}^2)(6.4 \times 10^6 \text{ m})^2}{6.7 \times 10^{-11} \frac{\text{N}\cdot\text{m}^2}{\text{kg}^2}} \approx 6 \times 10^{24} \text{ kg}$$

Example 4-12: The mass of Mars is about 1/10 the mass of Earth, and the radius of Mars is about half that of Earth. Is the value of g on the surface of Mars less than, greater than, or equal to the value of g on Earth?

Solution: We'll use the formula $g = GM/r^2$ to compare the two values of g:

$$\frac{g_{\text{Mars}}}{g_{\text{Earth}}} = \frac{G\frac{M_{\text{Mars}}}{r_{\text{Mars}}^2}}{G\frac{M_{\text{Earth}}}{r_{\text{Earth}}^2}} = \frac{M_{\text{Mars}}}{M_{\text{Earth}}} \cdot \left(\frac{r_{\text{Earth}}}{r_{\text{Mars}}}\right)^2 = \frac{1}{10} \cdot 2^2 = 0.4$$

Therefore, the value of g on Mars is only about 40% of its value here.

Example 4-13: A long, flat, frictionless table is set up on the surface of the moon (where $g = 1.6$ m/s^2). An object whose mass on Earth is 4 kg is also transported there.

a) What is the object's mass on the moon?
b) What is the object's weight on the moon?
c) If we drop this object from a height of $h = 20$ m, with what speed will it strike the lunar surface?
d) If we wish to push this object across the table to give it an acceleration of 3 m/s^2, how much force must we exert? Would this force be different if the table and object were back on Earth?

Solution:

a) The mass is the same, 4 kg.
b) The weight of the object on the moon is $w = m \cdot g_{\text{moon}} = (4 \text{ kg})(1.6 \text{ m/s}^2) = 6.4$ N. Notice that the object's weight on the moon is different from its weight on Earth.
c) Calling *down* the positive direction and using Big Five #5 with $v_0 = 0$ and $a = g_{\text{moon}} = 1.6$ m/s^2, we find that

$$v^2 = v_0^2 + 2ad \rightarrow v^2 = 2gh \rightarrow v = \sqrt{2gh} = \sqrt{2(1.6 \text{ m/s}^2)(20 \text{ m})} = 8 \text{ m/s}$$

d) Using $F = ma$, we get $F = (4 \text{ kg})(3 \text{ m/s}^2) = 12$ N. Since Newton's second law depends only on mass (not on weight, because there's no g in Newton's second law), we'd need this same force even if the object and table were back on Earth.

Example 4-14: A satellite is orbiting the earth at an altitude equal to 3 times the earth's radius. If the satellite weighs 144,000 N on the surface of the earth, what is the gravitational force on the satellite while it's in orbit?

Solution: Let R be the radius of the earth. If the satellite's *altitude*, h, is $3R$, then its distance *from the center* of the earth is $R + h = R + 3R = 4R$. Therefore, the distance from the earth's center has increased by a factor of 4, not 3. Since Newton's law of gravitation is an inverse-square law, the fact that r has increased by a factor of 4 means that F_{grav} has decreased by a factor of $4^2 = 16$. The gravitational force on the satellite while it's in orbit is therefore $\frac{1}{16}(144{,}000 \text{ N}) = 9{,}000$ N.

4.3 FRICTION

Some of the examples in the preceding sections described a frictionless surface. Of course, there's no such thing as a truly frictionless surface, but when a problem uses a term like *frictionless*, it simply means that friction is so weak that it can be neglected. Having frictionless surfaces also made those examples easier, so we could become comfortable with Newton's laws while first learning to apply them. However, there are cases in which friction cannot be ignored, so we need to learn how to handle such situations.

When two materials are in contact, there's an electrical attraction between the atoms of one surface with those of the other; this attraction will make it difficult to slide one object relative to the other. In addition, if the surfaces aren't perfectly smooth, the roughness will also increase the force required to slide the objects against each other. **Friction** is the term we use for the combination of these effects. Fortunately, the forces due to all those intermolecular forces and to the interactions of surface irregularities can be expressed by a single equation.

The OAT will expect you to know about two big categories of friction; they're called **static friction** and **kinetic** (or **sliding**) **friction.**[1] When there's no relative motion between the surfaces that are in contact (that is, when there's no sliding) we have static friction; when there *is* relative motion between the surfaces (that is, when there *is* sliding) we have kinetic friction.

Now, in order to state the equations we'll use to figure out these frictional forces, we first need to discuss another contact force, the one known as the normal force.

Place a book on a flat table. Assuming that the book isn't too heavy and the tabletop isn't made of, say, tissue paper, the book will remain supported by the table. One force acting on the book is the downward gravitational force. If this were the only force acting on the book, then the book would fall through the table. Hence, there must be an upward force acting on the book that cancels out the book's weight. This supporting force, which acts perpendicular to the tabletop, is called the **normal force.** It's called the *normal* force because it is, by definition, perpendicular to the surface that exerts it. The word *normal* means *perpendicular.* We'll denote the normal force by **N** or by $\mathbf{F}_N$. [Don't confuse **N** (or its magnitude, N) with the abbreviation for the newton, N.] In the case of an object simply lying on a flat surface, the magnitude of the normal force is just equal to the object's weight. As a result, the book feels a downward force of magnitude $w = mg$ and an upward force of magnitude $N = mg$, so the net force on the book is 0.

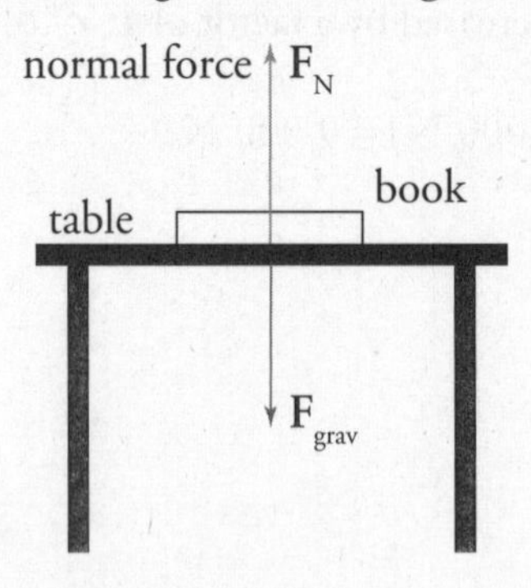

---

[1] Occasionally the OAT may refer to **rolling resistance.** Rolling resistance is not technically friction; it is the force that resists an object's rolling motion. Do not confuse rolling resistance with kinetic friction; an object can roll without sliding (or skidding), and any friction at the contact point between the object and the surface will then be static, not kinetic.

Example 4-15: Do the normal force and the gravitational force described in the preceding paragraph form an action–reaction pair?

Solution: No. While these forces *are* equal but opposite, they do not form an action–reaction pair, because they act on the same object (namely, the book). The forces in an action–reaction pair always act on different objects. So, while it's true that the forces in an action–reaction pair are always equal but opposite, it is not true that any pair of equal but opposite forces must always form an action–reaction pair. The reaction force to $\mathbf{F}_{\text{table-on-book}}$, which is the normal force, is $\mathbf{F}_{\text{book-on-table}}$. The reaction force to $\mathbf{F}_{\text{Earth-on-book}}$, which is the weight of the book, is $\mathbf{F}_{\text{book-on-Earth}}$. The force $\mathbf{F}_{\text{table-on-book}}$ is not the reaction to $\mathbf{F}_{\text{Earth-on-book}}$.

For an object on a horizontal surface that feels no other downward forces, the normal force will be equal to the weight of the object. However, there are many cases in which the normal force isn't equal to the weight of the object. For example, suppose we place a book against a vertical wall and push on the book with a horizontal force **F**. Then the magnitude of the normal force exerted by the wall will be equal to F, which may certainly be different from the weight of the book. Here's another example (which we'll look at in more detail in the next section): If we place a book on an inclined plane (e.g., a ramp) then the normal force exerted by the ramp on the book will not be equal to the weight of the book. What we can say is the general definition of the normal force: *The normal force is the perpendicular component of the contact force exerted by a surface on an object.*

We had to discuss the normal force here, because the force of friction exerted by a surface on an object in contact is related to the normal force. In the case of sliding (kinetic) friction, the magnitude of the force of friction is directly proportional to the magnitude of the normal force. The constant of proportionality depends on what the surface is made of and what the object is made of; this constant is called the **coefficient of kinetic friction**, denoted by μ_k (the Greek letter *mu*, with subscript k), where the k denotes kinetic friction. For every pair of surfaces, the coefficient μ_k is an experimentally determined positive number with no units, and the greater its value, the greater the force of kinetic friction. For example, the value of μ_k for rubber-soled shoes on ice is only about 0.1, while for rubber-soled shoes on wood, the value of μ_k is much higher; it's about 0.7 for your sneakers, but could be greater than 1 if you walk around in rock-climbing shoes.

Notice carefully that this is *not* a vector equation. It is only an equation giving the *magnitude* of $\mathbf{F}_f$ in terms of the *magnitude* of $\mathbf{F}_N$.

Force of Kinetic Friction

$$F_f = \mu_k F_N$$

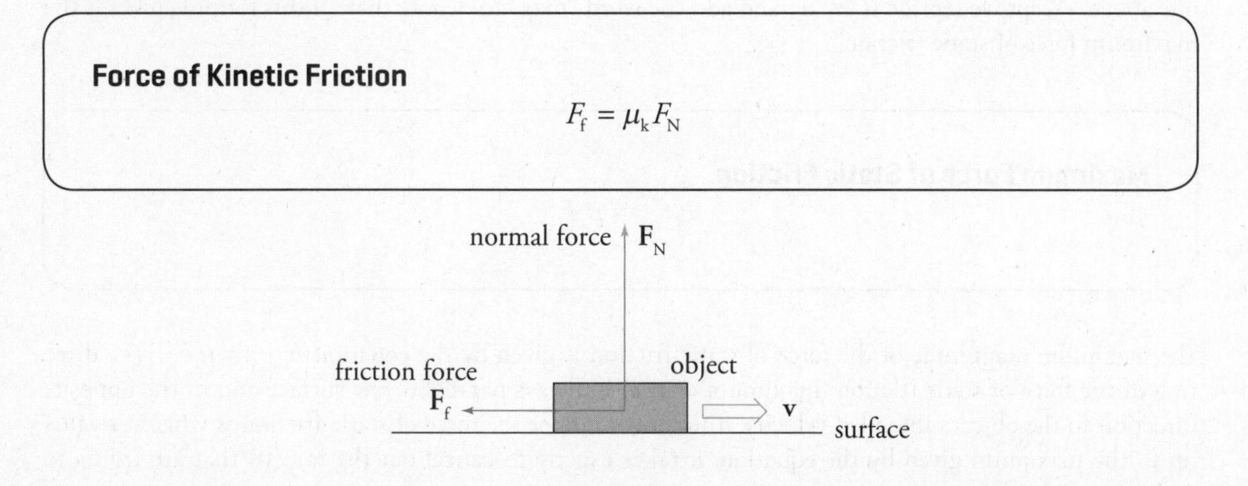

The magnitude of the force of kinetic friction is given by the equation $F_f = \mu_k F_N$. The direction of the force of kinetic friction is always parallel to the surface and in the opposite direction to the object's velocity (relative to the surface).

Example 4-16: A book of mass $m = 2$ kg slides across a flat tabletop. If the coefficient of kinetic friction between the book and table is 0.4, what's the magnitude of the force of kinetic friction on the book?

Solution: Because the magnitude of the normal force is $F_N = mg = (2 \text{ kg})(10 \text{ m/s}^2) = 20$ N, the magnitude of the force of kinetic friction is $F_f = \mu_k F_N = (0.4)(20 \text{ N}) = 8$ N.

The formula for static friction is similar to the one for kinetic friction, but there are two important differences. First, given a pair of surfaces, there's a **maximum coefficient of static friction** between them, μ_s (the subscript *s* now denotes static friction), and on the OAT, it's always greater than the coefficient of kinetic friction. This is equivalent to saying that, in general, static friction is capable of being stronger than kinetic friction. To illustrate this, imagine there's a heavy crate sitting on the floor and you want to push the crate across the room. You walk up to the crate and push on it, harder and harder until, finally, it "gives" and starts sliding. Once the crate is sliding, it's easier to keep it sliding than it was to get it started in the first place. The friction that resisted your initial push to get the crate moving was static friction. Because it was easier to keep it sliding than it was to get it started sliding, kinetic friction must be weaker than the maximum static friction force.

The second difference between the formula for kinetic friction and the one for static friction is that there's actually no general formula for the force of static friction. All we have is a formula for the *maximum* force of static friction. It's important that you understand this distinction. Let's go back to that heavy crate sitting on the floor. Let's say you know by previous experience that it'll take 400 N of force on your part to get that crate sliding. So, what if you push with a force of 100 N? Well, obviously, the crate won't move. Therefore, there must be another 100 N acting on the crate, opposite to your push, to make the net force on the crate zero. Okay, what if you now push on the crate with a force of 200 N? The crate still won't move, so there must now be another 200 N acting on the crate, opposite to your push, to make the net force on the crate zero. Whatever force you exert on the crate, as long as it's less than 400 N, will cause the force of static friction to cancel you out. Static friction is capable of supplying any necessary force, but only up to a certain maximum. That's why we can't write down a general formula for the force of static friction, only a formula for the maximum force of static friction. The formula looks just like the one above, except we replace μ_k by μ_s, and add the word "max" to denote that all this formula gives is the maximum force of static friction.

Maximum Force of Static Friction

$$F_{f,\text{max}} = \mu_s F_N$$

The maximum magnitude of the force of static friction is given by the equation $F_{f,\text{max}} = \mu_s F_N$. The direction of the force of static friction (maximum or not) is always parallel to the surface and in the opposite direction to the object's intended velocity. The magnitude of the force of static friction is whatever value, up to the maximum given by the equation, it takes exactly to cancel out the force(s) that are trying to make the object slide.

Example 4-17: A crate that weighs 1000 N rests on a horizontal floor. The coefficient of static friction between the crate and the floor is 0.4. If you push on the crate with a force of 250 N, what is the magnitude of the force of static friction?

Solution: The answer is not 400 N. The *maximum* force of static friction that the floor could exert on the crate is $F_{f,\,max} = \mu_s F_N$ = (0.4)(1000 N) = 400 N. However, if you exert a force of only 250 N on the crate, then static friction will only be 250 N. (Just imagine what would happen to the crate if you pushed on it with a force of 250 N and the floor pushed it back toward you with a force of 400 N!)

Example 4-18: You push a 50 kg block of wood across a flat concrete driveway, exerting a constant force of 300 N. If the coefficient of kinetic friction between the wood and concrete is 0.5, what will be the acceleration of the block?

Solution: The normal force acting on the block has magnitude $F_N = mg$ = (50 kg)(10 m/s²) = 500 N. Therefore, the force of kinetic friction acting on the sliding block has magnitude $F_f = \mu_k F_N$ = (0.5)(500 N) = 250 N. This means that the net force acting on the block (and parallel to the driveway) is equal to $F - F_f$ = (300 N) – (250 N) = 50 N. If F_{net} = 50 N and m = 50 kg, then $a = F_{net}/m$ = (50 N)/(50 kg) = 1 m/s².

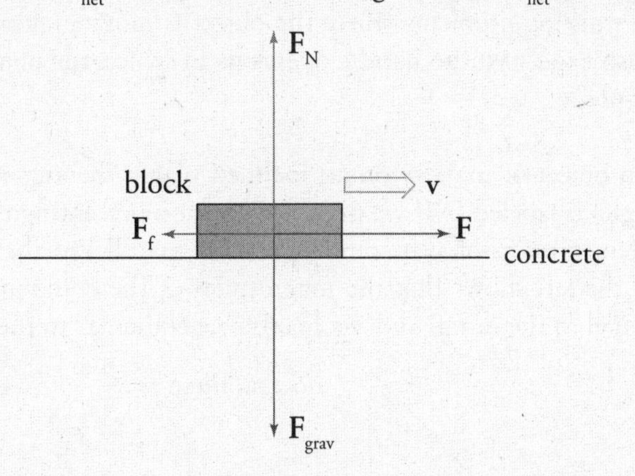

Example 4-19: Instead of pushing the block by a force that's parallel to the driveway, you wrap a rope around the block, sling the rope over your shoulder, and walk it across the driveway. If the rope makes an angle of 30° to the horizontal, and the tension in the rope is 300 N (the same force you exerted on the block in the last example), what will the block's acceleration be now?

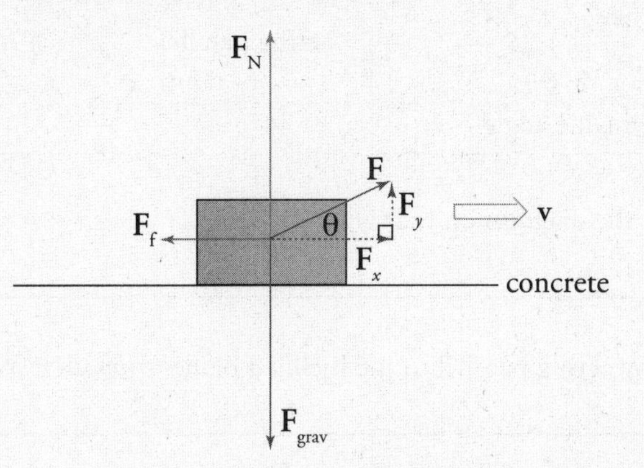

Solution: This is a tough question, but it uses a lot of the material we've covered so far. First, we'll need the normal force to find the friction force. The net vertical force on the block is 0 (because we're not lifting the block off the ground or watching it fall through the concrete). Therefore, $F_N + F_y = F_{grav}$, so $F_N = F_{grav} - F_y$. (Here's another example of the normal force not equaling the weight of the object.) Since $F_y = F \sin \theta = F \sin 30° = (300 \text{ N})(0.5) = 150$ N, we have $F_N = (500 \text{ N}) - (150 \text{ N}) = 350$ N. (Intuitively, the normal force is less than the weight of the block because the vertical component of the tension in the rope is "taking some of the pressure" off the surface.) Therefore, $F_f = \mu_k F_N = (0.5)(350 \text{ N}) = 175$ N. Now, the horizontal force that you provide is $F_x = F \cos \theta = F \cos 30° \approx (300 \text{ N})(0.85) = 255$ N. Therefore, the net force acting on the block, parallel to the driveway, is equal to $F_x - F_f = (255 \text{ N}) - (175 \text{ N}) = 80$ N. If $F_{net} = 80$ N and $m = 50$ kg, then $a = F_{net}/m = (80 \text{ N})/(50 \text{ kg}) = 1.6 \text{ m/s}^2$. (Notice that you get the block moving faster—even exerting the same force—by doing it this way!)

4.4 INCLINED PLANES

So far, we've had practice working problems where the object is moving along a flat, horizontal surface. However, the OAT will also expect you to handle questions in which the object is on a ramp, or, in fancier language, an **inclined plane**.

The figure below shows an object of mass m on an inclined plane; the angle the plane makes with the horizontal (the **incline angle**) is labeled θ. If we draw the vector representing the weight of the object, we notice that it can be written in terms of two components: one parallel to the ramp and one perpendicular to it. The diagram on the left shows that the magnitudes of the components of the object's weight, **w** = mg, are $mg \sin \theta$ (parallel to the ramp) and $mg \cos \theta$ (perpendicular to the ramp).

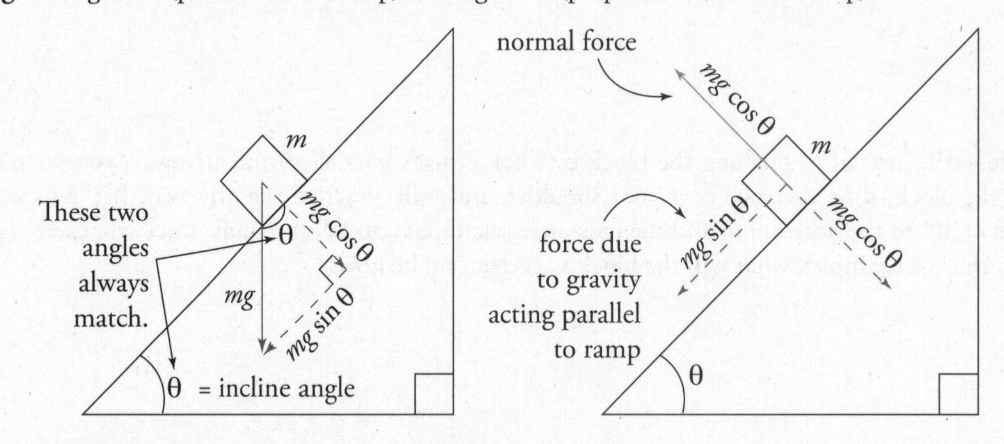

Therefore, as illustrated in the diagram on the right,

$$\text{the force due to gravity acting parallel to the inclined plane} = mg \sin \theta$$

where θ is measured between incline and horizontal. **You should memorize both of these facts.**

Incidentally, any time we see an angle in an OAT problem we'll probably be breaking a vector (say a force, a velocity, or an acceleration) into components. When we looked at projectile motion we broke the projectile's initial velocity into horizontal and vertical components; here, we're breaking the force of gravity into a component parallel to and one perpendicular to the surface of the incline. Why the difference? In general, the components you'll use will be vertical and horizontal, *unless* the object can only move along one possible line; in that case, the components to use will be the direction of (possible) travel (in this case, parallel to the incline), and the direction perpendicular to that.

Example 4-20: A block of mass $m = 4$ kg is placed at the top of a frictionless ramp of incline angle 30° and length 10 m.

a) What is the block's acceleration down the ramp?
b) How long will it take for the block to slide to the bottom?

Solution:

a) Because the force due to gravity acting parallel to the ramp is $F = mg \sin \theta$, the acceleration of the block down the ramp will be

$$a = \frac{F}{m} = \frac{mg\sin\theta}{m} = g\sin\theta = (10 \text{ m/s}^2)\sin 30° = 5 \text{ m/s}^2$$

b) Using Big Five #3 with $d = 10$ m, $v_0 = 0$, and $a = 5$ m/s², we find that

$$d = v_0 t + \frac{1}{2}at^2 = \frac{1}{2}at^2 \rightarrow t = \sqrt{\frac{2d}{a}} = \sqrt{\frac{2(10 \text{ m})}{5 \text{ m/s}^2}} = 2 \text{ s}$$

Notice that the block's mass was irrelevant to both of these questions. That's because all of the forces were directly proportional to mass, but so was the object's inertia; in effect, mass cancelled out of both sides of $F = ma$. This is common in problems in which the forces on an object are all functions of gravity.

Example 4-21: A block of mass m slides down a ramp of incline angle 60°. If the coefficient of kinetic friction between the block and the surface of the ramp is 0.2, what's the block's acceleration down the ramp?

Solution: There are now two forces acting parallel to the ramp: $mg \sin \theta$ (directed downward along the ramp) and F_f, the force of kinetic friction (directed upward along the ramp). Therefore, the net force down the ramp is $F_{net} = mg \sin \theta - F_f$. To find F_f, we multiply F_N by μ_k. Since $F_N = mg \cos \theta$, we have

$$F_{net} = mg\sin\theta - \mu_k mg\cos\theta$$

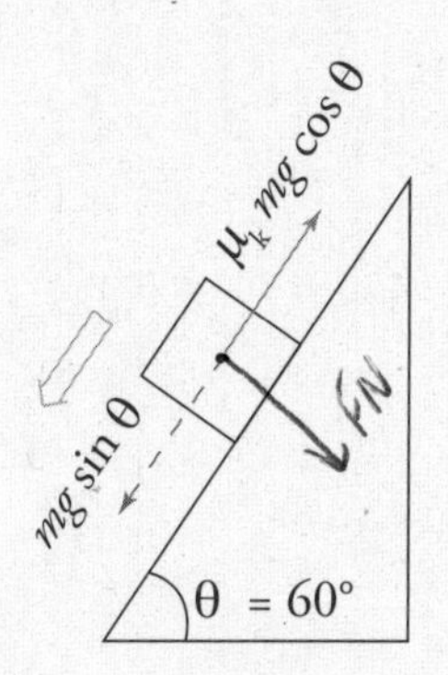

Dividing F_{net} by m gives us a:

$$a = \frac{F_{net}}{m} = \frac{mg\sin\theta - \mu_k mg\cos\theta}{m} = g(\sin\theta - \mu_k\cos\theta)$$

Putting in the numbers, we get

$$a = (10\text{ m/s}^2)(\sin 60° - 0.2\cos 60°) \approx (10\text{ m/s}^2)(0.85 - 0.2\cdot\tfrac{1}{2}) = 7.5\text{ m/s}^2$$

Example 4-22: A block of mass m is placed on a ramp of incline angle θ. If the block doesn't slide down, find the relationship between μ_s (the coefficient of static friction) and θ.

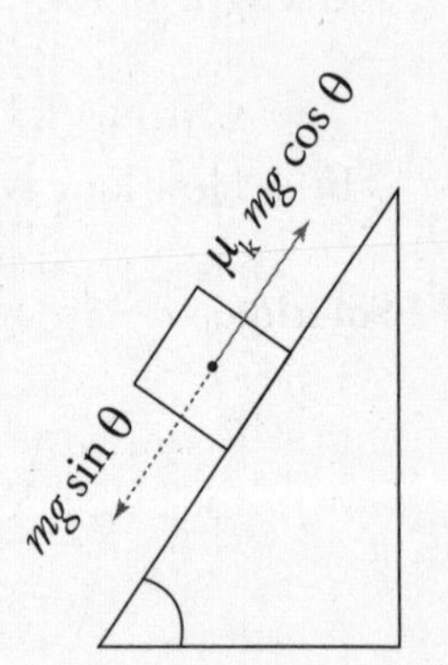

Solution: If the block doesn't slide, then static friction is strong enough to withstand the pull of gravity acting downward parallel to the ramp. This means that the *maximum* force of static friction must be greater than or equal to $mg\sin\theta$. Since $F_{f(static), max} = \mu_s F_N$, and $F_N = mg\cos\theta$, we have $F_{f(static), max} = \mu_s mg\cos\theta$. Therefore,

$$F_{f(static)\ max} \geq mg\sin\theta$$

$$\mu_s mg\cos\theta \geq mg\sin\theta$$

$$\mu_s g\cos\theta \geq g\sin\theta$$

$$\mu_s \geq \frac{\sin\theta}{\cos\theta}$$

$$\therefore \mu_s \geq \tan\theta$$

4.5 PULLEYS

A **pulley** is a device that changes the direction of the **tension** (the force exerted by a stretched string, cord, or rope) that pulls on the object that the string is attached to. (We'll use $\mathbf{F}_T$ or **T** to denote a tension force.) For example, in the picture below, if we pull *down* on the string on the right with a force of magnitude F_T, then the tension force on the left side of the pulley will pull *up* on the block with the same magnitude of force, F_T.

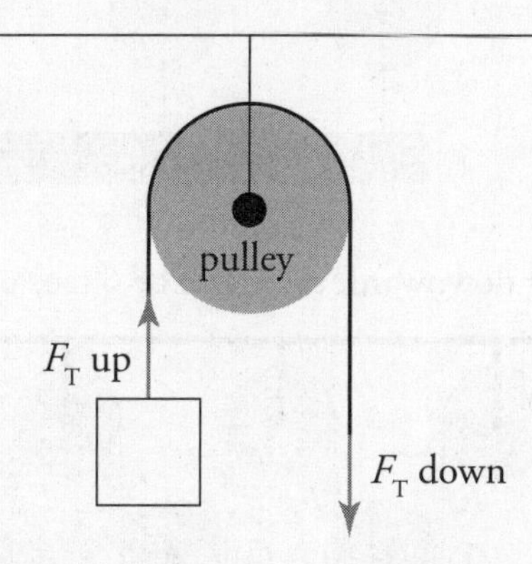

Pulleys can also be used to decrease the force necessary to lift an object. For example, consider the pulley system illustrated on the left below. If we pull down on the string on the right with a force of magnitude F_T, then we'll create a tension force of magnitude F_T throughout the entire string. As a result, there will be *two* tension forces, each of magnitude F_T, pulling up to lift the block (and the bottom pulley, too, but we assume that the pulleys are massless; that is, the mass of any pulley is small enough that it can be ignored). Therefore, we only need to exert half as much force to lift the block! This simple observation, that a pulley system (with massless, frictionless pulleys) causes a constant tension to exist through the entire string, which can lead to multiple tension forces pulling on an object, is the key to many OAT problems on pulleys.

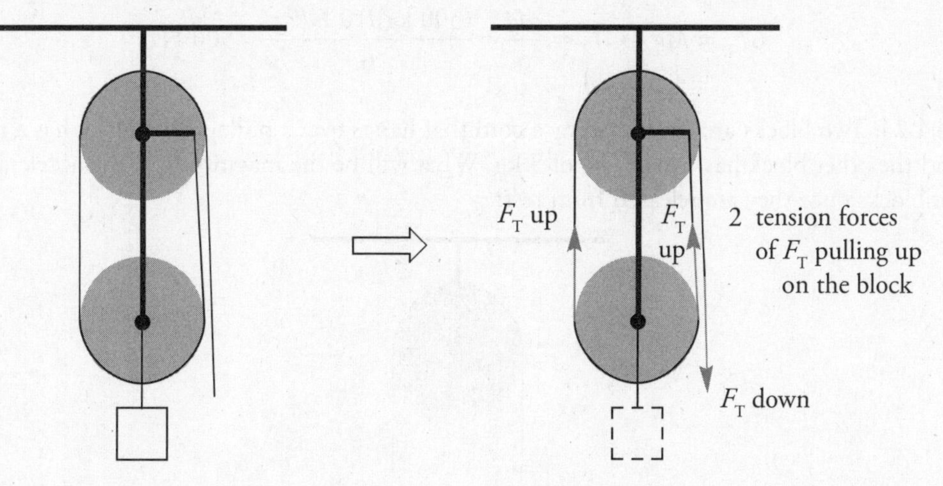

Pulley systems like this multiply our force by however many strings are pulling on the object.

Notice carefully that the tension force is applied wherever a string (or rope, or cable, or whatever) comes in contact with a pulley, which means that there will often be *two* tension forces on a single pulley, one on each side. You can see this in the right-hand diagram on the previous page.

4.5

Example 4-23: In the figure below, how much force would we need to exert on the free end of the cord in order to lift the plank (mass $M = 300$ kg) with constant velocity? (Ignore the masses of the pulleys.)

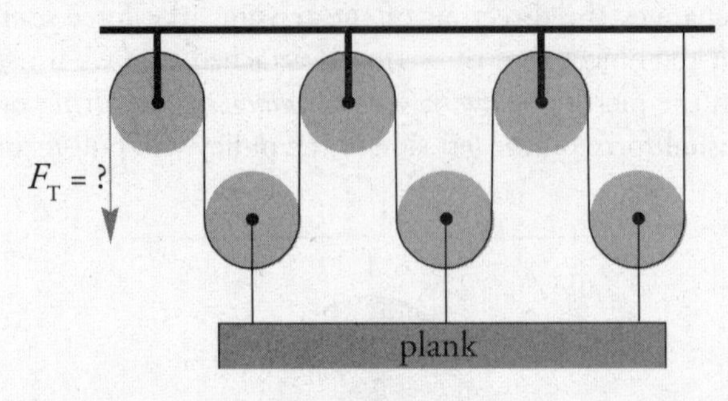

Solution: As a result of our pulling downward, there will be 6 tension forces pulling up on the plank:

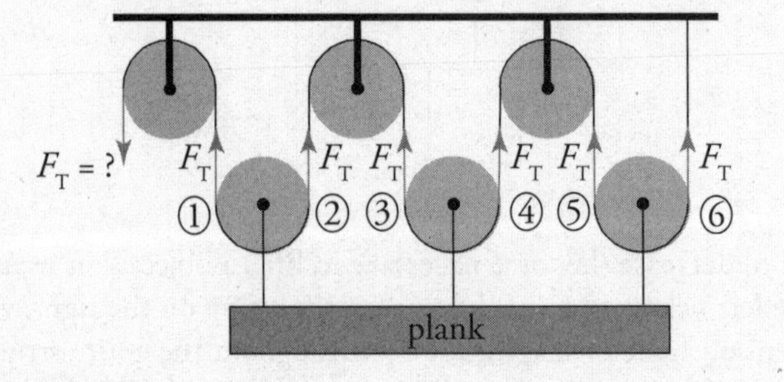

In order to lift with constant velocity (acceleration = zero), we require the net force on the plank to be zero. Therefore, the total of all the tension forces pulling up, $6F_T$, must balance the weight of the plank downward, Mg. This gives us

$$6F_T = Mg \to F_T = \frac{Mg}{6} = \frac{(300 \text{ kg})(10 \text{ N/kg})}{6} = 500 \text{ N}$$

Example 4-24: Two blocks are connected by a cord that hangs over a pulley. One block has a mass, M, of 10 kg, and the other block has a mass, m, of 5 kg. What will be the magnitude of the acceleration of the system of blocks once they are released from rest?

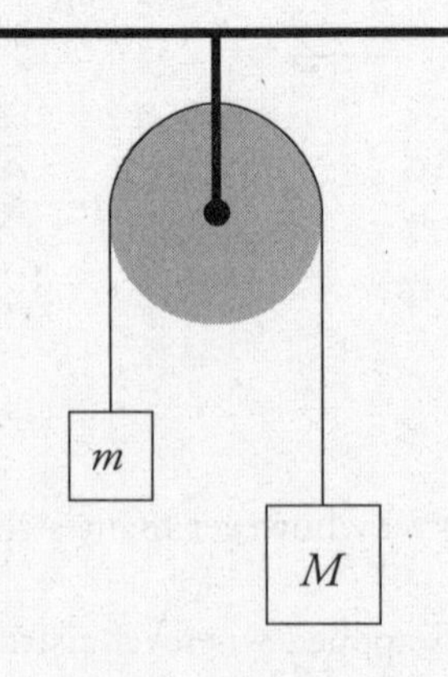

Solution: We'll solve this by a step-by-step approach using a **force diagram**. To apply Newton's second law, $\mathbf{F}_{net} = m\mathbf{a}$, to any problem, we follow these steps:

Step 1: Draw all the forces that act *on* the object. (That is, draw the force diagram.)
Step 2: Choose a direction to call *positive* (simply take the direction of the object's motion to be positive; it's almost always the easiest, most natural decision).
Step 3: Find $\mathbf{F}_{net}$ and set it equal to $m\mathbf{a}$.

We have effectively done these steps in the solutions to the examples we have seen already, but now that we have a situation involving two accelerating objects, it is even more important to make sure that we have a systematic plan of attack. When you have more than one object to worry about, just make sure that the Step-2 decision you make for one object is compatible with the Step-2 decision you make for the other one(s). On the left below are the force diagrams for the blocks on the pulley. Notice that we call *up* the positive direction for *m* (because that's where it's going), and we call *down* the positive direction for *M* (because that's where *it's* going); these decisions are compatible, because when *m* moves in its positive direction, so does *M*.

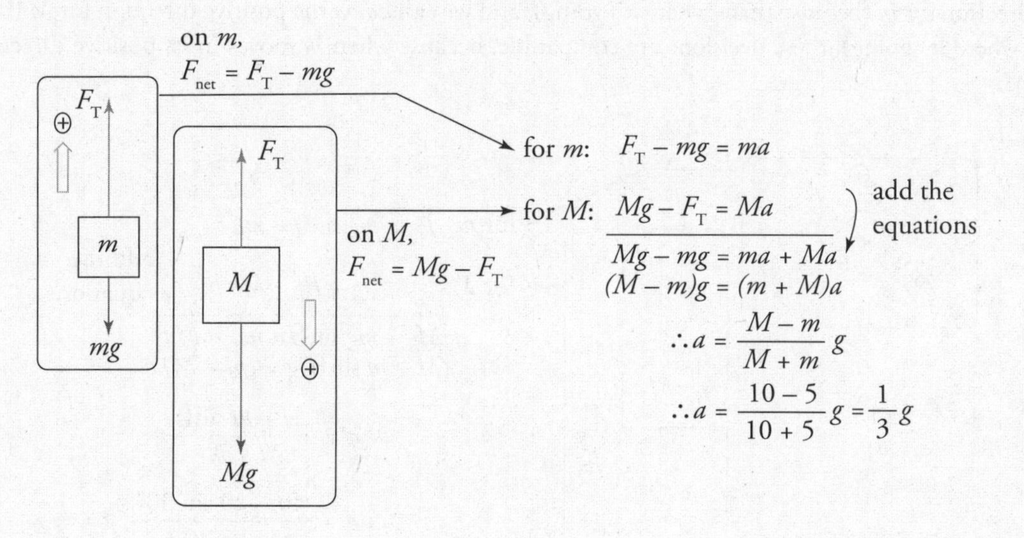

Because *up* is the positive direction for little *m*, the force F_T on *m* is positive and the force *mg* is negative; therefore, for little *m*, we have $F_{net} = F_T + (-mg) = F_T - mg$. Since *down* is the positive direction for big *M*, the force *Mg* on *M* is positive and the force F_T is negative; therefore, for big *M*, we have $F_{net} = Mg + (-F_T) = Mg - F_T$. On the right above, we've written down F_{net} = mass × acceleration for each block. There are two equations, but we have two unknowns (F_T and *a*), so we *need* two equations. To solve the equations, the trick is simply to *add the equations*. Notice that this makes the F_T's drop out, so all we're left with is one unknown, *a*, which we can solve for immediately. The calculation shown above gives $a = g/3$, so we get $a = 3.3 \text{ m/s}^2$.

If the question had asked for the tension in the cord, we could now use the value we found for *a* and plug it back into either of our two equations (we'd get the same answer no matter which one we used). Using $F_T - mg = ma$, we'd find that

$$F_T = ma + mg = m(a + g) = m(\tfrac{1}{3}g + g) = \tfrac{4}{3}mg = \tfrac{4}{3}(5 \text{ kg})(10 \text{ N/kg}) = 67 \text{ N}$$

Example 4-25: In the figure below, the block of mass m slides up a frictionless inclined plane, pulled by another block of mass M that is falling. If $\theta = 30°$, $m = 20$ kg, and $M = 40$ kg, what's the acceleration of the block on the ramp?

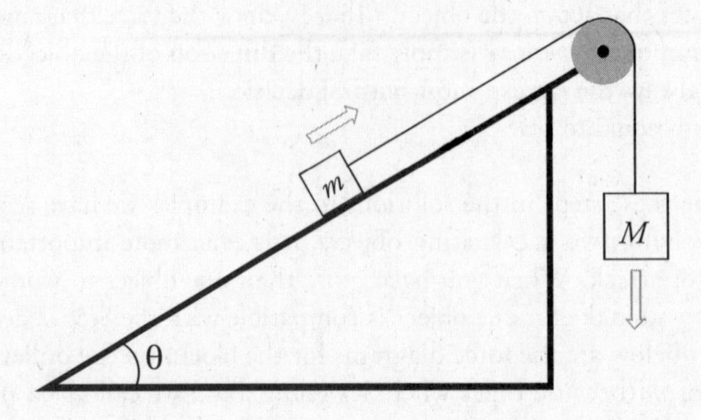

Solution: On the left below are the force diagrams for the blocks. Notice that we call *up the ramp* the positive direction for m (because that's where it's going), and we call *down* the positive direction for M (because that's where *it's* going); these decisions are compatible, because when m moves in its positive direction, so does M.

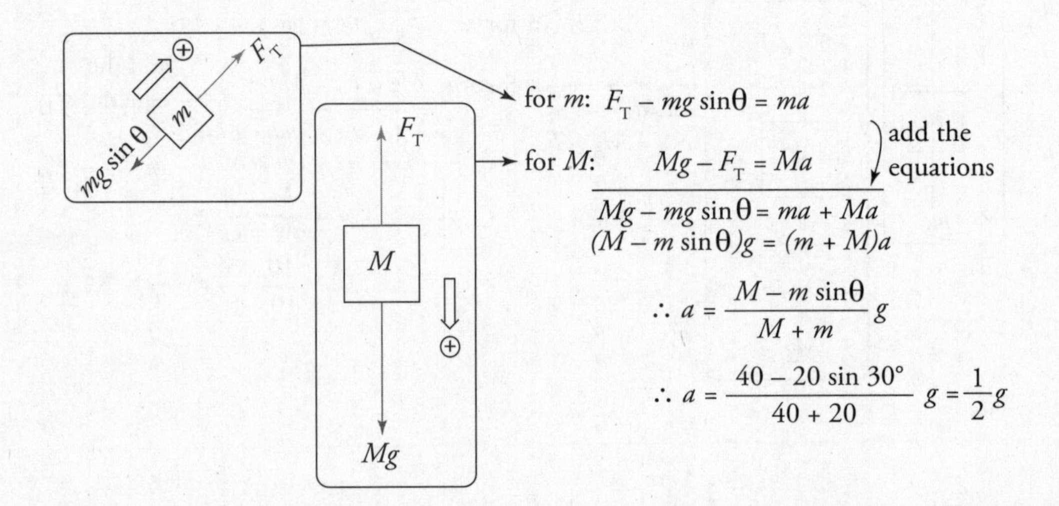

Because *up the ramp* is the positive direction for little m, the force F_T on m is positive and the force due to gravity along the ramp, $mg\sin\theta$, is negative; therefore, for little m, we have $F_{net} = F_T + (-mg\sin\theta) = F_T - mg\sin\theta$. Since *down* is the positive direction for big M, the force Mg on M is positive and the force F_T is negative; therefore, for big M, we have $F_{net} = Mg + (-F_T) = Mg - F_T$. On the right above, we've written down F_{net} = mass × acceleration for each block. As in the preceding example, there are two equations (and two unknowns, F_T and a). Again using the trick of adding the equations, the F_T's drop out, and all we're left with is one unknown, a, to solve for. The calculation shown above gives $a = g/2$, so we get $a = 5\text{ m/s}^2$.

Summary of Formulas

Newton's Laws:

First law: $\mathbf{F}_{net} = 0 \Leftrightarrow v = \text{constant}$

Second law: $\mathbf{F}_{net} = ma$

Third law: $\mathbf{F}_{1\text{-on-}2} = -\mathbf{F}_{2\text{-on-}1}$

Weight: $\mathbf{w} = m\mathbf{g}$

Gravitational force: $F_{grav} = G\frac{Mm}{r^2}$ given that $w = F_{grav}$, we get $g = G\frac{M}{r^2}$.

Kinetic friction: $F_f = \mu_k F_N$

Static friction: $F_{f,max} = \mu_s F_N$

$\mu_{s,\ max} > \mu k$

Direction of friction is opposite to the direction of motion (or intended direction of motion).

Force due to gravity acting parallel to inclined plane: $mg \sin \theta$

Force due to gravity acting perpendicular to inclined plane: $mg \cos \theta$, where θ is measured between incline and horizontal.

Chapter 5
Mechanics II

5.1 CENTER OF MASS

In the examples we looked at in the preceding chapter, objects were treated as though they were each a single particle. In fact, in the step-by-step solution to one of the pulley problems, we drew a force diagram showing all the forces acting on the objects in the system. To make that step go faster, we sometimes just represent each object by a dot and draw the force arrows on the dot. For example, the force diagram in the solution to Example 4-24 could have been drawn like this:

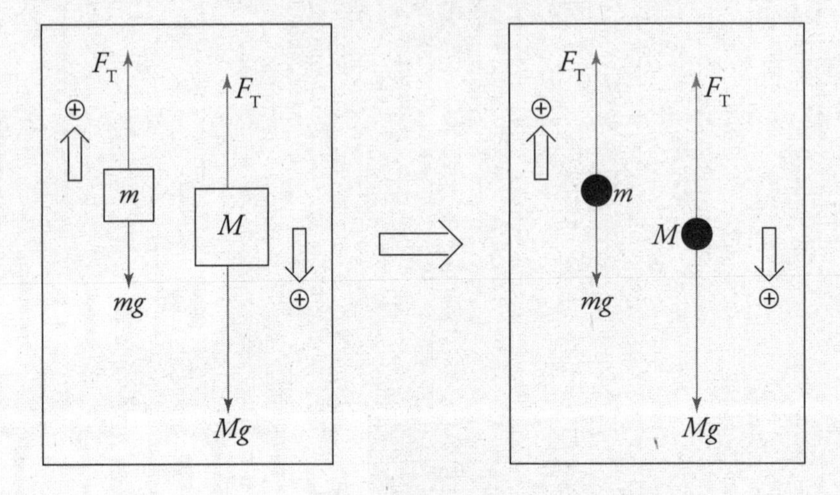

Each dot really denotes the *center of mass* of the object, which we'll now describe and define.

Imagine the following series of experiments. You walk into a large room with a friend, a hammer, and a glow-in-the dark (phosphorescent) sticker. After shining light on the sticker (so that it will glow), stick it on the metal head of the hammer. Hand the hammer to your friend, stand back, and turn off the light. Ask your friend to flip and toss the hammer across the room so that you can watch its trajectory. You'll see only the glow-in-the-dark sticker, and it will, in general, trace out some complicated loopy path as the hammer tumbles and flies through the air.

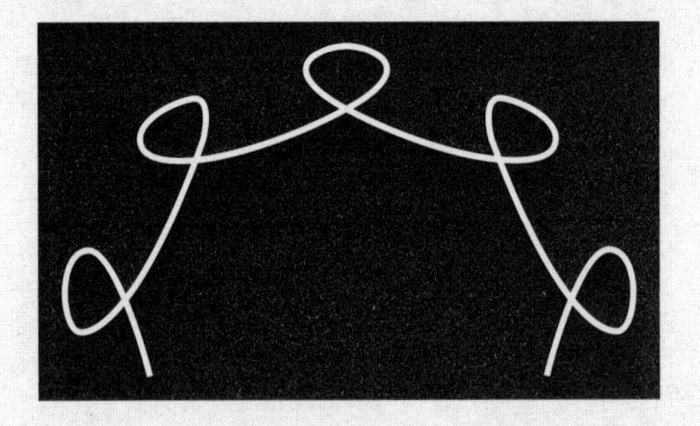

Repeat the experiment with the sticker attached to the end of the handle of the hammer. Once again, when your friend flips and tosses the hammer across the room so that you can watch it face on, you'll see only the glow-in-the-dark sticker, and it'll trace out another complicated loopy path.

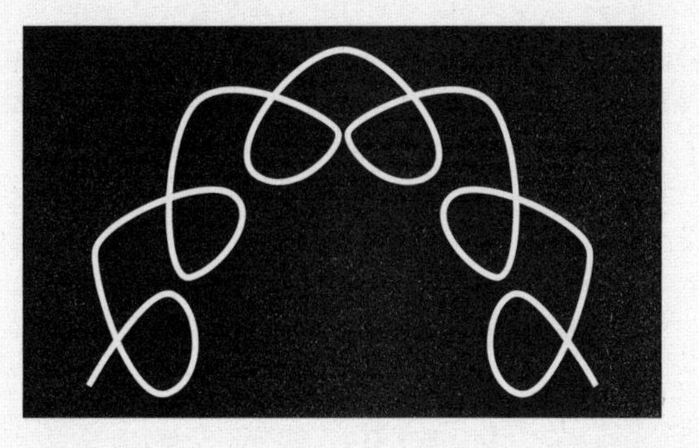

Now let's try this one more time, but rather than attaching the sticker at some random spot on the hammer, first find the point where the hammer just balances on the tip of your finger. Put the sticker on that spot and hand the hammer to your friend. Turn off the light, and watch as the hammer is tossed across the room. This time you'll see the sticker trace out a nice parabola, no loops.

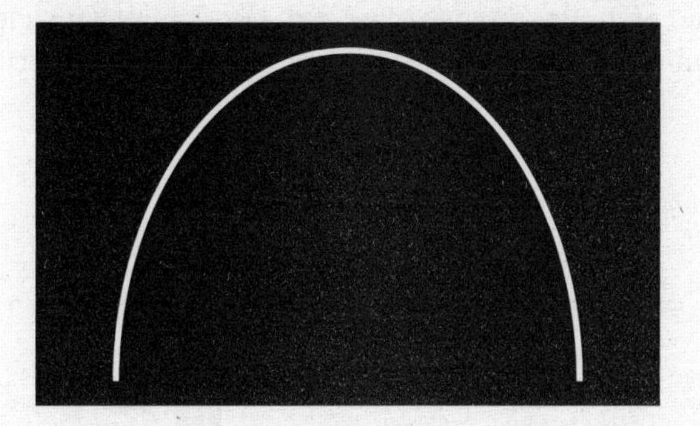

Apparently there was something special about the final location of the sticker. Most points on the hammer traced out complicated loopy trajectories, but this final point traced out a simple parabolic path, just as a single particle would. It is this one point that behaves as if the object (whether it's a block or a hammer or whatever) was a single particle. This special point is the **center of mass**. Another way of looking at it is to say that the center of mass is the point at which we could consider all the mass of the object to be concentrated. It's the dot in our simplified force diagrams.

For a simple object such as a sphere, block, or cylinder, whose density is constant (that is, for an object that's *homogeneous*), the center of mass is where you'd expect it to be—at its geometric center.

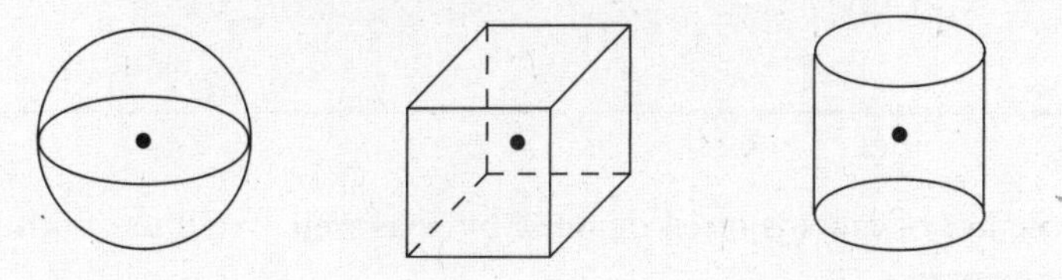

Note that in some cases, the center of mass isn't even located within the body of the object:

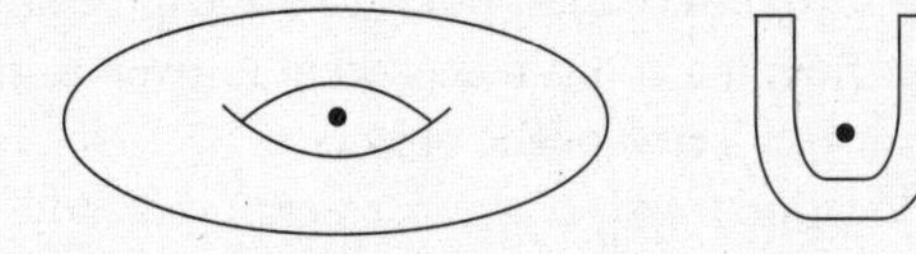

For a nonhomogeneous object, such as a hammer, whose density *does* vary from point to point, there's no single-step way mathematically to calculate the location of the center of mass.

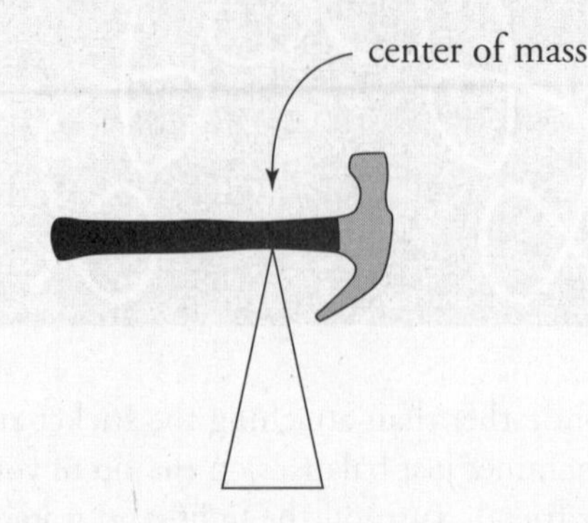

However, there is a simpler type of problem on which the OAT *will* expect you to locate the center of mass. The situation involves a series of masses arranged in a line. For example, imagine that you had a stick with several blocks hanging from it. Where should you attach a string to the stick so that this mobile would balance?

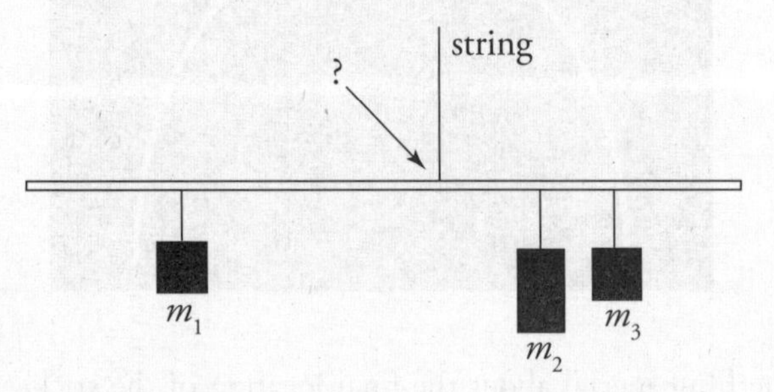

For a problem like this, in which each individual mass can be considered to be at a single point in space, here's the formula for the location of the center of mass:

Center of Mass for Point Masses

$$x_{CM} = \frac{m_1x_1 + m_2x_2 + m_3x_3 \ldots}{m_1 + m_2 + m_3 \ldots}$$

(The location of the center of mass is often denoted by $\bar{x}$ as well. We'll use both notations.) To use this formula, follow these steps:

Step 1: Choose an origin (a reference point to call $x = 0$). The locations of the objects will be measured relative to this point. Often the easiest point to use will be at the location of the left-hand mass, but any point is fine; if a coordinate system is given in the problem, use it.
Step 2: Determine the locations (x_1, x_2, x_3, etc.) of the objects.
Step 3: Multiply each mass by its location (m_1x_1, m_2x_2, m_3x_3, etc.) then add.
Step 4: Divide by the total mass ($m_1 + m_2 + m_3 + \ldots$).

Example 5-1: In the figure below, three blocks hang below a massless meter stick. Block m_1 hangs from the *20 cm* mark, block m_2 hangs from the *70 cm* mark, and block m_3 hangs from the *80 cm* mark. If $m_1 = 2$ kg, $m_2 = 5$ kg, and $m_2 = 3$ kg, at what mark on the meter stick should a string be attached so that this system would hang horizontally?

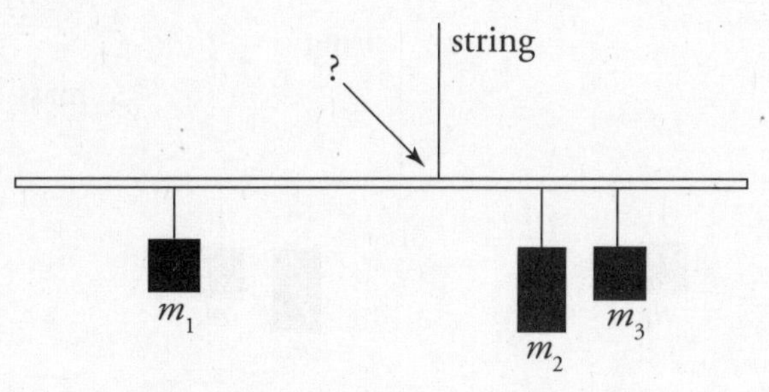

Solution: The first step is to choose an origin, a reference point to call $x = 0$. We are free to choose our zero mark anywhere we want, but the simplest choice here is the one implicitly mentioned in the question itself. The question wants to know at what mark on the meter stick we should attach the string; in other words, how far from the left end of the meter stick should we attach the string? Since the question asks essentially, "How far from the *left end*...?" the best place to choose our zero mark is at the *left end*. We now can write $x_1 = 20$ cm, $x_2 = 70$ cm, and $x_3 = 80$ cm. Using the formula above, we find that

$$\begin{aligned} x_{\text{CM}} &= \frac{m_1x_1 + m_2x_2 + m_3x_3}{m_1 + m_2 + m_3} \\ &= \frac{(2\text{ kg})(20\text{ cm}) + (5\text{ kg})(70\text{ cm}) + (3\text{ kg})(80\text{ cm})}{(2\text{ kg}) + (5\text{ kg}) + (3\text{ kg})} \\ &= \frac{630\text{ kg}\cdot\text{cm}}{10\text{ kg}} \\ \therefore x_{\text{CM}} &= 63\text{ cm} \end{aligned}$$

What if we had instead chosen the center of the meter stick (the *50 cm* mark) to be our origin? In that case, we would have found $x_1 = -30$ cm (because m_1 hangs from the *20 cm* mark, and *20 cm* is 30 cm to the *left*—hence the minus sign—of *50 cm*), $x_2 = 20$ cm, and $x_3 = 30$ cm. The formula would have told us that

$$\begin{aligned} x_{\text{CM}} &= \frac{m_1x_1 + m_2x_2 + m_3x_3}{m_1 + m_2 + m_3} \\ &= \frac{(2\text{ kg})(-30\text{ cm}) + (5\text{ kg})(20\text{ cm}) + (3\text{ kg})(30\text{ cm})}{(2\text{ kg}) + (5\text{ kg}) + (3\text{ kg})} \\ &= \frac{130\text{ kg}\cdot\text{cm}}{10\text{ kg}} \\ \therefore x_{\text{CM}} &= 13\text{ cm} \end{aligned}$$

Well, 13 cm to the *right* (because x_{CM} is *positive*) of the *50 cm* mark is the *63 cm* mark, the same answer we found before.

Example 5-2: In the figure below, three blocks hang below a uniform (homogeneous) meter stick of mass 3 kg. Block m_1 hangs from the *20 cm* mark, block m_2 hangs from the *70 cm* mark, and block m_3 hangs from the *80 cm* mark. If $m_1 = 2$ kg, $m_2 = 5$ kg, and $m_3 = 3$ kg, at what mark on the meter stick should a string be attached so that this system would hang without tipping?

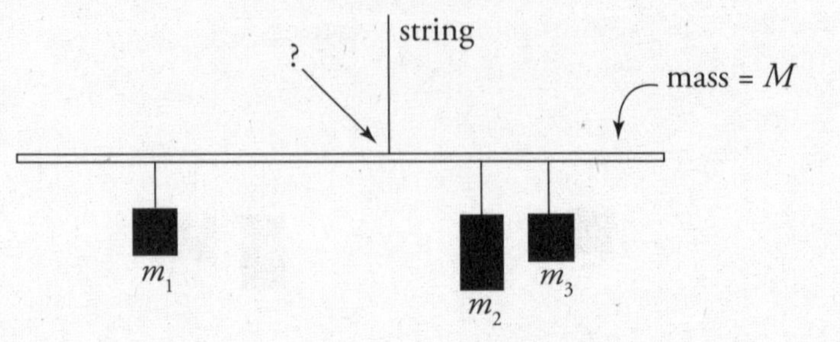

Solution: Does the mass of the stick (even if the stick is homogeneous) need to be taken into account? Well, let's see. If we were to include the mass of the stick (let's call it M) in the formula for the center of mass, it would seem that we'd just add it in the denominator, but what do we do in the numerator? What x would we multiply M by? The answer is: the stick's own center of mass! Since the stick is homogeneous, its center of mass (by itself) would be at its geometric center—that is, at the *50 cm* mark. So, with $M = 3$ kg and $X = 50$ cm, we'd find that

$$\begin{aligned} x_{CM} &= \frac{m_1x_1 + m_2x_2 + m_3x_3 + MX}{m_1 + m_2 + m_3 + M} \\ &= \frac{(2 \text{ kg})(20 \text{ cm}) + (5 \text{ kg})(70 \text{ cm}) + (3 \text{ kg})(80 \text{ cm}) + (3 \text{ kg})(50 \text{ cm})}{(2 \text{ kg}) + (5 \text{ kg}) + (3 \text{ kg}) + (3 \text{ kg})} \\ &= \frac{780 \text{ kg}\cdot\text{cm}}{13 \text{ kg}} \end{aligned}$$

$$\therefore x_{CM} = 60 \text{ cm}$$

Notice that this is a different location from what we found if the stick's mass could be neglected. Therefore, the mass of the stick *does* need to be included, even if it's homogeneous.

What if we had instead chosen the center of the meter stick (the *50 cm* mark) to be our origin? In that case, we would have had $X = 0$ for the location of M, and the formula would have told us that

$$\begin{aligned} x_{CM} &= \frac{m_1x_1 + m_2x_2 + m_3x_3 + MX}{m_1 + m_2 + m_3 + M} \\ &= \frac{(2 \text{ kg})(-30 \text{ cm}) + (5 \text{ kg})(20 \text{ cm}) + (3 \text{ kg})(30 \text{ cm}) + (3 \text{ kg})(0 \text{ cm})}{(2 \text{ kg}) + (5 \text{ kg}) + (3 \text{ kg}) + (3 \text{ kg})} \\ &= \frac{130 \text{ kg}\cdot\text{cm}}{13 \text{ kg}} \end{aligned}$$

$$\therefore x_{CM} = 10 \text{ cm}$$

Well, 10 cm to the right of the *50 cm* mark is the *60 cm* mark; the same answer we found before.

Example 5-3: An ammonia molecule (NH_3) contains 3 hydrogen atoms that are positioned at the vertices of an equilateral triangle. The nitrogen atom lies 38 pm (1 pm = 1 picometer = 10^{-12} m) directly above the center of this triangle. If the N:H mass ratio is 14:1, how far below the N atom is the center of mass of the molecule?

Solution: The objects in this system (the four atoms) are not arranged in a line, so how can we hope to determine the center of mass? The key to the answer is to realize that we don't need to include all four of these objects in a single calculation; we can divide the problem into stages. Since the three H atoms have equal masses and are symmetrically arranged at the corners of an equilateral triangle, the center of mass of just these 3 H's is at their geometric center: namely, the center of the triangle. Therefore, by definition of center of mass, the 3 H atoms behave as if all their mass were concentrated at the center of the triangle. This now turns the problem into computing the center of mass of 2 objects (which obviously lie on a line): the 3 H atoms at the center of the triangle and the N atom:

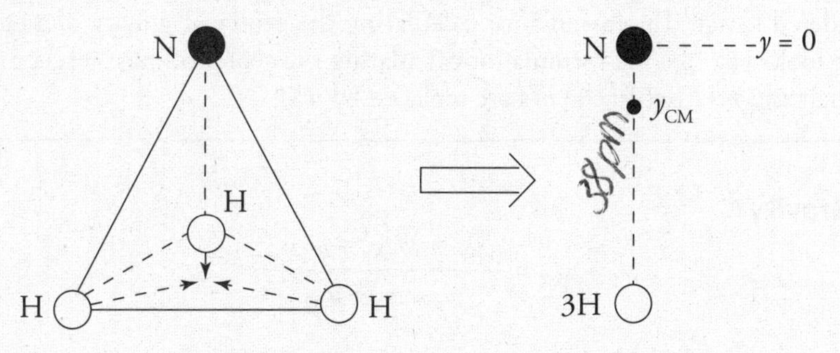

Because the question asks for the center of mass of the molecule relative to the N atom, we'll let the position of the N atom be our zero mark. (It's labeled y in the diagram on the right simply because the way the system is drawn, the objects are arranged along a *vertical* line.) The formula now gives us

$$
\begin{aligned}
y_{CM} &= \frac{m_N y_N + m_{3H} y_{3H}}{m_N + m_{3H}} \\
&= \frac{(14)(0\text{ cm}) + (3\cdot 1)(38\text{ pm})}{(14)+(3\cdot 1)} \\
&= \frac{114\text{ pm}}{17} \\
\therefore y_{CM} &\approx 7\text{ pm}
\end{aligned}
$$

Therefore, the center of mass of the NH_3 molecule is 7/38, or about 1/6 of the way down from the nitrogen atom toward the plane of the hydrogens. Because the nitrogen atom is more massive than the hydrogens, we expect the center of mass to not be at the geometric center but, rather, much closer to the nitrogen atom. (This is just like the balancing point of the hammer: Since the metal head is much heavier [because it's denser] than the rest of the hammer, we expect the hammer's center of mass to be not at the geometric center, but, instead, closer to the heavier end.)

You may have noticed in Example 5-2 that we applied the point mass formula to a system that didn't include only point masses: The stick's mass was spread along its entire length. What we did in that problem is what we can *always* do with a collection of homogenous (i.e., constant density) masses: First, find the center of mass of each piece; second, apply the point mass formula, assuming that each piece's mass is concentrated at its own center of mass.

It's possible (though unlikely) that on the OAT you'll have to find the center of mass of a two-dimensional collection of masses. In Example 5-3 on the previous page, we were able to simplify the problem to reduce it to a single dimension, but that might not always be the case. If you can't simplify the problem in this way, do what we always do with multidimensional problems: break it into components, and consider the components separately. In other words, first find the center of mass in, say, the x-direction, using only the x-components of position; then do the same in the y-direction.

Center of Gravity

If the gravitational field is uniform throughout a system, then the center of gravity is the same as the center of mass. The **center of gravity (CG)** is the point at which the total gravitational force on the system can be considered to act. The formula for calculating the center of gravity of a collection of objects arranged in a line looks just like the formula for calculating the center of mass, except the object's masses are replaced by their *weights* (that is, the m's are replaced by w's):

Center of Gravity

$$x_{CG} = \frac{w_1x_1 + w_2x_2 + w_3x_3 \ldots}{w_1 + w_2 + w_3 \ldots}$$

It's now easy to see why the center of gravity is the same as the center of mass if g is constant, because the g's cancel:

$$\begin{aligned} x_{CG} &= \frac{w_1x_1 + w_2x_2 + w_3x_3 \ldots}{w_1 + w_2 + w_3 \ldots} \\ &= \frac{(m_1g)x_1 + (m_2g)x_2 + (m_3g)x_3 \ldots}{m_1g + m_2g + m_3g \ldots} \\ &= \frac{g(m_1x_1 + m_2x_2 + m_3x_3 \ldots)}{g(m_1 + m_2 + m_3 \ldots)} \\ &= \frac{m_1x_1 + m_2x_2 + m_3x_3 \ldots}{m_1 + m_2 + m_3 \ldots} \end{aligned}$$

$$\therefore x_{CG} = x_{CM}$$

Example 5-4: A long homogeneous plank of weight 30 N supports two blocks: one of weight 120 N that is 8 m to the left of the plank's midpoint, and another of weight 40 N that is 5 m to the right of the plank's midpoint. Where's the center of gravity of this system?

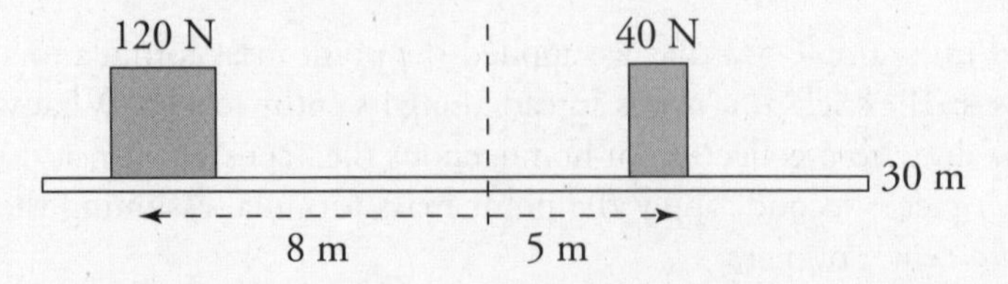

Solution: Choosing the midpoint of the plank to be $x = 0$, we have

$$\begin{aligned} x_{CG} &= \frac{w_1x_1 + w_2x_2 + WX}{w_1 + w_2 + W} \\ &= \frac{(120 \text{ N})(-8 \text{ m}) + (40 \text{ N})(5 \text{ m}) + (30 \text{ N})(0 \text{ m})}{(120 \text{ N}) + (40 \text{ N}) + (30 \text{ N})} \\ &= \frac{-760 \text{ N·m}}{190 \text{ N}} \\ \therefore x_{CG} &= -4 \text{ m} \end{aligned}$$

Therefore, the center of gravity (as well as the center of mass) is 4 m to the left of the plank's midpoint.

On the OAT, you can almost always assume that as in the example above, the center of mass is the same as the center of gravity. The only exception would be if the gravitational field was specifically defined as being nonuniform within the space of the object, and this would be very rare on the OAT.

5.2 UNIFORM CIRCULAR MOTION

So far, we've analyzed motion that takes place along a straight line (horizontal, vertical, or slanted) or along a parabola. The OAT will also require that you know how to analyze an object that moves in a circular path.

The title of this section is Uniform Circular Motion (often abbreviated UCM). What does *uniform* mean here? When we talk about uniform acceleration, we mean constant acceleration; uniform density means constant density; *uniform* is a term used in physics to denote something that remains constant. What property of an object undergoing uniform circular motion is constant? The radius of its path is constant, but that's already in the definition of *circular*, so it must be something else.

An object moving in a circular path is said to execute

uniform circular motion

if its *speed* is constant.

Notice right away that this does *not* mean the object's *velocity* is constant. Velocity is a vector: It has both speed and direction. If an object is moving in a circular path, then it's constantly turning, so its direction is constantly changing. A changing direction, even at constant speed, automatically means a changing velocity. An object's velocity vector is always tangent to its path, regardless of the shape of the path (parabola, circle, figure-8, or whatever) so in the figure below, you can see that the object will have a different velocity vector at every point on the circle, even though the magnitudes of these vectors are all the same.

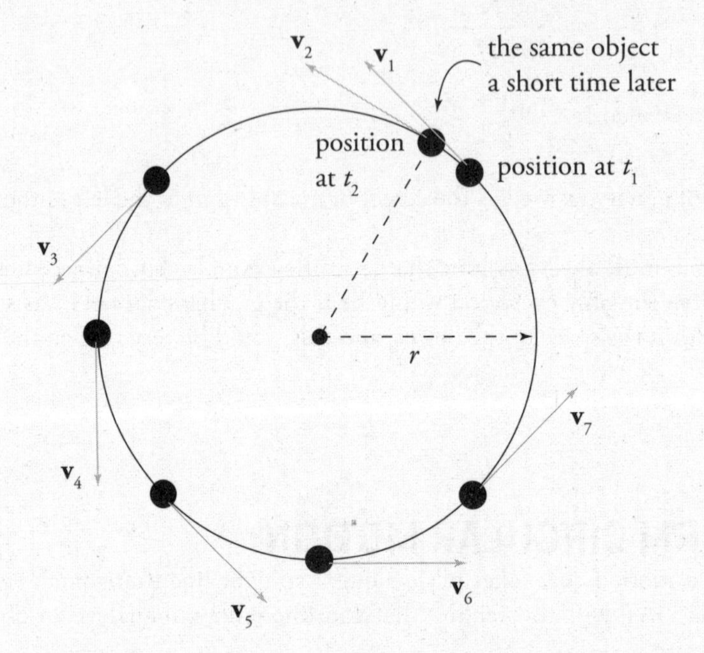

The first thing that should come to mind when you see an object's velocity changing is that the object is experiencing acceleration. The acceleration of an object undergoing uniform circular motion is not affecting the *speed* of the object; this acceleration is only changing the direction of the velocity in order to keep the object moving in a circle.

In the figure below, the velocity vectors of the object are drawn at two close points in its path; they're labeled $\mathbf{v}_1$ and $\mathbf{v}_2$. By definition, the direction of the acceleration is the same as the direction of the velocity change (remember the definition: $\mathbf{a} = \Delta\mathbf{v}/\Delta t$). So, the acceleration of the object has the same direction as $\Delta\mathbf{v} = \mathbf{v}_2 - \mathbf{v}_1$. Notice that $\mathbf{v}_2 - \mathbf{v}_1$, which is $\mathbf{v}_2 + (-\mathbf{v}_1)$, points toward the center of the circle. Therefore, the acceleration of the object always points toward the center of the circle. (This will be true no matter where on the circle we look.)

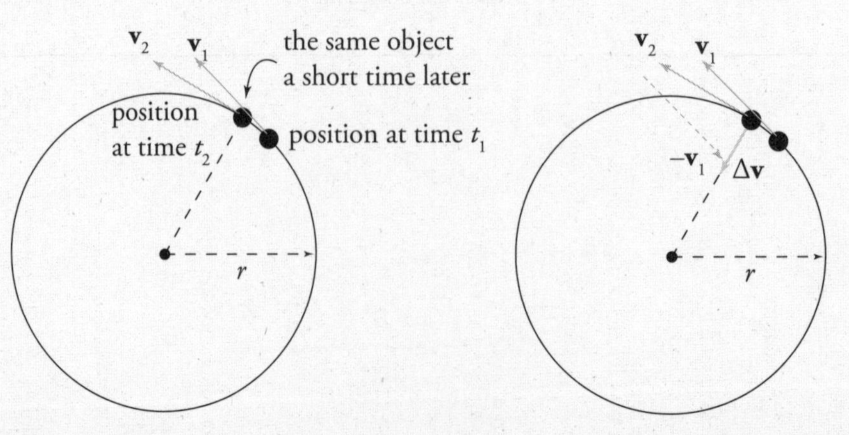

The acceleration of an object undergoing uniform circular motion always points toward the center of the circle. The term **centripetal** (from the Latin, meaning *to seek the center*) is therefore used to describe the acceleration of an object undergoing UCM. We'll denote centripetal acceleration by $\mathbf{a}_c$.

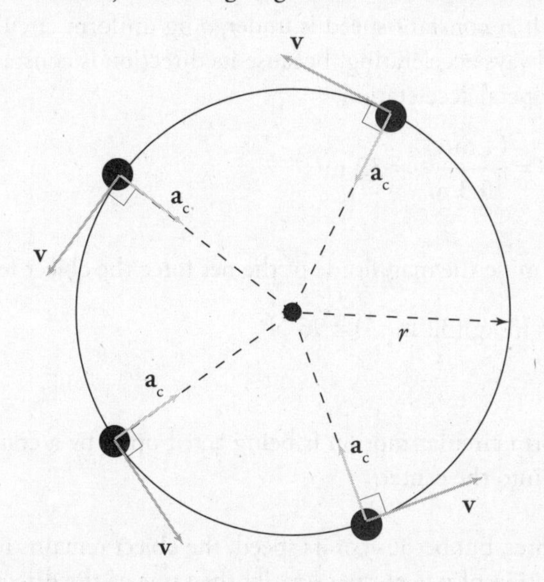

Since **v** is always tangent to the circle, and $\mathbf{a}_c$ always points to the center of the circle, **v** and $\mathbf{a}_c$ are always perpendicular to each other at any position of the object.

(*Note*: In the figure above, all the velocity vectors are different—because they point in different directions—so they really shouldn't all be labeled by the same **v**. The same is true for the centripetal acceleration vectors. However, adding subscripts to distinguish all the **v** vectors and all the $\mathbf{a}_c$ vectors would have made the picture look too confusing.)

We now know the *direction* of the centripetal acceleration at any point on the circle; what is its *magnitude*? If v is the speed of the object and r is the radius of the circular path, then the magnitude of the centripetal acceleration, a_c, is v^2/r.

Magnitude of Centripetal Acceleration

$$a_c = \frac{v^2}{r}$$

If an object is accelerating, then it must be feeling a force (after all, $\mathbf{F}_{net} = m\mathbf{a}$, so you can't have an acceleration without a force). Since $\mathbf{F}_{net}$ and **a** always point in the same direction, no matter what the path of the object, the net force on an object undergoing UCM must, like **a**, point toward the center. So, guess what we call it? **Centripetal force** (denoted $\mathbf{F}_c$). This is the *net* force directed toward the center that acts on an object to make it execute uniform circular motion. And since $F_{net} = ma$, we'll have $\mathbf{F}_c = m\mathbf{a}_c$ and $F_c = ma_c$, so the magnitude of the centripetal force is mv^2/r, where m is the mass of the object that's moving around the circle.

Magnitude of Centripetal Force

$$F_c = ma_c = \frac{mv^2}{r}$$

Example 5-5: An object of mass 3 kg moves at a constant speed of 4 m/s in a circular path of radius 0.5 m. What is the magnitude of its acceleration? What is the magnitude of the net force on the object?

Solution: An object moving in a circular path at constant speed is undergoing uniform circular motion. Although its speed is constant, the object is always accelerating, because its direction is constantly changing. The acceleration of the object is the centripetal acceleration,

$$a_c = \frac{v^2}{r} = \frac{(4\ \text{m/s})^2}{0.5\ \text{m}} = 32\ \text{m/s}^2$$

From Newton's second law, we can now determine the magnitude of the net force the object feels:

$$F_c = ma_c = (3\ \text{kg})(32\ \text{m/s}^2) = 96\ \text{N}$$

Example 5-6: If an object undergoing uniform circular motion is being acted upon by a constant force toward the center, why doesn't the object fall into the center?

Solution: Actually, it *is* falling toward the center, but because of its speed, the object remains in a circular orbit around the center. Remember: the direction of **v** is not necessarily the same as the direction of $\mathbf{F}_{net}$. So, just because $\mathbf{F}_{net}$ points toward the center does not mean that **v** must point toward the center. It's the direction of the *acceleration*, not the velocity, that always matches the direction of $\mathbf{F}_{net}$. Let's look at the motion of the object at a certain point in its circular path:

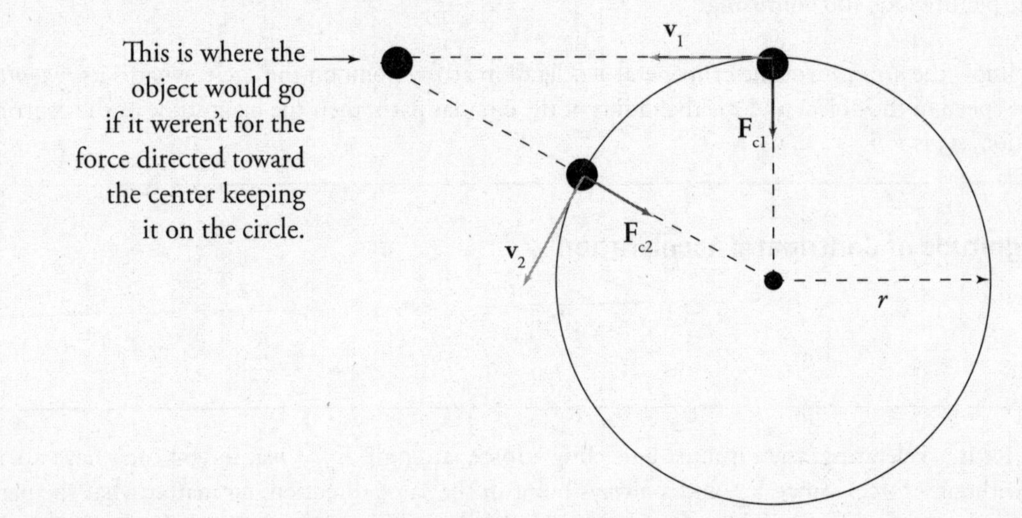

In this figure, the net force on the object at Position 1 points downward (toward the center of the circle). Therefore, it's telling $\mathbf{v}_1$ to move downward a little, so that at the next moment, at Position 2, the velocity will point downward slightly. Notice that this is just what we want in order to keep the object traveling in a circle! If it weren't for this force pointing toward the center (that is, if the centripetal force were suddenly removed), then the object's velocity wouldn't change. It would not continue to move in a circle but would instead fly off in a straight line, tangent to the circle at the point where the force was removed.

Example 5-7: How would the net force on an object undergoing uniform circular motion have to change if the object's speed doubled?

Solution: Centripetal force, mv^2/r, is proportional to the *square* of the speed. So, if the object's speed increased by a factor of 2, then the magnitude of $\mathbf{F}_c$ would have to increase by a factor of $2^2 = 4$.

Solving circular motion problems often involves something more than simply using the formulas $a_c = v^2/r$ or $F_c = mv^2/r$. The key to solving such problems is to answer this question:

What provides the centripetal force?

In other words, what force(s) act in the dimension toward the center of the circle?

Centripetal force is not some new kind of force like gravity or tension. It's simply the name for the net force directed toward the center of the circular path. The vector sum of forces such as gravity and tension is what gets *called* centripetal force, when those forces, or components of them, are directed toward the center of the circle. When drawing a force diagram for an object undergoing UCM, here are a couple of tips:

1. Do not add a force called $\mathbf{F}_c$ in your picture; forces such as gravity, tension, normal force, etc. *do* go in your picture, but $\mathbf{F}_c$ doesn't. Remember, $\mathbf{F}_c$ is what the forces toward the center have to add up to.
2. Always call *toward the center* the positive direction. Any forces toward the center are then positive forces, and any forces directed away from the center are negative. You'll need this to find F_{net} and then set the result equal to F_c.

Example 5-8: The moon orbits the earth in a (nearly) circular path at (nearly) constant speed. If M is the mass of the earth, m is the mass of the moon, and r is the moon's orbit radius, find an expression for the moon's orbit speed.

Solution: We begin by answering the question, *What provides the centripetal force?* The answer is the gravitational pull by the earth. We now simply translate our answer into an equation, like this:

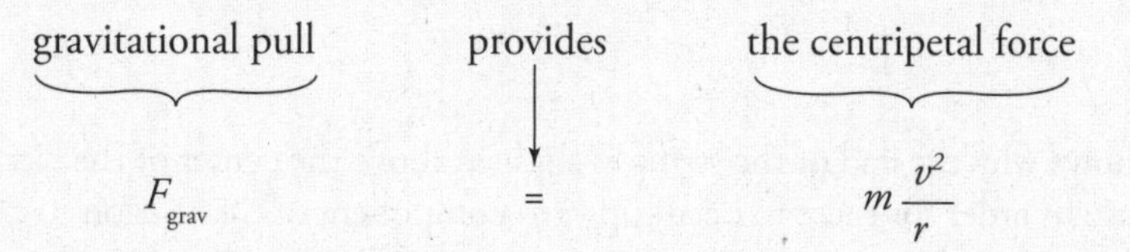

Since we know $F_{grav} = GMm/r^2$, we get

$$F_{grav} = F_c \rightarrow G\frac{Mm}{r^2} = m\frac{v^2}{r} \rightarrow G\frac{M}{r} = v^2 \rightarrow \therefore v = \sqrt{G\frac{M}{r}}$$

Notice that the mass of the moon, m, cancels out. So, any object orbiting at the same distance from the earth as the moon must move at the same speed as the moon.

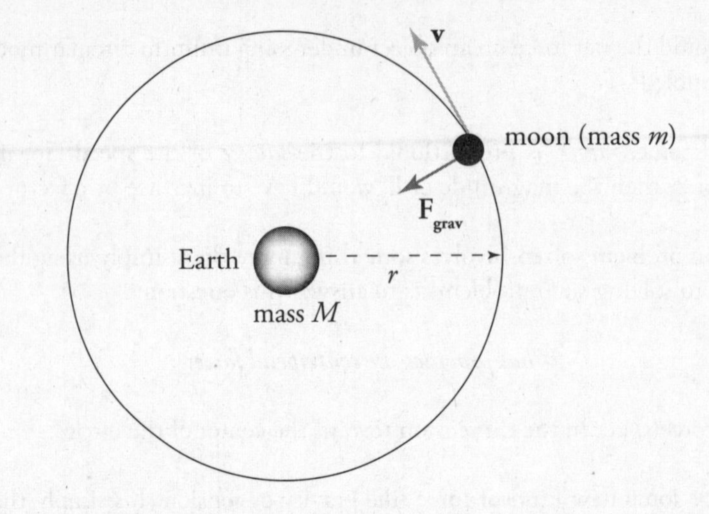

Example 5-9: A string is tied around a rock of mass 0.2 kg, and the rock is then whirled at a constant speed v in a horizontal circle of radius 0.4 m, as shown in the figure below. If sin θ = 0.4 and cos θ = 0.9, what's v?

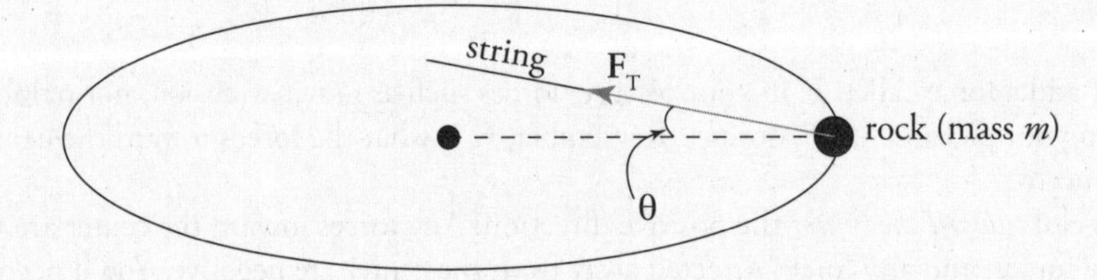

Solution: First, let's draw a bigger force diagram:

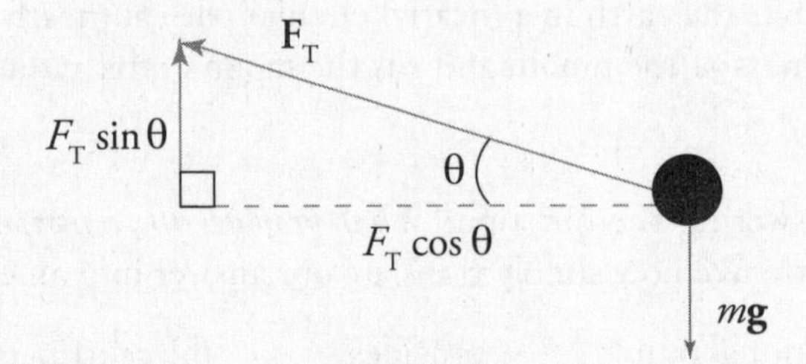

(This figure also shows why the end of the string is slightly above the center of the circle. The string has to point upward a little in order for there to be an upward component of the tension to cancel out the weight of the rock and allow the rock to revolve in a *horizontal* circle.) Because the rock is moving in a horizontal circle and not accelerating vertically, we know that the net vertical force must be zero. Therefore, the vertical component of the string's tension, $F_y = F_T \sin\theta$, must balance out the weight of the rock, mg:

$$F_T \sin\theta = mg$$

From this, we can figure out that

$$F_{\mathrm{T}} = \frac{mg}{\sin\theta} = \frac{(0.2\text{ kg})(10\text{ N/kg})}{0.4} = 5\text{ N}$$

Now, let's look at the circular motion: *What provides the centripetal force?* As the diagram shows, there's only one force directed toward the center of the circle (namely, the horizontal component of the tension, $F_x = F_{\mathrm{T}} \cos\theta$) so this must be it:

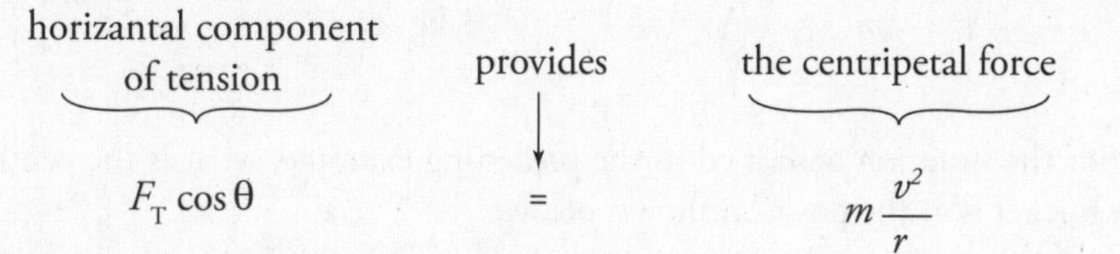

We now just plug in the value we found for F_{T} to get v:

$$F_{\mathrm{T}} \cos\theta = m\frac{v^2}{r} \rightarrow v = \sqrt{\frac{rF_{\mathrm{T}}\cos\theta}{m}} = \sqrt{\frac{(0.4\,\text{m})(5\,\text{N})(0.9)}{0.2\,\text{kg}}} = 3\text{ m/s}$$

Example 5-10: A rope of length 60 cm is tied to the handle of a bucket (whose mass is 3 kg), and the bucket is then whirled in a vertical circle. At the bottom of its path, the tension in the rope is 50 N. What is the speed of the bucket at this point?

Solution: First, let's draw a diagram.

$\mathbf{F}_{\mathrm{T}}$

$\mathbf{v}$

$\mathbf{w} = mg$

Because we call *toward the center* the positive direction when doing circular motion problems, we see that the tension, $\mathbf{F}_{\mathrm{T}}$, is a positive force, and the bucket's weight, $\mathbf{w}$, is a negative force. (Because $\mathbf{w}$ points *away* from the center, we count it as negative.) Therefore, the net force on the bucket at this point is $F_{\mathrm{T}} - w$. Because the net force directed toward the center is called the centripetal force, we'd write

$$F_{\mathrm{T}} - w = F_{\mathrm{c}}$$

Because $w = mg$ and $F_c = mv^2/r$, this equation becomes

$$F_T - mg = m\frac{v^2}{r}$$

We now just use this equation and the numbers we were given to figure out v, realizing that the radius of the circle is equal to the length of the rope (so $r = 0.6$ m):

$$v = \sqrt{\frac{r(F_T - mg)}{m}} = \sqrt{\frac{(0.6\text{ m})[50\text{ N} - (3\text{ kg})(10\text{ N/kg})]}{3\text{ kg}}} = 2\text{ m/s}$$

Example 5-11: For the situation described in the preceding example, what is the centripetal force on the bucket when the bucket is at the position shown below?

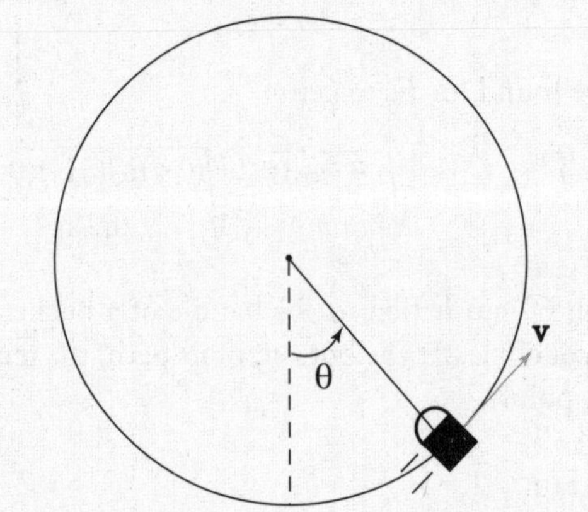

Solution: Here's the force diagram:

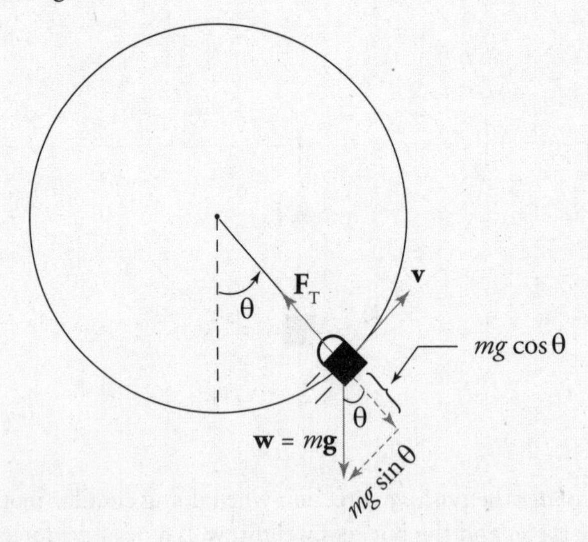

Because there's a force of F_T pointing toward the center and a force of $mg\cos\theta$ pointing *away* from the center, the net force toward the center of the circle (which is the centripetal force) is

$$F_{\substack{\text{net}\\ \text{toward center}}} = F_c = F_T - mg\cos\theta$$

Let's examine this situation a little more closely. Notice that at the position of the bucket shown, we also have a force component *tangent* to the circle ($mg\sin\theta$), which *opposes* the direction of the bucket's velocity. As a result, the bucket's speed will be reduced. Centripetal acceleration only makes an object turn so that it moves in a circular path; it does not change the speed. **Tangential** acceleration, on the other hand, *does* change the speed. Therefore, the bucket's speed will decrease as it rises to the top of the circle, and we wouldn't call the entire motion of the bucket "uniform." However, even if the speed of an object moving in a circle changes, there will always be a component of the net force that points toward the center of the circle; this is the centripetal force. The mathematical translation of the statement "the net force toward the center provides the centripetal force" becomes

$$F_T - mg\cos\theta = m\frac{v^2}{r} \rightarrow F_T = m\frac{v^2}{r} + mg\cos\theta$$

Because v decreases as the bucket rises (because of the downward tangential force, $mg\sin\theta$) and since $\cos\theta$ decreases as the bucket rises (because the angle θ increases from 0° to 180°), this final equation for F_T shows us that the tension in the rope will decrease as the bucket rises.

It's not often that we need to worry about both centripetal and tangential acceleration in an OAT problem, but the example above shows how to deal with it when we do encounter such a situation: Ignore the tangential components of force and acceleration when calculating the centripetal force and acceleration. This is really just another example of the general principle: In OAT-level physics, you can always consider the components of motion separately.

5.3 TORQUE

We can tie a rope to a bucket and make it move in a circular path, but how would we make the bucket itself spin? One way would be to grab the handle and then rotate our hand, or we could place our hands on opposite sides of the bucket and then, by moving our hands in opposite directions, rotate the bucket. In order to make an object's center of mass accelerate, we need to exert a force. In order to make an object *spin*, we need to exert a *torque*.

Torque is the measure of a force's effectiveness at making an object spin or rotate. (More precisely, it's the measure of a force's effectiveness at making an object *accelerate* rotationally.) If an object is initially at rest, and then it starts to spin, something must have exerted a torque. And if an object is already spinning, something would have to exert a torque to get it to stop spinning. In this section, we'll begin by looking at two different (but entirely equivalent) ways of figuring out torque.

All systems that can spin or rotate have a "center" of turning. This is the point that does not move while the remainder of the object is rotating, effectively becoming the center of the circle. There are many terms used to describe this point, including **pivot point** and **fulcrum**.

Let's say we want to tighten a bolt with a wrench. The figure below illustrates the situation.

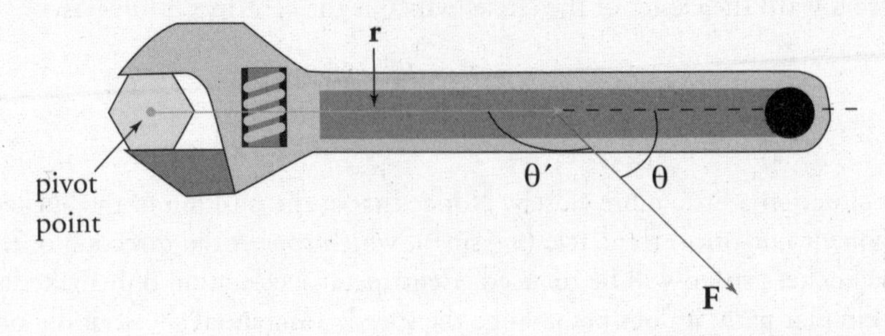

If we applied the force **F** to the wrench, would we make the wrench and the bolt rotate? Yes, because this force **F** has *torque.* (Notice: Torque is not a force; it's a property of a force.) To say how *much* torque **F** provides, we need a couple of preliminary definitions. First, the vector from the center of rotation (the **pivot point**) to the point of application of the force is called the **radius vector**, **r**. The angle between the vectors **r** and **F** is called θ. Now notice in the figure above that the angle between the vectors **r** and **F** at the point where they actually meet is denoted by θ'. This is because the angle between two vectors is actually the angle they make *when they start at the same point.* But in the figure, the vector **r** starts at the pivot point (which is where **r** always starts), and **F** starts at the *end* of **r** (which is where **F** always starts). One way to find the correct angle between these vectors is to imagine sliding **r** over so that it does start where **F** starts; the dashed line in the figure shows the line along which such a translated **r** vector would lie and the resulting correct angle θ. However, all this fuss about which angle is the correct one doesn't really matter, as you'll soon see.

The amount of torque a force **F** provides depends on three things: the magnitude of **F**, the length of **r**, and the angle θ.

Torque

$$\tau = rF\sin\theta$$

(The letter we use for torque is τ, the Greek letter *tau.*) From this equation, we can immediately figure out the unit of torque:

$$[\tau] = [r][F] = \text{m}\cdot\text{N} = \text{N}\cdot\text{m}$$

There's no special name for this unit; it's just a newton-meter.[1]

For example, let's say that $F = 20$ N, $r = 10$ cm, and $\theta = 30°$. Then the torque provided by this force would be $\tau = rF\sin\theta = (0.1\text{ m})(20\text{ N})\sin 30° = 1$ N·m. Notice that if we had instead used θ', we would have gotten the same answer, since $\theta' = 150°$ and $\sin 150° = \sin 30°$. This is why we don't have to worry about

---

[1] In Chapter 6 we'll encounter another newton-meter and rename it the joule. What's the difference? Torque has a direction, like a vector (though technically it's what's called a pseudovector), while the joule, a unit of energy, is a scalar. For the OAT, there's no need to worry about this; just calculate torque in newton-meters, and then label it clockwise or counterclockwise.

which angle, θ or θ′, is the true angle between **r** and **F** when we calculate torque, because **r** and **F** will always be *supplements* (they'll add up to 180°) and the sine of an angle is always equal to the sine of its supplement. Therefore, $\tau = rF \sin\theta = rF \sin\theta'$.

Look at this force on the wrench:

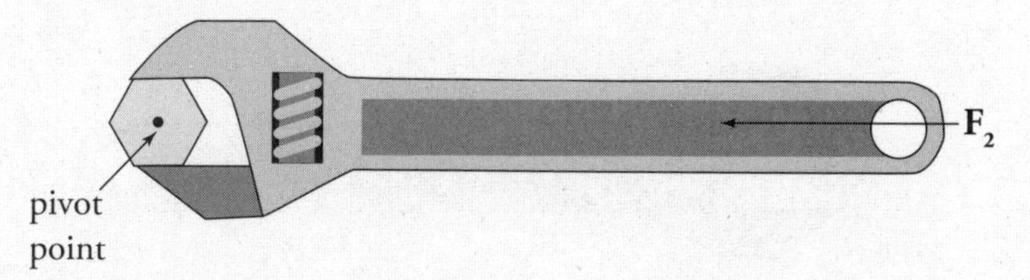

Our intuition tells us that this force would not make the wrench (or bolt) rotate. Therefore, we expect that this force has zero torque. Using the definition, we can see that this is true. If we were to draw the **r** vector from the pivot to the point where F_2 is applied, we'd see that the value of sin θ is 0, so $\tau_2 = 0$. Forces with no torque (like this one) cannot increase (or decrease) the rotational speed of an object.

How about this force on the wrench?

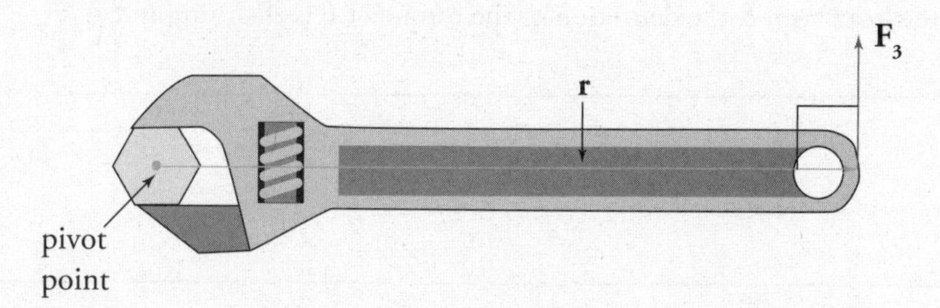

The force F_3 is perpendicular to its **r** vector, so θ = 90° and sin θ = 1, its maximum value. Therefore, when r ⊥ F, we get the maximum torque for a given r and F, and the equation for torque gives us simply $\tau_3 = rF_3$. (This situation is very common, by the way.)

$$\text{If } \mathrm{r} \perp \mathrm{F}, \text{ then } \tau = rF.$$

The force F_3 above would produce counterclockwise rotation, so we say that it produces a **counterclockwise (CCW)** torque. The force F_4 below would produce clockwise rotation, so we say it produces a **clockwise (CW)** torque.

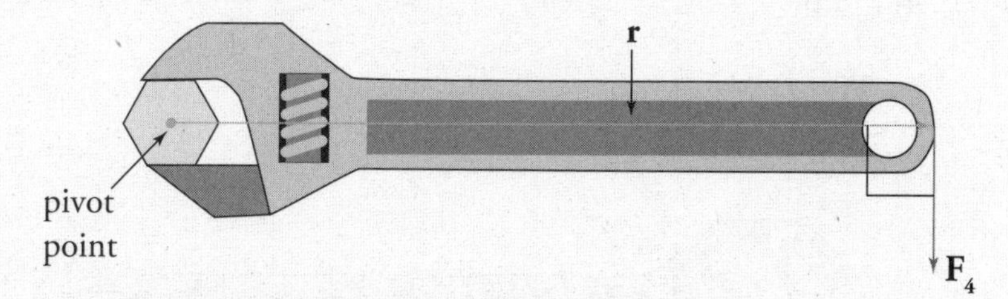

If $F_3 = F_4$, then these forces produce the same amount of torque, but one is clockwise and the other is counterclockwise. If we want to distinguish between them mathematically, we can say that $\tau_3 = +rF_3$ and $\tau_4 = -rF_4$, since it's customary to specify CCW rotation as positive and CW as negative.

The other method for calculating torque, which gives the same answer as the method we've just described, is based on the *lever arm* of a force. Let's look again at the first picture of our wrench:

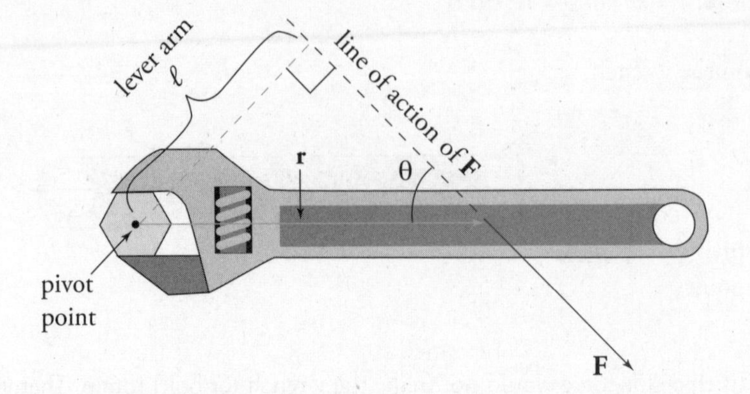

This time, however, rather than measuring the distance from the pivot to the *point* where the force is applied (the length r), we'll measure the shortest distance from the pivot to the *line* along which **F** is applied. This distance, which is always perpendicular to the line of action of F, is called the **lever arm** of F, written as ℓ or l.

Once we know the lever arm, ℓ, the definition of the torque of **F** is then simply $\tau = \ell F$.

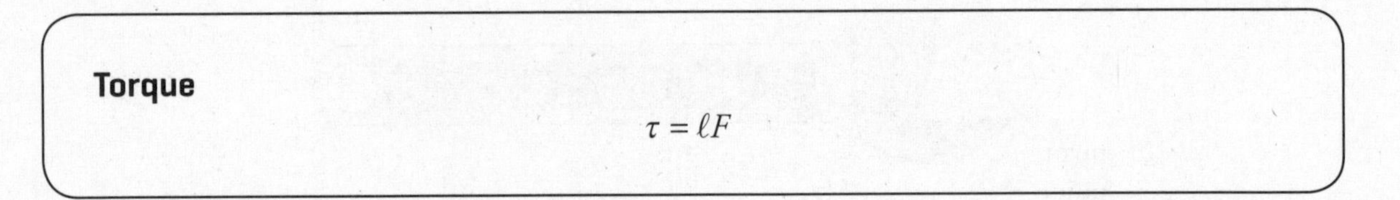

Torque

$$\tau = \ell F$$

To see that this gives the same value for the torque as the formula $\tau = rF\sin\theta$, just notice that in the picture on the preceding page (bottom), the lever arm, ℓ, is the side opposite the angle θ in a right triangle whose hypotenuse is r; therefore, $\ell = r\sin\theta$. So, $\tau = \ell F$ is the same as $\tau = (r\sin\theta)F$. Because you can use either formula for calculating the torque, use whichever one is more convenient in a particular problem. In general, it's convenient to use the lever arm method if the length of the lever arm is obvious from the situation; otherwise, use $\tau = rF\sin\theta$.

For the force $\mathbf{F}_5$ shown below, our intuition tells us that this force would not make the wrench (or bolt) rotate. Therefore, we expect that this force has zero torque. Using the definition of lever arm, we can see that this is true. The line of action of $\mathbf{F}_5$ passes right through the pivot point, so the level arm of the force is zero, and $\tau_5 = \ell_5 F_5 = (0)F_5 = 0$.

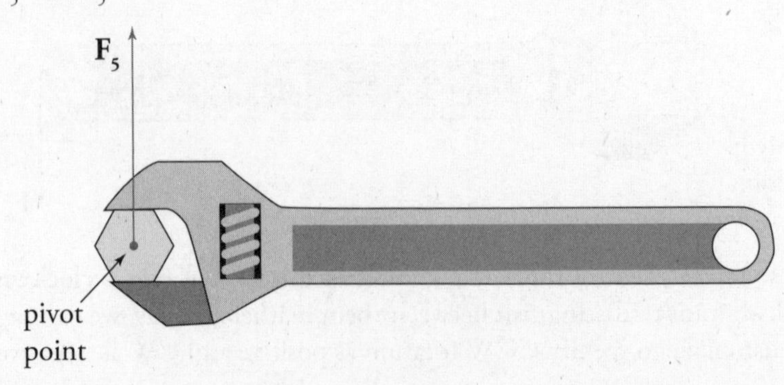

In general, if a force acts at the pivot or along a line through the pivot, then its torque is zero.

Example 5-12: A square metal plate (of side length s) rests on a flat table, and we exert a force **F** at one corner, parallel to one of the sides, as shown below. What is the torque of this force? (Use the center of the plate as the pivot point.)

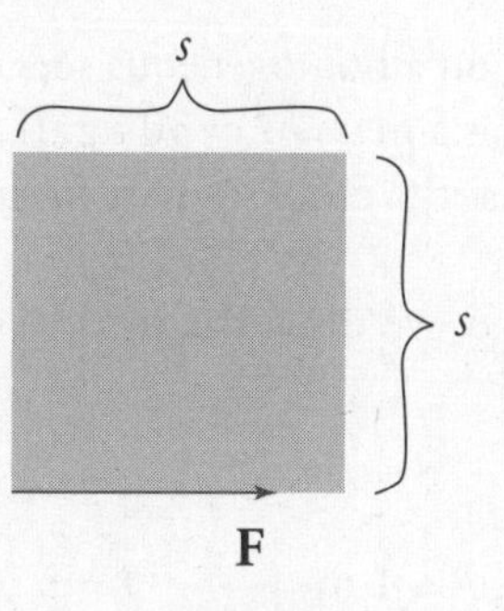

Solution: We'll calculate the torque of **F** by two different methods: first using the formula $\tau = rF\sin\theta$, and then using the formula $\tau = \ell F$.

Method 1. We draw in the **r** vector, which points from the pivot to the point where the force is applied. The angle between **r** and **F** can be taken to be $\theta = 45°$. If s is the length of each side of the square, then the length of **r** is $\frac{1}{2}s\sqrt{2}$ (because r is the hypotenuse of a 45°-45° right triangle, it's $\sqrt{2}$ times the length of each leg).

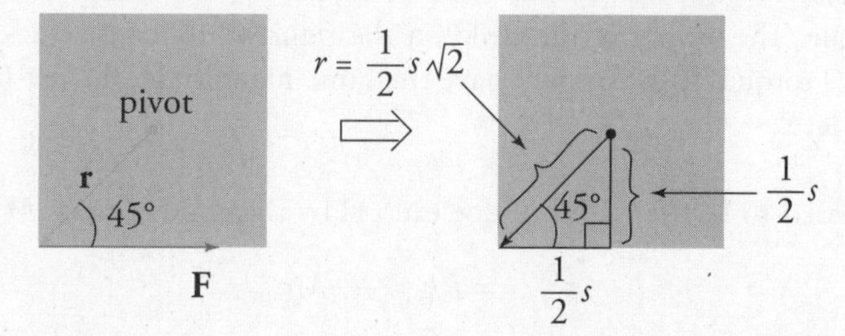

This gives $\tau = rF\sin\theta = \left(\frac{1}{2}s\sqrt{2}\right)(F)\sin 45° = \left(\frac{1}{2}s\sqrt{2}\right)(F)\left(\frac{\sqrt{2}}{2}\right) = \frac{1}{2}sF$.

Method 2. The line of action of the force **F** is simply the bottom side of the square. The perpendicular distance from the pivot to the side of the square is half the length of the square, $\frac{1}{2}s$, so this is the lever arm, ℓ.

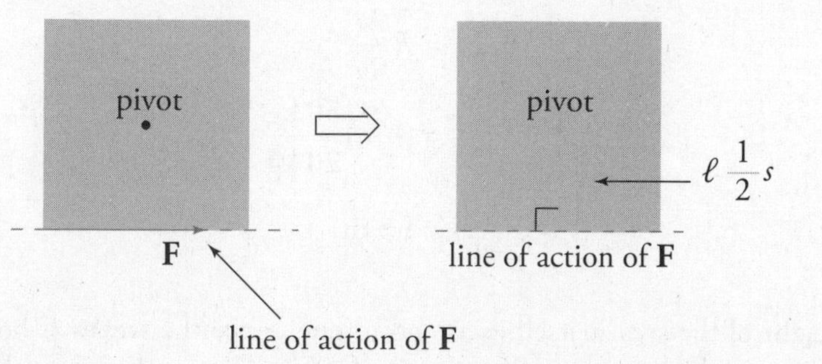

Therefore, $\tau = \ell F = \frac{1}{2}sF$.

In this situation, the formula using the lever arm is the easier way to calculate the torque. That's because you can look at the diagram and see the length of the lever arm right away. If you find yourself having to *calculate* the length of the lever arm, you probably should just be using $\tau = rF \sin \theta$.

Example 5-13: Two children are sitting on a homogeneous seesaw that pivots at its center. One child has a mass m of 20 kg, and the other child has a mass M of 30 kg. If the child of mass M sits 1 m to the left of center, how far to the right of center must the child of mass m sit in order to keep the seesaw level?

Solution: In the figure on the next page, we draw the force vectors acting on the seesaw; these are the weights of the children.

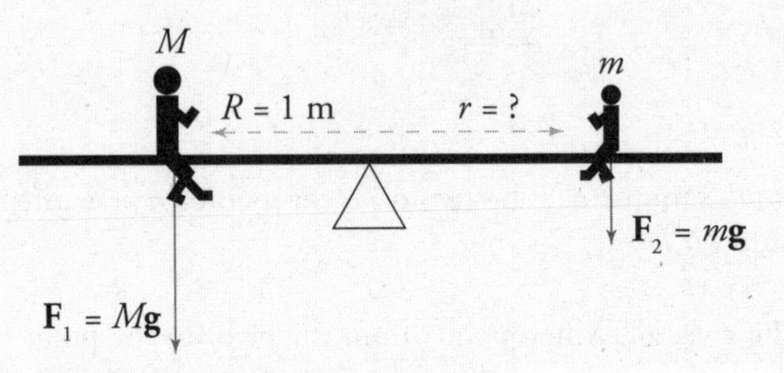

In order for the seesaw to balance, each child must produce the same amount of torque. The weight of the child on the left produces a torque that would cause counterclockwise rotation, so we'll call it a counterclockwise (CCW) torque. The weight of the child on the right would cause clockwise rotation, so we'll call it a clockwise (CW) torque. If the torques have the same magnitude, the net torque will be zero and the seesaw will remain level.

Because $\mathbf{F}_1$ is perpendicular to $\mathbf{R}$, the CCW torque exerted by the child of mass M is

$$\tau_{\text{CCW}} = RF_1 = R \cdot Mg$$

and because $\mathbf{F}_2$ is perpendicular to $\mathbf{r}$, the CW torque exerted by the child of mass m is

$$\tau_{\text{CW}} = rF_2 = r \cdot mg$$

Setting these equal to each other (to balance the torques) will give us r:

$$\begin{aligned} \tau_{\text{CW}} &= \tau_{\text{CCW}} \\ r \cdot mg &= R \cdot Mg \\ r &= R\frac{M}{m} \\ &= (1 \text{ m})\frac{30 \text{ kg}}{20 \text{ kg}} \\ \therefore r &= 1.5 \text{ m} \end{aligned}$$

Notice that the weight of the seesaw itself exerts no torque. Since the seesaw is homogeneous, its center of gravity is at its center, which is where the pivot is; if a force acts *at* the pivot, then its r is zero, so the torque of the force is zero.

If you're thinking we could just have solved for the distance at which the center of mass of the system was at the fulcrum (pivot point) of the seesaw, you're right; we get the same answer either way.

Example 5-14: In the figure below, three blocks hang below a massless meter stick. Block m_1 hangs from the *20 cm* mark, block m_2 hangs from the *70 cm* mark, and block m_3 hangs from the *80 cm* mark. If m_1 = 2 kg, m_2 = 5 kg, and m_3 = 3 kg, at what mark on the meter stick should a string be attached so that this system would hang horizontally?

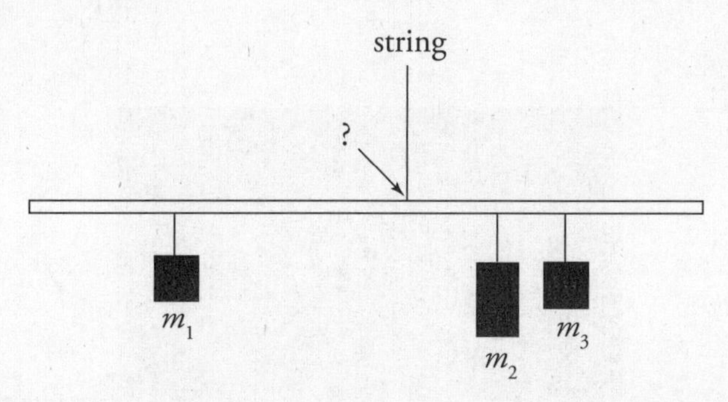

Solution: Look familiar? This is the same example we solved in the Center of Mass section. Let's see how we can answer this same question by balancing the torques. Let the pivot be the point where the string is attached to the stick. (Consider that the string is attached at the *x* cm mark, so that it's *x* cm from the left end of the stick.) Then the weight of mass m_1 produces a counterclockwise torque (τ_1), and the weights of m_2 and of m_3 each produce a clockwise torque (τ_2 and τ_3). If the counterclockwise torque (τ_1) balances the total clockwise torque ($\tau_2 + \tau_3$), the stick will remain level.

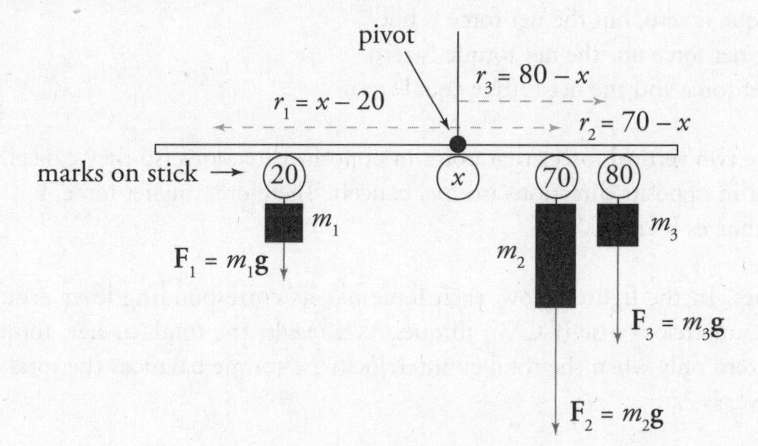

For each force, we need to find its corresponding *r*. For $\mathbf{F}_1$, we have r_1 = (*x* – 20) cm; for $\mathbf{F}_2$, we have r_2 = (70 – *x*) cm; and for $\mathbf{F}_3$, we have r_3 = (80 – *x*) cm. The equation that balances the torques is

$$\tau_{\text{CCW}} = \tau_{\text{CW}}$$
$$r_1 \cdot m_1 g = r_2 \cdot m_2 g + r_3 \cdot m_3 g$$
$$r_1 m_1 = r_2 m_2 + r_3 m_3$$
$$(x - 20)(2\text{ kg}) = (70 - x)(5\text{ kg}) + (80 - x)(3\text{ kg})$$
$$\therefore x = 63\text{ cm}$$

This is the same answer we found before. (By the way, the torque exerted by the tension in the string is equal to zero [which is why we ignored it] because the tension acts *at* the pivot.)

Example 5-15: A homogeneous rectangular sheet of metal lies on a flat table and is able to rotate around an axis through its center, perpendicular to the table. Four forces, all of the same magnitude, are exerted on the sheet as shown below:

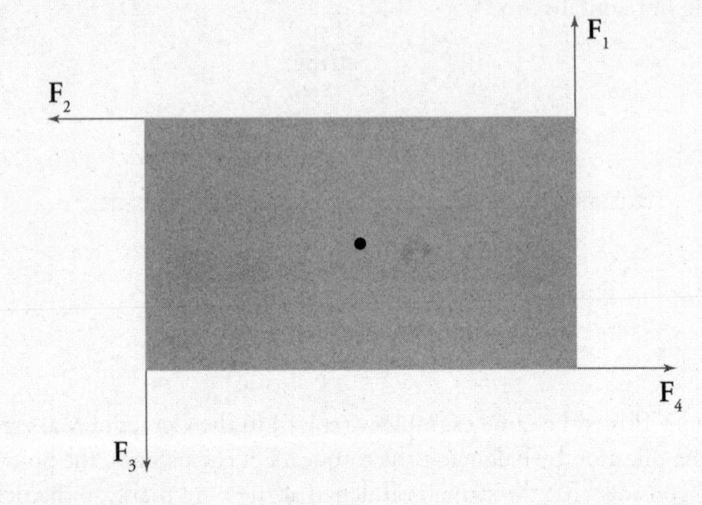

Which one of the following statements is true?

A. The net force is zero, but the net torque is not.
B. The net torque is zero, but the net force is not.
C. Neither the net force nor the net torque is zero.
D. Both the net force and the net torque equal zero.

Solution: There are two vertical forces that point in opposite directions (so they cancel), and two horizontal forces that point in opposite directions (so *they* cancel). Therefore, the net force, $\mathbf{F}_{net} = \mathbf{F}_1 + \mathbf{F}_2 + \mathbf{F}_3 + \mathbf{F}_4$, is zero. Eliminate choices B and C.

Now for the torques. In the figure below, each force has its corresponding lever arm. Notice that each force produces a counterclockwise (CCW) torque. As a result, the total, or net, torque cannot be zero. (The net torque is zero only when the total counterclockwise torque balances the total clockwise torque.) Therefore, the answer is A.

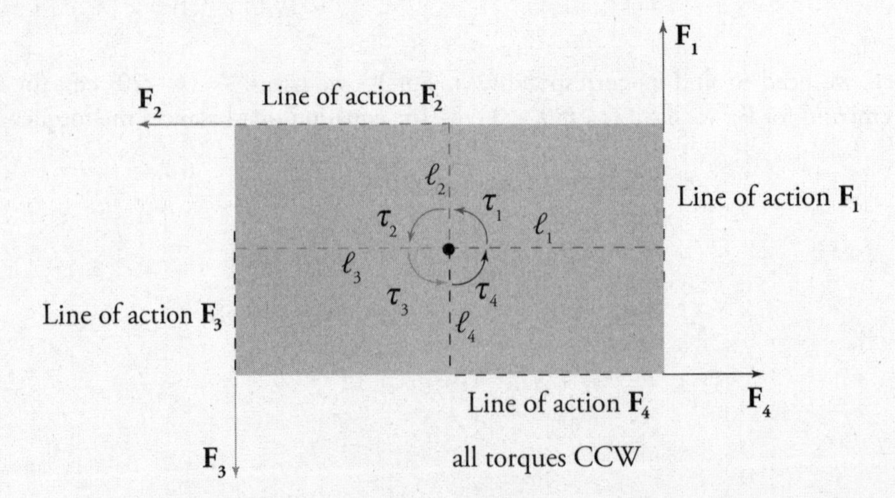

5.4 EQUILIBRIUM

As it's used in physics, the term **equilibrium** means *zero acceleration*. Notice that this does not mean zero velocity. As long as the velocity of the system remains constant (no change in speed or direction), then we can say that the system is in equilibrium. If the velocity happens to be zero, then we say the system is in **static** equilibrium.

There are actually two kinds of equilibrium, because there are two kinds of acceleration. There's *translational* equilibrium and *rotational* equilibrium. A system is said to be in **translational equilibrium** if the forces cancel; if $F_{net} = 0$, then the translational acceleration (a) is zero. A system is in **rotational equilibrium** if the torques cancel; if $\tau_{net} = 0$, then the rotational acceleration (denoted by α, the Greek letter *alpha*) is zero. If the term *equilibrium* is used without specifying which type, then it's assumed that the system is in *both* translational and rotational equilibrium.

Example 5-13 (the children on the seesaw) and Example 5-14 (the blocks balancing on the stick) both involved systems in equilibrium. In each case, we balanced the torques to ensure rotational equilibrium. We didn't explicitly analyze the translational equilibrium, but in the example of the children on the seesaw, the normal force exerted upward by the pivot balanced the total weight of the children, and in the example of the blocks hanging from the stick, the upward tension in the supporting string balanced the total weight of the blocks.

We'll now look at a couple of other examples of systems in equilibrium.

Example 5-16: A barber pole of mass 10 kg hangs from the end of a homogeneous rod of mass 40 kg that sticks out horizontally from the side of a vertical wall. The end of the rod, where the barber pole is attached, is connected to the upper part of the wall by a taut cable. For the angle θ, it is known that $\sin\theta = 0.6$ and $\cos\theta = 0.8$.

a) What's the tension in the cable?
b) What force is exerted by the wall on the rod?

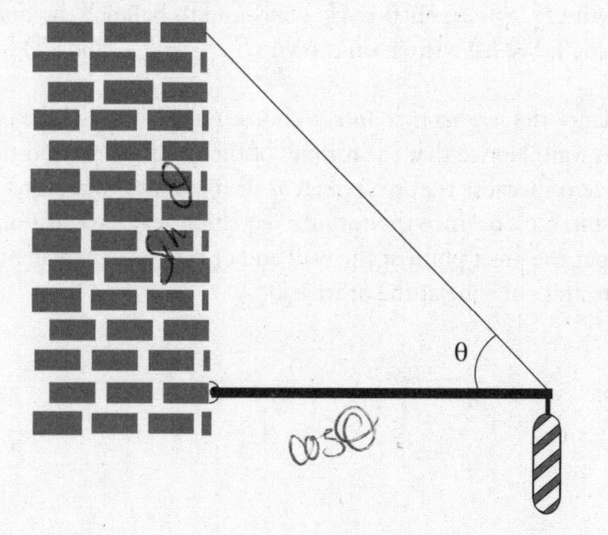

5.4

Solution:

a) First, let's draw a diagram of all the forces acting on the rod.

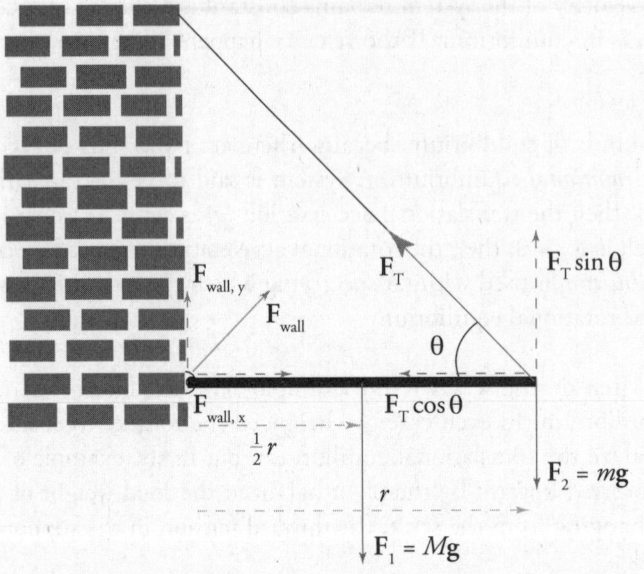

Notice that because the rod is in contact with the wall, the wall is exerting a force on the rod. However, at the start of the problem, we have no way of knowing what this force looks like (in other words, what either its magnitude or its direction are), so we break the force F_{wall} into a horizontal component and a vertical component. We do the same with the tension force, F_T, (which must act along the direction of the cable), and we can write these components as $F_{T,x} = F_T \cos\theta$ and $F_{T,y} = F_T \sin\theta$.

The system is in static equilibrium, so there must be no net torque and no net force. If we try to balance out all the forces, we find that we have too many unknowns. To balance the vertical forces, we'd write $F_{wall,y} + F_T \sin\theta = Mg + mg$, and to balance the horizontal forces, we'd write $F_{wall,x} = F_T \cos\theta$. We have three unknown ($F_{wall,x}$, $F_{wall,y}$, and F_T) but only two equations.

The trick is to balance the *torques* first and to choose our pivot to be the point of contact between the rod and wall. Notice that the torques of the components and the force exerted by the wall will both be zero (because they're applied *at* the pivot), so they won't even appear in the equation. As a result, our "balance-the-torques" equation will have just one unknown, F_T. That's why we chose to put the pivot point at the wall end of the rod: There are two unknown force components there, and only one at the other end.

So, with our pivot so chosen, we have three forces exerting torque: $\mathbf{F}_{T,y}$ produces a counterclockwise torque, and each of the weight vectors, $M\mathbf{g}$ and $m\mathbf{g}$, produces a clockwise torque. These torques balance to keep the rod level.

$$\begin{aligned}\tau_{\text{CCW}} &= \tau_{\text{CW}} \\ r \cdot F_T \sin\theta &= \tfrac{1}{2} r \cdot Mg + r \cdot mg \\ F_T \sin\theta &= \tfrac{1}{2} Mg + mg \\ F_T &= \frac{(\frac{1}{2}M + m)g}{\sin\theta} \\ &= \frac{(\frac{1}{2} \cdot 40 \text{ kg} + 10 \text{ kg})(10 \text{ N/kg})}{0.6} \\ \therefore F_T &= 500 \text{ N}\end{aligned}$$

b) Now that we've answered part (a) and found F_T, the tension in the cable, we can now find $F_{\text{wall}, x}$ and $F_{\text{wall}, y}$. We use the "balance-the-horizontal-forces" equation, $F_{\text{wall}, x} = F_T \cos\theta$, to get

$$F_{\text{wall},x} = F_T \cos\theta = (500 \text{ N})(0.8) = 400 \text{ N}$$

Then we use the "balance-the-vertical-forces" equation to find $F_{\text{wall}, y}$:

$$\begin{aligned}F_{\text{wall},y} + F_T \sin\theta &= Mg + mg \\ F_{\text{wall},y} &= Mg + mg - F_T \sin\theta \\ &= (40 \text{ kg})(10 \text{ N/kg}) + (10 \text{ kg})(10 \text{ N/kg}) - (500 \text{ N})(0.6) \\ \therefore F_{\text{wall},y} &= 200 \text{ N}\end{aligned}$$

Finally, the magnitude of the force exerted by the wall on the rod can be found using the Pythagorean theorem:

$$(F_{\text{wall}})^2 = (F_{\text{wall},x})^2 + (F_{\text{wall},y})^2 \rightarrow F_{\text{wall}} = \sqrt{(F_{\text{wall},x})^2 + (F_{\text{wall},y})^2} \rightarrow F_{\text{wall}} = \sqrt{(400\text{N})^2 + (200\text{N})^2} \approx 447\text{N}$$

Whew! Let's now look at a problem that's more OAT-like in terms of the amount of calculation:

Example 5-17: In the figure below, a block of mass 40 kg is held in place by two ropes exerting equal tension forces. If $\cos\theta = 2/3$, what's the tension in each rope?

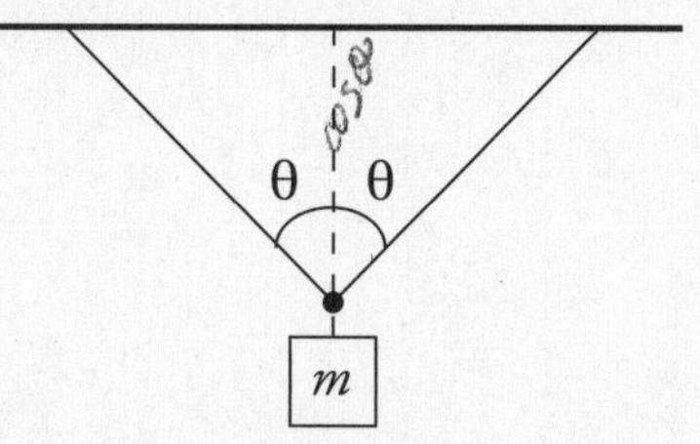

Solution: At the point where the mass is attached to the two ropes, we balance the forces. The horizontal forces automatically balance (we have $F_T \sin\theta$ pointing to the left and $F_T \sin\theta$ pointing to the right). For the vertical forces, we notice that there's the vertical component of the tension in the left-hand rope plus the vertical component of the tension in the right-hand rope ($F_T \cos\theta + F_T \cos\theta = 2F_T \cos\theta$), to balance out the weight of the block, *mg*. This gives us:

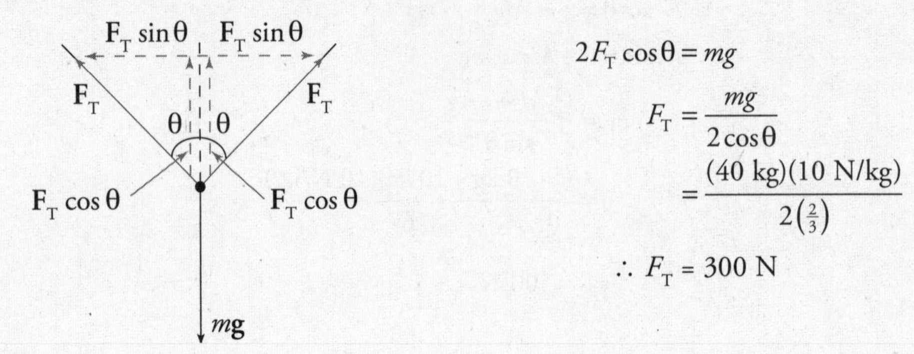

$$2F_T \cos\theta = mg$$

$$F_T = \frac{mg}{2\cos\theta}$$

$$= \frac{(40\text{ kg})(10\text{ N/kg})}{2\left(\frac{2}{3}\right)}$$

$$\therefore F_T = 300\text{ N}$$

Summary of Formulas

Center of mass: $x_{CM} = \frac{m_1x_1 + m_2x_2 + m_3x_3 \cdots}{m_1 + m_2 + m_3 \cdots}$

Center of gravity: $x_{CG} = \frac{w_1x_1 + w_2x_2 + w_3x_3 \cdots}{w_1 + w_2 + w_3 \cdots}$

in uniform gravitational field (g constant), $x_{CM} = x_{CG}$

Centripetal acceleration: $a_c = \frac{v^2}{r}$ (directed toward center of circle)

Centripetal force: $F_c = ma_c = \frac{mv^2}{r}$

$F_c = F_{\text{net towards center}}$

Torque: $\tau = rF\sin\theta$ (θ = angle between **r** and **F**)

$\tau = \ell F$ (ℓ = lever arm of force)

Equilibrium: $F_{net} = 0$ (translational equilibrium)

$\tau_{net} = 0$ (rotational equilibrium)

static equilibrium means:

$F_{net} = 0$

$\tau_{net} = 0$

$\mathbf{v} = 0$

Chapter 6
Mechanics III

6.1 WORK

Imagine a constant force **F** pushing a crate through a displacement **d**, as shown below:

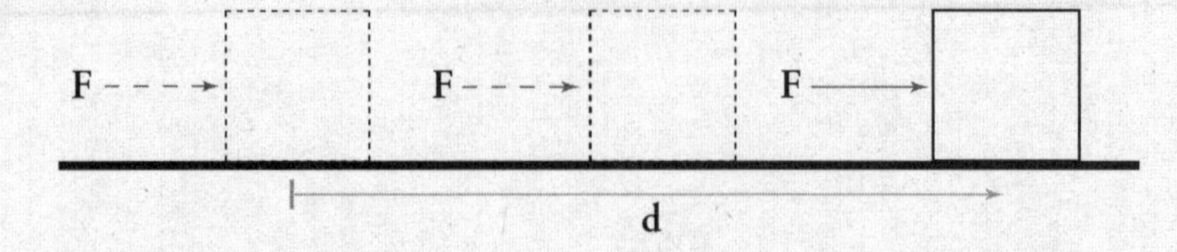

(Notice that the force **F** here doesn't just act momentarily at the initial position of the crate, with the crate then sliding across the floor with **F** removed; the force **F** is assumed to act constantly over the entire displacement.) We say that the **work** done by **F** is the product of F and d: Work $W = Fd$.

For example, if the magnitude of **F** is 20 N and the magnitude of **d** is 5 m, then the work done by the force **F** in the situation pictured above is (20 N)(5 m) = 100 N·m. When it's used to measure work, the newton-meter (N·m) is renamed the **joule**, abbreviated J. Therefore, we have $W = 100$ J.

The situation pictured above is quite special, however, because the vectors **F** and **d** point in the same direction. What if **F** and **d** do not point in the same direction? For example, what if we tie one end of a rope around the crate, sling the other end over our shoulder and pull the crate across the floor? Then our force **F** (which is actually the tension in the rope) will be at an angle to the displacement:

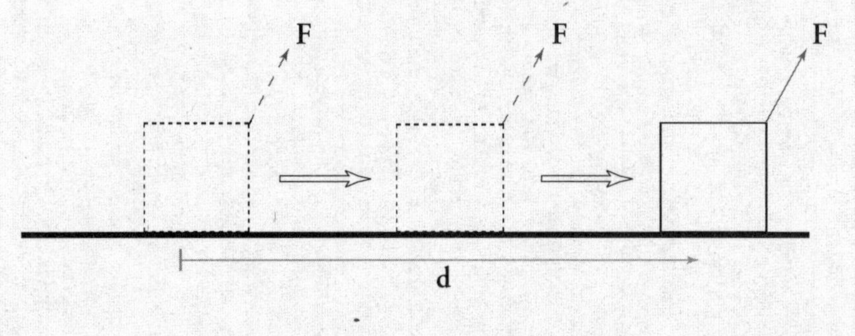

In this case, the work done by **F** is not the product of F and d. It's only the component of the force in the direction of **d** that does work. If θ is the angle between **F** and **d**, then the component of **F** that's parallel to **d** has magnitude $F \cos \theta$. Therefore, the work done by **F** is $(F \cos \theta)(d)$.

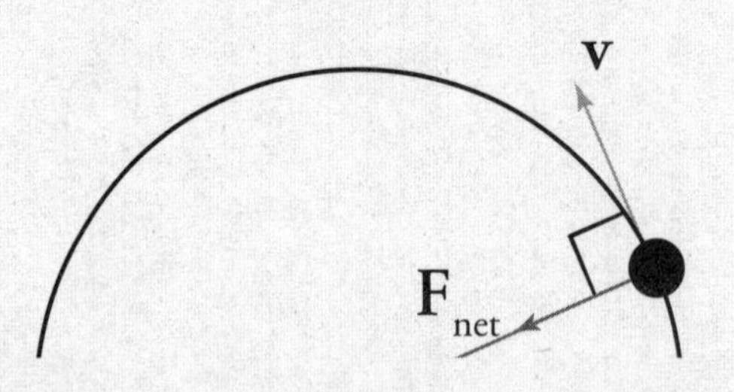

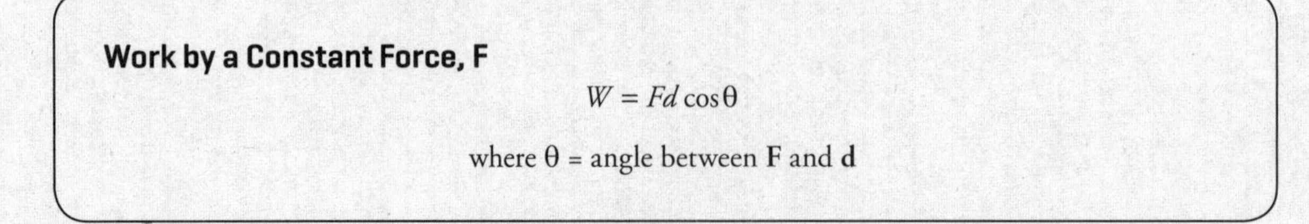

Work by a Constant Force, F

$$W = Fd \cos\theta$$

where θ = angle between **F** and **d**

Notice that the formula $W = Fd \cos \theta$ includes the formula $W = Fd$ as a special case. After all, if **F** and **d** do point in the same direction, then $\theta = 0$, and $\cos \theta = \cos 0 = 1$, so $Fd \cos \theta$ becomes Fd. Therefore, the formula $W = Fd \cos \theta$ covers all cases of a constant force **F** acting through a displacement **d**.

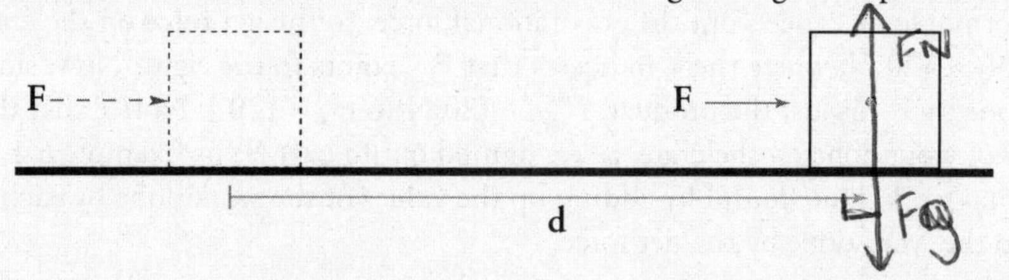

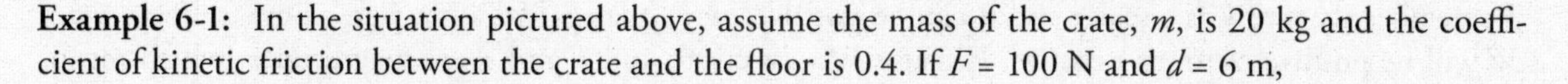

Example 6-1: In the situation pictured above, assume the mass of the crate, m, is 20 kg and the coefficient of kinetic friction between the crate and the floor is 0.4. If $F = 100$ N and $d = 6$ m,

a) How much work is done by **F**?
b) How much work is done by the normal force?
c) How much work is done by gravity?
d) How much work is done by the force of friction?
e) What is the total work done on the crate?

Solution:

a) Because **F** is parallel to **d**, the work done by **F** is simply $Fd = (100\text{ N})(6\text{ m}) = 600$ J.
b) The normal force is perpendicular to the floor, and to **d**. Since the angle between $\mathbf{F}_N$ and **d** is $\theta = 90°$, and $\cos 90° = 0$, the work done by $\mathbf{F}_N$ is zero.
c) The gravitational force is also perpendicular to the floor, and to **d**. Because the angle between $\mathbf{F}_{grav}$ and **d** is $\theta = 90°$, and $\cos 90° = 0$, the work done by $\mathbf{F}_{grav}$ is zero, too.
d) First, since $F_N = mg = (20\text{ kg})(10\text{ N/kg}) = 200$ N, we have $F_f = \mu_k F_N = (0.4)(200\text{ N}) = 80$ N. However, the direction of the vector $\mathbf{F}_f$ is opposite to the direction of **d**, so the angle between $\mathbf{F}_f$ and **d** is $\theta = 180°$. Because $\cos 180° = -1$, the work done by the friction force is (80 N)(6 m)(–1) = –480 J.
e) To find the total work done on the crate, we just add up the work done by each of the forces that acts on the crate. In this case, then, we'd have

$$W_{\text{total}} = W_{\text{by F}} + W_{\text{by F}_N} + W_{\text{by F}_{\text{grav}}} + W_{\text{by F}_f} = (600\text{ J}) + (0\text{ J}) + (0\text{ J}) + (-480\text{ J}) = 120\text{ J}$$

Here are a couple of things to notice about Example 6-1:

1) Although work depends on two vectors for its definition (namely, **F** and **d**), work itself is *not* a vector. *Work is a scalar.* W may be positive, negative, or zero, but work has no direction.
2) In this example, there were four forces acting on the crate: the pushing force **F**, gravity, the normal force, and friction. Each force does its own amount of work, which is why each part had to specify for which force we wanted the work. Only in the last part, where the total work is desired, can we omit the specific force we're looking at (because we're considering them all).

Example 6-2: In the situation described in Example 6-1, what is the net force on the crate? How much work is done by $\mathbf{F}_{net}$?

Solution: The normal force cancels out the gravitational force, so the net force on the crate is just $\mathbf{F} + \mathbf{F}_f$ = (100 N) + (–80 N) = +20 N, where the + indicates that $\mathbf{F}_{net}$ points to the right. Now, since $\mathbf{F}_{net}$ is parallel to **d**, the work done by $\mathbf{F}_{net}$ is just the product, $F_{net}d$ = (20 N)(6 m) = 120 J. Notice that this is the same as the total amount of work done on the crate, as we figured out in part (e) of Example 6-1. This wasn't a coincidence. The total work done (found by adding up the values of the work done by each force separately) is always equal to the work done by the net force.

Remember that work is a scalar and it can be positive, zero, or negative. Now here's how to know *when* W will be positive, zero, or negative. Because $W = Fd \cos \theta$, and F and d are magnitudes (which means they're positive), the sign of W depends entirely on the sign of $\cos \theta$.

The diagrams below show the three cases.

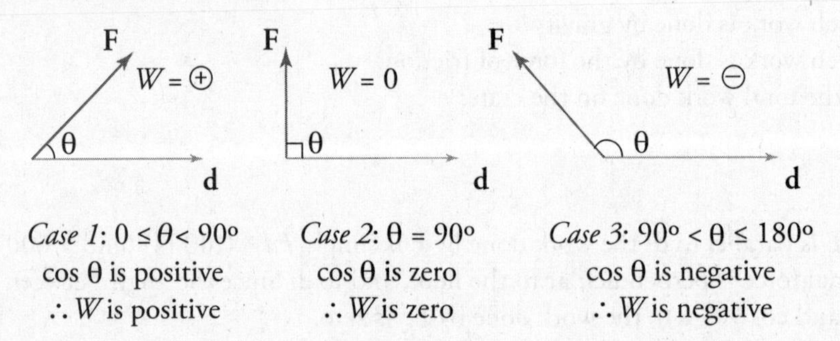

Case 1: $0 \leq \theta < 90°$
$\cos \theta$ is positive
$\therefore W$ is positive

Case 2: $\theta = 90°$
$\cos \theta$ is zero
$\therefore W$ is zero

Case 3: $90° < \theta \leq 180°$
$\cos \theta$ is negative
$\therefore W$ is negative

In Case 1, the angle between **F** and **d** is less than 90° (an acute angle); since the cosine of such an angle is positive, the work done by this force will be positive.

In Case 2, the angle between **F** and **d** is 90°; since the cosine of 90° is zero, the work done by this force will be zero.

In Case 3, the angle between **F** and **d** is greater than 90° (an obtuse angle); since the cosine of such an angle is negative, the work done by this force will be negative.

Example 6-1 illustrated all three cases. The force that pushed the crate across the floor did positive work; gravity and the normal force did zero work; and sliding friction did negative work.

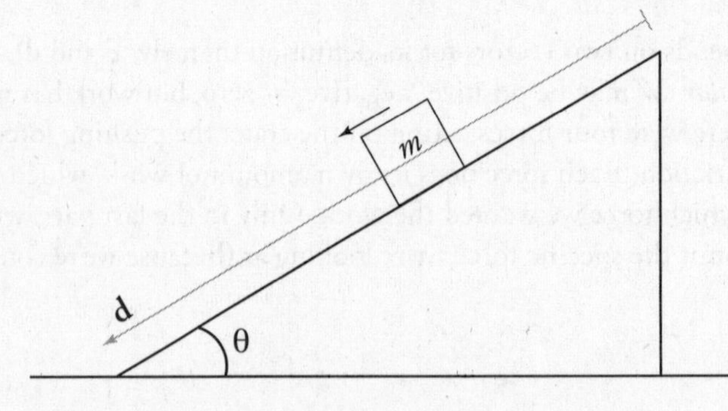

Example 6-3: In the situation pictured on the previous page, assume the mass of the block, m, is 20 kg and the coefficient of kinetic friction between the block and the ramp is 0.4. If d = 10 m and θ = 30°,

a) How much work is done by the normal force?
b) How much work is done by the force of friction?
c) How much work is done by gravity?
d) What is the total work done on the block?

Solution:

a) The normal force is perpendicular to the ramp, and to **d**. Since the angle between $\mathbf{F}_N$ and **d** is $\theta = 90°$, and cos 90° = 0, the work done by $\mathbf{F}_N$ is zero. Forces acting perpendicular to the direction of travel always do zero work.

b) First, we know that since the block is on a ramp, we'll have $F_N = mg \cos \theta$, where θ is the incline angle of the ramp. The magnitude of $\mathbf{F}_f$, the force of kinetic friction, is $\mu_k F_N$, so we get F_f = (0.4)(20 kg)(10 N/kg) cos 30°, which is approximately (0.4)(200 N)(0.85) = 68 N. Now, since the vectors $\mathbf{F}_f$ and **d** point in opposite directions (because **d** points down the ramp and $\mathbf{F}_f$ points up the ramp), the work done by $\mathbf{F}_f$ will be $-F_f d$ = –(68 N)(10 m) = –680 J.

c) There are two ways we can answer this part. One way is to remember that the force due to gravity acting parallel to the ramp is $mg \sin \theta$, where θ is the incline angle. Since this component of the gravitational force is parallel to **d**, we can simply multiply $mg \sin \theta$ by d to find the work done by gravity: $W = (mg \sin \theta)(d)$ = (20 kg)(10 N/kg)(sin 30°)(10 m) = 1000 J. Here's another way: The force $\mathbf{F}_{grav} = m\mathbf{g}$ points straight down, and the angle between $\mathbf{F}_{grav}$ and **d** is β, where β is the angle shown below. It's the complement of the incline angle θ; that is, $\beta = 90° - \theta$.

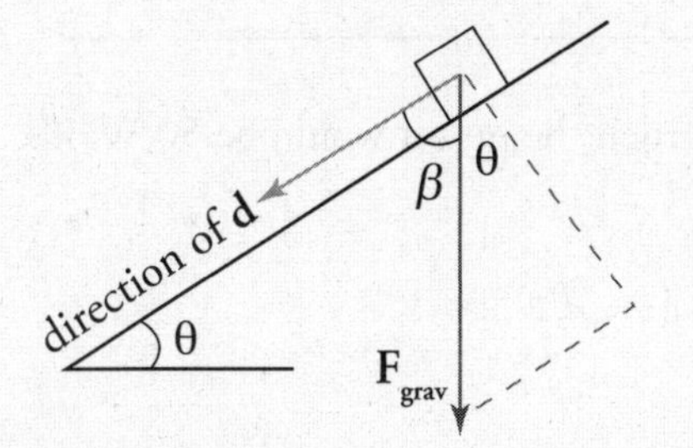

Since θ = 30°, we have β = 60°. Therefore, the work done by $\mathbf{F}_{grav}$ is $F_{grav} d \cos \beta = mgd \cos \beta$ = (20 kg)(10 N/kg)(10 m) (cos 60°) = 1000 J. You need to be very careful here; the formula for work reads, "$W = Fd \cos \theta$," but the θ in this formula is *not* the same as the θ labeled in the figure. The angle in the formula for W is the angle between **F** and **d**, and this is not the same as the incline angle.

d) To find the total work done on the block, we just add up the work done by each of the forces that acts on the block. In this case, then, we'd have

$$W_{total} = W_{\text{by } F_N} + W_{\text{by } F_f} + W_{\text{by } F_{grav}} = (0\text{ J}) + (-680\text{ J}) + (1000\text{ J}) = 320\text{ J}$$

6.2 POWER

Power measures how fast work gets done. For example, if a force does 100 J of work in 20 seconds, then work is being done at a *rate* of

$$\frac{100\text{ J}}{20\text{ s}} = 5\text{ J/s}$$

This is the power.

We use the letter P to denote power, and from the sample calculation above, we can see that the unit of power is the joule-per-second. This unit has its own name: the **watt**, abbreviated W. Therefore, power is measured in watts: $[P]$ = J/s = W. (Don't confuse the abbreviation for the watt, W, with the usual variable used for work, W.)

The term *watt* makes most of us think of light bulbs, but the watt is used to measure the power of anything, not just light bulbs. After all, should the unit *horsepower* make us think that only horses can provide power? By the way, 1 hp (1 horsepower) is equal to about 750 W.

The sample calculation above also shows us how we should define P in general:

Power

$$P = \frac{\text{work}}{\text{time}} = \frac{W}{t}$$

What if 100 J of work is done over a time interval of just 2 seconds? Then the power would be 50 W; it's easy to see that the faster work gets done, the greater the power.

A handy formula that you can also use to calculate P uses the fact that $v = d/t$:

$$P = \frac{W}{t} = \frac{Fd}{t} = F\frac{d}{t} = Fv \rightarrow P = Fv$$

(We're assuming here that **F** is parallel to **d**, so that $W = Fd$, and that the object's speed, v, is constant.) To see how this formula would be used, let's answer this question: How much power must be provided to a toy rocket of mass 50 kg to keep it moving upward at a constant speed of 40 m/s? Ignoring air resistance, the engine thrust must provide an upward force that's equal to the weight of the rocket: $F = mg$ = (50 kg)(10 N/kg) = 500 N. Therefore, $P = Fv$ = (500 N)(40 m/s) = 20,000 W = 20 kW.

From the definition of power, we can see that

$$W = Pt$$

This equation is used as often on the OAT as the definition $P = W/t$. For example, if a machine has a power output of 200 W, how much work can it do in 1 hour? Multiplying power by time (and remembering to change 1 hour into (60)(60) = 3600 seconds) gives the work:

$$W = Pt = (200\,\text{W})(3600\,\text{s}) = 720{,}000\,\text{J} = 720\,\text{kJ}$$

Example 6-4: A force of magnitude 40 N pushes on an object of mass 8 kg through a displacement of 5 m for 10 seconds. What's the power provided by this force?

Solution: Power is equal to work divided by time, so

$$P = \frac{W}{t} = \frac{Fd}{t} = \frac{(40\,\text{N})(5\,\text{m})}{10\,\text{s}} = 20\,\text{W}$$

Example 6-5: You're lifting bricks, each with a mass of 2 kg, from the floor up to a shelf that is 1.5 m high.

a) How much work do you perform lifting each brick?
b) If you can place 20 bricks on the shelf every minute, what is your power output?

Solution:

a) The force you must provide to lift a brick is equal to the weight of the brick, which is mg = (2 kg)(10 N/kg) = 20 N. Since this force must act over a distance of 1.5 m to lift it up to the shelf, the work required is $W = Fd$ = (20 N)(1.5 m) = 30 J.
b) If you can place 20 bricks on the shelf every 60 seconds, then on average you're lifting one brick every 3 seconds. If the work performed in 3 seconds is 30 J—as we found in part (a)—then your power output is

$$P = \frac{W}{t} = \frac{30\,\text{J}}{3\,\text{s}} = 10\,\text{W}$$

Example 6-6: A car of mass 2000 kg accelerates from rest to a speed of 30 m/s in 9 seconds. Given that the engine does a total of 900,000 J of work, what is the average power output of the car's engine?

Solution: Since we're given the amount of work done and the time interval, we can find the average power output of the engine simply by dividing work by time:

$$P = \frac{W}{t} = \frac{900{,}000\ \text{J}}{9\ \text{s}} = 100{,}000\ \text{W} = 100\ \text{kW}$$

Notice that neither the mass of the car, nor its final speed, were needed to answer the question because the required information (work and time) were given.

Example 6-7: One month, your electric bill states that you used 500 kWh of electricity, at a cost of 8¢ per kWh. What is a kWh, and how much is your electric bill that month?

Solution: A kilowatt (kW) is a thousand watts; it's a unit of power. An hour (h) is a time interval. Therefore, a kilowatt-hour, kWh, obtained by multiplying power times time, Pt, has units of work. (1 kWh = (1000 W)(3600 s) = 3.6×10^6 J = 3.6 MJ.) The electric company performed 500 kWh of work pushing and pulling the electrons within the wires in your home to make electrical devices function, at a cost to you of (500 kWh)(8¢/kWh) = $40.

6.3 KINETIC ENERGY

An intuitive way to describe **energy** is that it's the ability to do work. Objects that move have this ability, since they can crash into something and thus exert a force over a distance. Therefore, objects that move have energy; specifically, we say they have **kinetic energy**, the energy due to motion.

To figure out how much kinetic energy a moving object has, imagine that an object of mass m is initially at rest (and thus has no kinetic energy). To get it moving, we have to exert a force **F** on it, over some distance d. (Let's assume, to keep things simple, that **F** points in the same direction as **d**.) How fast will the object be moving as a result? The acceleration is a constant $a = F/m$, so, using Big Five #5, we get

$$v^2 = v_0^2 + 2ad \rightarrow v^2 = 2ad \rightarrow v^2 = 2\frac{F}{m}d$$

Therefore, the final speed, v, will be $\sqrt{2Fd/m}$

Now let's do a little algebra and rewrite the last equation above like this:

$$Fd = \tfrac{1}{2}mv^2$$

We recognize the product Fd as the work done by the force. So, we did work on the object to get it moving, and now because it's moving, it has kinetic energy. How much kinetic energy? This last equation tells us that we should consider the amount of kinetic energy to be $\frac{1}{2}mv^2$.

Kinetic Energy

$$KE = \tfrac{1}{2}mv^2$$

In words, this definition says that the kinetic energy of an object whose mass is m and whose speed is v is equal to one-half m times the square of the speed. Since $\frac{1}{2}mv^2$ is equal to the work Fd, we see right away that the unit of KE should also be the joule. In addition, like work, kinetic energy is a scalar.

Example 6-8: An object of mass 10 kg moves with a velocity of 4 m/s to the north. What is its kinetic energy? What would happen to the kinetic energy if the speed of the object doubled?

Solution: Kinetic energy is a scalar that cares only about the speed of an object; the direction of the object's velocity is irrelevant. So we find that

$$KE = \tfrac{1}{2}mv^2 = \tfrac{1}{2}(10\,\text{kg})(4\text{ m/s})^2 = 80\,\text{J}$$

Because KE is proportional to v^2, if v were to increase by a factor of 2 then KE would increase by a factor of $2^2 = 4$.

The Work-Energy Theorem

The use of Big Five #5 shown above (to motivate the definition $KE = \frac{1}{2}mv^2$) assumed that the initial speed of the object was zero. But what if the initial speed wasn't zero? Then we'd have

$$\begin{aligned} v^2 = v_0^2 + 2ad \rightarrow v^2 - v_0^2 = 2ad \rightarrow \quad & v^2 - v_0^2 = 2\frac{F}{m}d \\ & \tfrac{1}{2}m(v^2 - v_0^2) = Fd \\ & Fd = \tfrac{1}{2}mv^2 - \tfrac{1}{2}mv_0^2 \\ & W = KE_{\text{final}} - KE_{\text{initial}} \end{aligned}$$

In other words, the total work done on the object is equal to the change in its kinetic energy. This fact is important enough that it's given a name:

Work-Energy Theorem

$$W_{\text{total}} = \Delta KE$$

This formula gives you another way to calculate work. You don't even need to know the force or the displacement! If you know the change in an object's kinetic energy, then you automatically know the total amount of work that was done on it.

Look back at the set of three diagrams showing when the work done by a force is positive, zero, or negative. In Case 1, the force is pulling in roughly the same direction as the object's displacement (more formally, the force **F** has a component that's in the same direction as **d**). We can think of such a force as "helping" the object move, and therefore causing its speed to increase. Is this consistent with the work-energy theorem? Yes. This was the case of positive work being done, and according to the work-energy theorem, positive work would automatically imply a positive change in kinetic energy. If the kinetic energy increases, then the speed increases.

In Case 3, the force is pulling in roughly the opposite direction from the object's displacement (more formally, the force **F** has a component that's in the opposite direction from **d**). We can think of such a force as "hindering" the object's motion, and therefore causing its speed to decrease. This is also consistent with the work-energy theorem because Case 3 was the case of negative work being done, and according to the work-energy theorem, negative work automatically implies a negative change in kinetic energy. If the kinetic energy decreases, then the speed decreases.

Example 6-9: An object of mass 10 kg whose initial speed is 4 m/s is accelerated until it achieves a final speed of 9 m/s.

a) How much work was done on this object?
b) If the acceleration took place over a displacement **d** of magnitude 13 m, and the force **F** exerted on it was constant and parallel to **d**, what was F?

Solution:

a) Although neither **F** nor **d** is given, we can still figure out the work done by using the work-energy theorem:

$$\begin{aligned} W_{\text{total}} &= \Delta KE \\ &= KE_{\text{f}} - KE_{\text{i}} \\ &= \tfrac{1}{2}mv^2 - \tfrac{1}{2}mv_0^2 \\ &= \tfrac{1}{2}m(v^2 - v_0^2) \\ &= \tfrac{1}{2}(10 \text{ kg})\left[(9 \text{ m/s})^2 - (4 \text{ m/s})^2\right] \end{aligned}$$

$$\therefore W = 325 \text{ J}$$

b) Because **F** is parallel to **d**, we know that $W = Fd$. We just found W in part (a), and since we now know d, we can find F:

$$W = Fd \rightarrow F = \frac{W}{d} = \frac{325\,\text{J}}{13\,\text{m}} = 25\,\text{N}$$

Example 6-10: An object of mass 10 kg is moving at a speed of 9 m/s. How much work must be done on this object in order to stop it?

Solution: Once again, we're asked to find W without being given **F** and **d**, so we use the work-energy theorem. If we want to stop the object, we want to bring its final kinetic energy to zero. Therefore,

$$\begin{aligned} W &= \Delta KE \\ &= \tfrac{1}{2}mv^2 - \tfrac{1}{2}mv_0^2 \\ &= 0 - \tfrac{1}{2}mv_0^2 \\ &= -\tfrac{1}{2}(10 \text{ kg})(9 \text{ m/s})^2 \\ \therefore W &= -405 \text{ J} \end{aligned}$$

The work that must be done on the object has to be negative, because only negative work causes a decrease in speed.

Example 6-11: An object of mass 3 kg is undergoing uniform circular motion. The object's speed is 4 m/s, and the radius of the path is 0.5 m.

a) What's the magnitude of the net force on the object?
b) How much work is done by the net force during each revolution of the object?

Solution:

a) The net force on an object undergoing uniform circular motion (UCM) is the centripetal force:

$$F_c = m\frac{v^2}{r} = (3\,\text{kg})\frac{(4 \text{ m/s})^2}{0.5 \text{ m}} = 96\,\text{N}$$

b) We can answer this part in two ways. The centripetal force points toward the center of the circular path, so it's always perpendicular to the object's velocity:

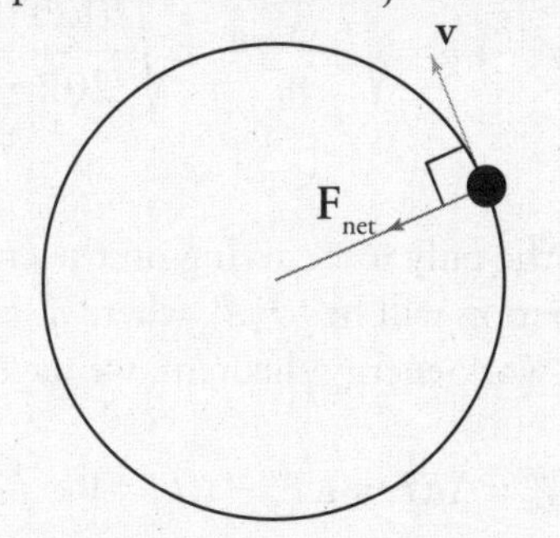

The work done by a force that's perpendicular to an object's motion is *zero* (remember Case 2 depicted in Section 6.1 (example 6-2): $\mathbf{F} \perp \mathbf{d}$ means $W = 0$).

Another way is to use the work-energy theorem. Since the object's speed is constant, its kinetic energy is constant, too. No change in kinetic energy means no work is being done.

Example 6-12: A box of mass 4 kg is initially at rest on a frictionless horizontal surface. A horizontal force **F** of magnitude 32 N is exerted on the object and then removed. If the speed of the object is then 2 m/s, over what distance did **F** act?

Solution: By the work-energy theorem, the work done by **F** was

$$W = \Delta KE = KE_f - KE_i = KE_f = \tfrac{1}{2}mv^2 = \tfrac{1}{2}(4\text{ kg})(2\text{ m/s})^2 = 8\text{ J}$$

The question now is, "Given that **F** is parallel to **d** (so $W = Fd$), what's d?"

$$W = Fd \rightarrow d = \frac{W}{F} = \frac{8\text{ J}}{32\text{ N}} = 0.25\text{ m}$$

Example 6-13: Consider the block described in Example 6-3. If the initial speed of the block was zero, what is the block's speed when it reaches the bottom of the ramp?

Solution: We figured out in part (d) of that example that the total work done on the block was 320 J. By the work-energy theorem, we find that

$$W = \Delta KE = KE_f - KE_i = KE_f = \tfrac{1}{2}mv^2 \rightarrow v = \sqrt{\frac{2\,W_{\text{total}}}{\text{m}}} = \sqrt{\frac{2(320\text{ J})}{20\text{ kg}}} = \sqrt{32\text{ m}^2/\text{s}^2} \approx 5.6\text{ m/s}$$

Example 6-14: Consider the crate described in Example 6-1.

a) If the initial speed of the crate was zero, what was the speed once the force **F** was removed after acting through the given displacement **d**?
b) How far would the crate slide before coming to rest?

Solution:

a) We figured out in part (e) of that example that the total work done on the crate was 120 J. The work-energy theorem then tells us that

$$W = \Delta KE = KE_f - KE_i = KE_f = \tfrac{1}{2}mv^2 \rightarrow v = \sqrt{\frac{2\,W_{\text{total}}}{m}} = \sqrt{\frac{2(120\text{ J})}{20\text{ kg}}} = \sqrt{12\text{ m}^2/\text{s}^2} \approx 3.5\text{ m/s}$$

b) Once the force **F** is removed, the only force acting on the crate that doesn't do zero work is friction. The work done by friction will be $-F_f d'$, where d' is the distance the crate will slide before coming to rest. By the work-energy theorem, we have

$$\begin{aligned} W = \Delta KE = KE_f - KE_i &= 0 - KE_i \\ -KE_i &= -F_f d' \\ F_f d' &= KE_i \\ d' &= \frac{KE_i}{F_f} \end{aligned}$$

Since the crate had 120 J of kinetic energy right when the force **F** was removed, and using the equation $F_f = \mu_k F_N = \mu_k mg$, we get

$$d' = \frac{KE_i}{F_f} = \frac{KE_i}{\mu_k mg} = \frac{120\text{ J}}{(0.4)(20\text{ kg})(10\text{ N/kg})} = 1.5\text{ m}$$

6.4 POTENTIAL ENERGY

In the preceding section, we defined kinetic energy as the energy an object has due to its motion. **Potential energy** is the energy an object has by virtue of its *position*. There are different "kinds" of potential energy because there are different kinds of forces. For example, in our study of OAT physics, we'll look at three types of potential energy: gravitational, electrical, and elastic. In this chapter, we'll study the first of these: *gravitational* potential energy.

Imagine a brick lying on the ground. Now, pick it up and place it on a shelf. You've just changed the position of the brick, and, since potential energy is the energy an object has by virtue of its position, you might expect that you've changed the brick's potential energy as well. You did. The brick's gravitational potential energy has been changed, because its position in a gravitational field has changed.

Now, let's be more specific. By *how much* did the brick's gravitational potential energy change? To find the answer, we need to look at the work done by the gravitational force (this is gravitational potential energy, after all). While the brick was being lifted, gravity did work on the brick. Let m be the mass of the brick, and let h be the height from the ground up to the shelf. The gravitational force on the brick is $\mathbf{F}_{grav} = m\mathbf{g}$, pointing downward; the displacement of the brick is h, upward.

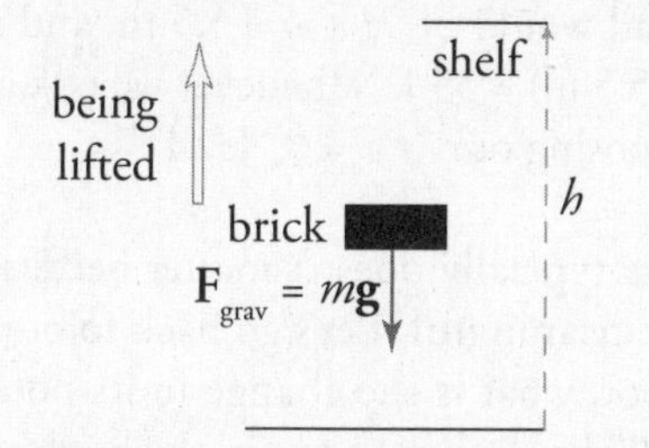

Because the force $\mathbf{F}_{grav}$ and the displacement $\mathbf{h}$ point in opposite directions, we know that the work done by $\mathbf{F}_{grav}$ will be the negative of F_{grav} times h: $W_{by\ F_{grav}} = -F_{grav}h = -mgh$. The change in gravitational potential energy is defined to be the opposite of the work done by the gravitational force:

$$\Delta PE_{grav} = -W_{by\ F_{grav}}$$

In this case, then, we have $\Delta PE_{grav} = -(-mgh) = mgh$. If the brick had *fallen* from the shelf to the floor, so that its height *decreased* by h, then we would have had $W_{by\ F_{grav}} = F_{grav}h = mgh$ and $\Delta PE_{grav} = -mgh$. In summary, then, we have

Change in Gravitational Potential Energy

$$\Delta PE_{grav} = \begin{cases} +mgh, & \text{if the height of } m \text{ is increased by } h \\ -mgh, & \text{if the height of } m \text{ is decreased by } h \end{cases}$$

where it's assumed that we're close enough to the surface of the earth that g can be considered a constant.

The formulas above give the *change* in the gravitational potential energy of an object of mass m. If we designate the ground as our "$PE_{grav} = 0$" level, then we can say that the gravitational potential energy of an object at height h is equal to mgh.

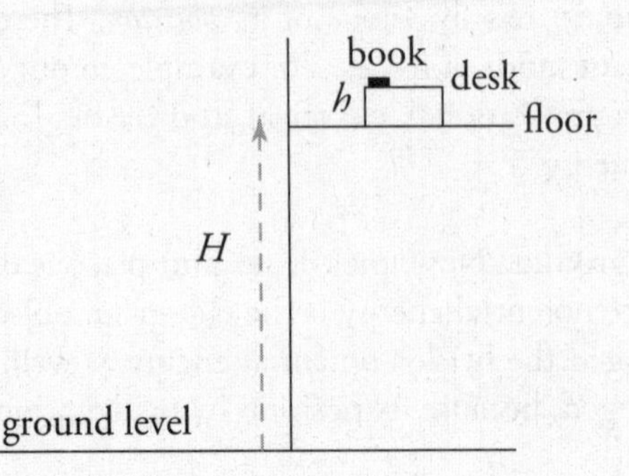

Potential energy is relative. Consider a book sitting on the desk in a second-floor office. Relative to the floor, the height of the book might be, say, half a meter. So, if the book has a mass of 1 kg, its gravitational potential energy is mgh = (1 kg)(10 N/kg)(0.5 m) = 5 J. But what if we were to measure the height of the book above the *ground*? Relative to the ground, the floor of the office might be at height H = 5 m, so the height of the book above the ground would be $H + h$ = 5.5 m, and the book's gravitational potential energy is $mg(H + h)$ = (1 kg)(10 N/kg)(5.5 m) = 55 J. Whenever we talk about "the" potential energy of an object, we must specify where we're choosing our "$PE = 0$" level.

The fact that potential energy is relative typically doesn't matter because it's only *changes* in potential energy that are important and physically meaningful. Let's go back to our book on the office desk example. If the book falls off the desk to the floor, what is the change in its potential energy? To the person who calls the floor of the office their "$PE = 0$" level, the change in the book's potential energy will be

$$\Delta PE_{grav} = PE_f - PE_i = 0 - mgh = -mgh = -(1\,\text{kg})(10\,\text{N/kg})(0.5\,\text{m}) = -5\,\text{J}$$

Now, to the person who calls the ground their "$PE = 0$" level, the change in the book's potential energy will be the same:

$$\Delta PE_{grav} = PE_f - PE_i = mgH - mg(H + h) = -mgh = -(1\,\text{kg})(10\,\text{N/kg})(0.5\,\text{m}) = -5\,\text{J}$$

Both people will always agree on the *change* in an object's potential energy, even if they disagree about what the potential energy *is* at a certain height (because they choose different "$PE = 0$" levels).

Example 6-15: A brick that weighs 25 N is lifted from the ground to a shelf that's 2 m high. What is its change in gravitational potential energy?

Solution: Because mg = 25 N, we have $\Delta PE_{grav} = mgh$ = (25 N)(2 m) = 50 J. Notice that since the brick was lifted *up*, its change in gravitational potential energy is *positive*.

Example 6-16: A 1 N apple in a tree is at height 4 m above the ground. The apple falls off its branch and lands on a branch that's only 1 m above the ground. What is the change in the apple's potential energy?

Solution: Because the apple *falls* through a distance of $h = 4 - 1 = 3$ m, the change in its gravitational potential energy is $-mgh = -(1\text{ N})(3\text{ m}) = -3$ J. We could also have answered the question like this: First, we choose, say, the ground to be our "$PE = 0$" level. Then the initial potential energy of the apple is $PE_i = mgh_i = (1\text{ N})(4\text{ m}) = 4$ J, and the final potential energy of the apple is $PE_f = mgh_f = (1\text{ N})(1\text{ m}) = 1$ J. The change in the potential energy is, therefore, $\Delta PE = PE_f - PE_i = (1\text{ J}) - (4\text{ J}) = -3$ J. Note that because the apple *falls*, the change in its gravitational potential energy must be *negative.*

Example 6-17: Which has more gravitational potential energy: an object of mass 2 kg at a height of 50 m, or an object of mass 50 kg at a height of 2 m? (Set $PE_{grav} = 0$ at the ground for both objects.)

Solution: Since the ground is the $PE_{grav} = 0$ level, then at height h an object's gravitational potential energy is $PE_{grav} = mgh$. The potential energy of the 2 kg object is

$$PE_1 = m_1 g h_1 = (2\,\text{kg})(10\text{ N/kg})(50\,\text{m}) = 1000\,\text{J}$$

and the potential energy of the 50 kg object is

$$PE_2 = m_2 g h_2 = (50\,\text{kg})(10\text{ N/kg})(2\,\text{m}) = 1000\,\text{J}$$

Therefore, these two objects have the *same* gravitational potential energy relative to the ground.

Gravity is a Conservative Force

Suppose we want to move a brick from the floor up to a shelf. One way we could do it would be to simply lift the brick straight up. Another way would be to set up a ramp and then push the brick up the ramp to the shelf. Let's figure out how much work gravity does in each of these cases. We'll assume that the brick has a mass of 3 kg and that the shelf is 2 m high.

The first case is easy. The gravitational force on the brick is $mg = (3\text{ kg})(10\text{ N/kg}) = 30$ N, directed straight downward. Since the displacement **h** of the brick is straight upward (that is, in the opposite direction from $\mathbf{F}_{grav}$), we know that the work done by gravity is negative F_{grav} times h:

$$W_{\text{by }F_{grav}} = -F_{grav}h = -(30\,\text{N})(2\,\text{m}) = -60\,\text{J}$$

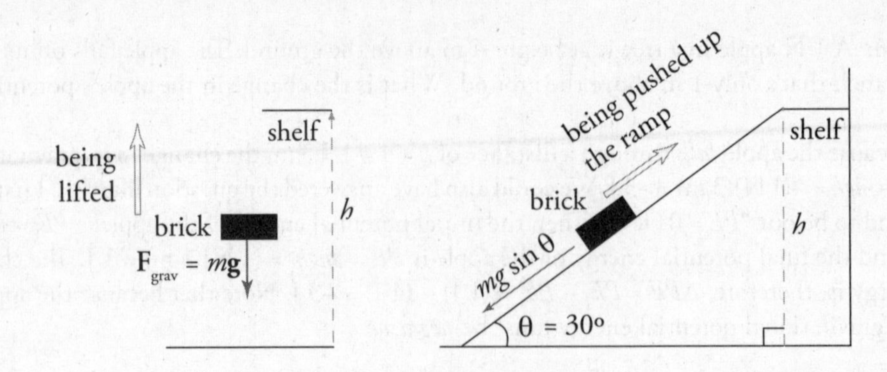

Now, let's look at the second case. Let's use a ramp whose incline angle θ is 30°. The gravitational force acting parallel to the ramp has magnitude $mg \sin \theta$, directed downward along the ramp. Because the displacement **d** is upward along the ramp (that is, in the opposite direction), we know the work done by gravity is negative, and equal to $-(mg \sin \theta)(d)$. Since the height of the shelf is $h = 2$ m, the length of the ramp (i.e., the hypotenuse of the right triangle) must be $d = h/(\sin \theta) = (2 \text{ m})/(\sin 30°) = 4$ m. Therefore, the work done by the gravitational force as the block is pushed up the ramp is

$$W_{\text{by } F_{grav}} = -(mg \sin \theta)(d) = -(30 \text{ N})(\sin 30°)(4 \text{ m}) = -(15 \text{ J})(4 \text{ m}) = -60 \text{ J}$$

This is the same answer as we found before! Since the change in the gravitational potential energy is defined to be the opposite of the work done by the gravitational force, $\Delta PE_{grav} = -W_{\text{by } F_{grav}}$, we can say that $\Delta PE_{grav} = -(-60 \text{ J}) = 60 \text{ J}$ in either case.

In the first case (lifting the brick straight upward), we exert a greater force over a smaller distance, while in the second case (moving the brick up a ramp), we exert a smaller force over a greater distance. However, the work done is the same in both cases.

These examples illustrate the following:

The work done by gravity

depends only on the initial and final heights of the object,

not on the path the object follows.

Another way of saying this is to state that gravity is a **conservative** force. (In fact, it is the conservative nature of the gravitational force that allows us to define gravitational potential energy.)

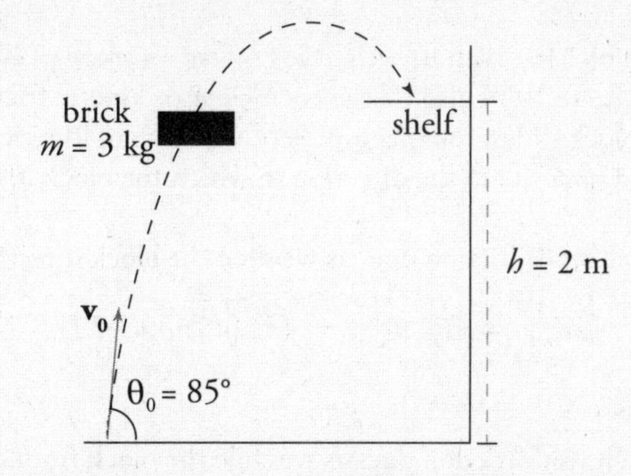

Example 6-18: In the situation pictured above, a brick is projected upward with an initial velocity $\mathbf{v}_0$ that makes an angle of 85° with the horizontal. The brick follows the path indicated and lands on the shelf. How much work did the gravitational force do on the brick?

Solution: The work done by gravity depends only on the initial and final positions of the object, not on the particular path the object takes. Since the initial height was $h_i = 0$ and the final height was $h_f = 2$ m, the change in the brick's gravitational potential energy is $\Delta PE_{grav} = mgh_f - mgh_i = mgh_f - 0 = mgh_f = (3 \text{ kg})(10 \text{ N/kg})(2 \text{ m}) = 60$ J. Therefore, the work done by the gravitational force is

$$W_{\text{by } F_{grav}} = -\Delta PE_{grav} = -60 \text{ J}$$

just as we found before.

Friction Is NOT a Conservative Force

Gravity is a conservative force because the work done by gravity depends only on the initial and final positions of the object, not on the path taken. We'll now show that friction is *not* a conservative force; the work done by kinetic friction *does* depend on the path taken.

Consider a flat tabletop and mark two points on it, A and B. We're going to slide a block from Point A to Point B along two different paths; the work done will be different for the two paths, which will show that friction is not a conservative force. The figure below shows the two points, A and B, separated by a distance of 5 m. Another way to get from A to B is to move from A to C and then from C to B; I've chosen a point C that's 3 m from A and 4 m from B.

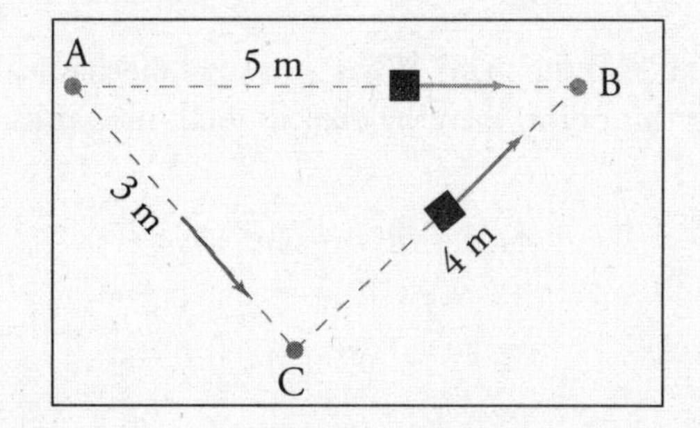

Assume the block has a mass of 1 kg; then its weight is $w = mg$ = (1 kg)(10 N/kg) = 10 N, so the normal force on the block has magnitude 10 N also. If the coefficient of kinetic friction between the block and tabletop is 0.4, then, as the block slides, the magnitude of the force of kinetic friction is $F_f = \mu_k F_N = (0.4)(10\text{ N}) = 4\text{ N}$, always directed opposite to the direction in which the block is sliding.

Let's first figure out how much work friction does as we slide the block directly from A to B:

$$W_{\substack{\text{by }\mathbf{F}_f\\ A\to B}} = -F_f \cdot d_{A\to B} = -(4\,\text{N})(5\,\text{m}) = -20\,\text{J}$$

Now let's figure out how much work friction does as we slide the block from A to B by way of C:

$$W_{\substack{\text{by }\mathbf{F}_f\\ A\to C\to B}} = W_{\substack{\text{by }\mathbf{F}_f\\ A\to C}} + W_{\substack{\text{by }\mathbf{F}_f\\ C\to B}} = (-F_f \cdot d_{A\to C}) + (-F_f \cdot d_{C\to B}) = (-4\,\text{N})(3\,\text{m}) + (-4\,\text{N})(4\,\text{m}) = -28\,\text{J}$$

Even though we started at A and ended at B in both cases, we got a different amount of work done by friction for two different paths from A to B. Therefore, friction is *not* a conservative force. This means that there's no such thing as "frictional potential energy," because potential energy can be defined only for conservative forces.

6.5 TOTAL MECHANICAL ENERGY

Now that we've defined kinetic energy and potential energy, we can define an object's **total mechanical energy**, E. It's just the sum of the object's kinetic energy and potential energy:

Total Mechanical Energy

$$E = KE + PE$$

For example, consider an object of mass m sitting on a shelf that's at height h above the floor. Then, relative to the floor (where we'll set PE_{grav} equal to 0), the object's total mechanical energy is

$$E = KE + PE = 0 + mgh = mgh$$

Now, what if this same object falls off the shelf? What is its total mechanical energy when its height is, say, $h/2$? If v is the object's speed at this point, then the object's total mechanical energy is

$$E = KE + PE = \frac{1}{2}mv^2 + mg\frac{h}{2}$$

Example 6-19: An object of mass m is projected straight upward with an initial speed of v_0 at time $t = 0$.

a) What is the object's total mechanical energy at time $t = 0$?
b) At what time t will the object reach its maximum height?
c) What is the maximum height?
d) What is the object's total mechanical energy at this point?

Solution:

a) If we take the object's height at $t = 0$ to be $h = 0$, then its initial total mechanical energy is

$$E = KE + PE = \frac{1}{2}mv_0^2 + mg(0) = \frac{1}{2}mv_0^2$$

b) When the object reaches the highest point in its vertical path, its velocity is 0. Using Big Five #2 with $a = -g$, we find that

$$v = v_0 + at \rightarrow 0 = v_0 + (-g)t \rightarrow t = \frac{v_0}{g}$$

c) Using Big Five #5, we can find the object's maximum height:

$$v^2 = v_0^2 + 2ad \rightarrow (0)^2 = v_0^2 + 2(-g)d \rightarrow d = -\frac{v_0^2}{2(-g)} = \frac{v_0^2}{2g}$$

d) The object's total mechanical energy at this point is

$$E = KE + PE = \tfrac{1}{2}mv^2 + mgh = \tfrac{1}{2}m(0)^2 + mg\left(\tfrac{v_0^2}{2g}\right) = 0 + m\tfrac{v_0^2}{2} = \tfrac{1}{2}mv_0^2$$

Notice in this example that the answer to part (d) is the same as the answer to part (a): the object's total mechanical energy at its highest point is the same as it was at the object's initial point. This illustrates a very important concept: the **Conservation of Total Mechanical Energy.** If the only forces acting on an object during its motion are conservative (that means, for example, *no friction*), then the object's total mechanical energy will remain throughout the motion. Pick any two positions (or times) during the object's motion; for example, we could pick the initial position (initial time) and the final position (final time). Then

$$E_i = E_f$$

Writing E as $KE + PE$, we have

Conservation of Total Mechanical Energy
(no outside forces)

$$KE_i + PE_i = KE_f + PE_f$$

Example 6-20: An object of mass m is projected straight upward with an initial speed of v_0 at time $t = 0$. Use Conservation of Total Mechanical Energy to find its maximum height.

Solution: If we take the object's height at $t = 0$ to be $h = 0$, then its initial total mechanical energy is

$$E = KE_i + PE_i = \tfrac{1}{2}mv_0^2 + mgh = \tfrac{1}{2}mv_0^2 + mg(0) = \tfrac{1}{2}mv_0^2$$

When the object reaches the highest point in its vertical path, its velocity is 0. Calling this height h, the object's total mechanical energy at this point is

$$E = KE_f + PE_f = \tfrac{1}{2}mv_0^2 + mgh = \tfrac{1}{2}m(0)^2 + mgh = mgh$$

Therefore, by Conservation of Total Mechanical Energy, we have

$$E_i = E_f$$

$$\frac{1}{2}mv_0^2 = mgh$$

$$\therefore h = \frac{v_0^2}{2g}$$

This is the same answer we found in Example 6-19(c) using the Big Five equations.

Another way to think about this problem is in terms of an energy *transfer*. At the moment the object was shot upward, it had only KE; at the top of its path, however, it has only PE. In other words, kinetic energy was transferred (or transformed) into gravitational potential energy:

$$KE \rightarrow PE \rightarrow \frac{1}{2}mv_0^2 = mgh \rightarrow \therefore h = \frac{v_0^2}{2g}$$

It can be very helpful to think of Conservation of Total Mechanical Energy in terms of energy transfers between KE and PE. (The OAT likes to ask questions about such energy transfers.)

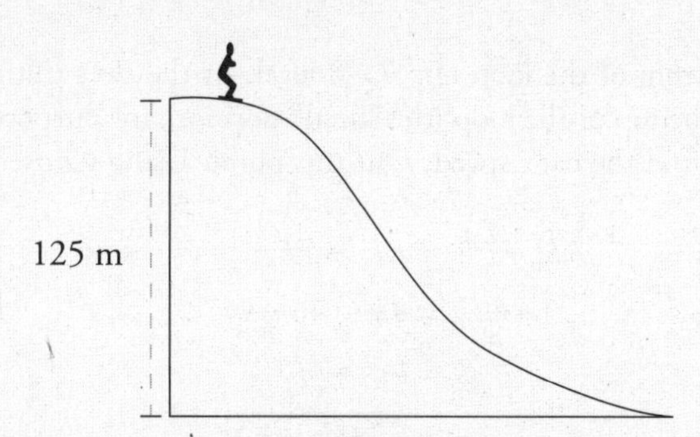

Example 6-21: A skier begins at rest at the top of a hill of height 125 m. If friction between her skis and the snow is negligible, what will be her speed at the bottom of the hill?

Solution: Let the bottom of the hill be $h = 0$, and call the top of the hill the skier's initial position and the bottom of the hill her final position. Then we have

$$KE_i + PE_i = KE_f + PE_f$$
$$0 + mgh = \tfrac{1}{2}mv^2 + 0$$
$$v = \sqrt{2gh}$$
$$= \sqrt{2(10\text{ m/s}^2)(125\text{ m})}$$
$$\therefore v = 50\text{ m/s}$$

We could also think about this problem in terms of an energy transfer. At the top of the hill, the skier had only *PE*; at the bottom of the hill, she has only *KE*. In other words, gravitational potential energy was transferred (or transformed) into kinetic energy:

$$PE \rightarrow KE \rightarrow \quad mgh = \tfrac{1}{2}mv_0^2 \quad \rightarrow \quad \therefore v = \sqrt{2gh}$$

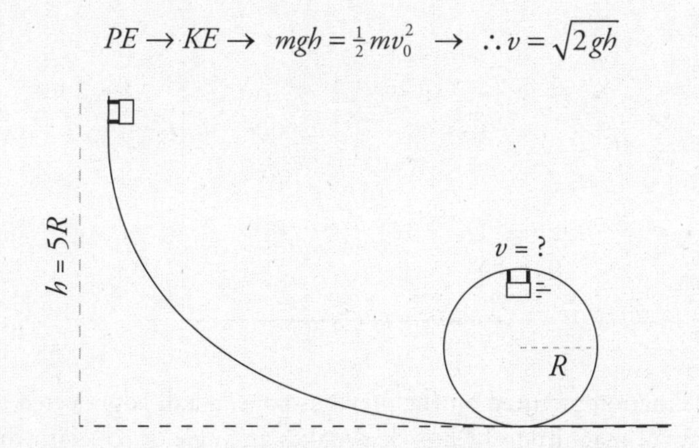

Example 6-22: A roller-coaster car drops from rest down the track and enters a loop. If the radius of the loop is R, and the initial height of the car is $5R$ above the bottom of the loop, how fast is the car going at the top of the loop? Assume that $R = 15$ m and ignore friction.

6.5

Solution: Let's call the bottom of the loop our $h = 0$ level. At the car's initial position, we have $h_i = 5R$ and $v_i = 0$ (so $KE_i = 0$). At the top of the loop (the "final" position, for purposes of this question), we have $h_f = 2R$. The question is to find the car's speed, v, at this point. Using Conservation of Total Mechanical Energy, we get

$$KE_i + PE_i = KE_f + PE_f$$

$$0 + mgh_i = \tfrac{1}{2}mv^2 + mgh_f$$

$$gh_i = \tfrac{1}{2}v^2 + gh_f$$

$$v = \sqrt{2g(h_i - h_f)}$$

$$= \sqrt{2g(5R - 2R)}$$

$$= \sqrt{2g \cdot 3R}$$

$$= \sqrt{2(10\text{ m/s}^2) \cdot 3(15\text{ m})}$$

$$\therefore v = 30\text{ m/s}$$

For extra practice, show that the car's speed when it's at the "9 o'clock" position within the loop is $\sqrt{1200\text{ m/s}} \approx 35\text{ m/s}$, and that the car's speed when it's at the bottom of the loop is $\sqrt{1500\text{ m/s}} \approx 39\text{ m/s}$.[1]

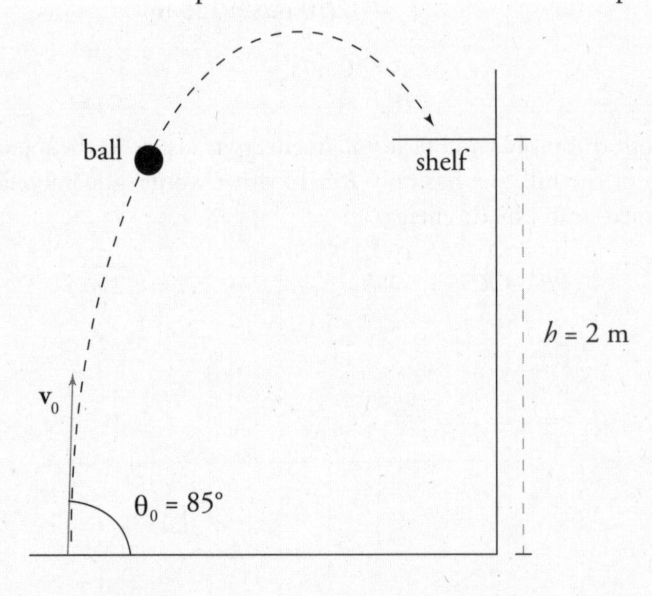

Example 6-23: In the situation pictured on the previous page, a ball is projected upward from the floor with initial velocity $\mathbf{v}_0$ of magnitude 12 m/s that makes an angle of 85° with the horizontal. The ball follows the path indicated and lands on the shelf. How fast is the ball traveling as it hits the shelf? (Ignore air resistance.)

[1] For even more practice, compute the centripetal acceleration at these points, and show that the amusement park operator is in danger of being sued. (As a benchmark, consider that fighter pilots with the benefit of pressurized suits risk blacking out at accelerations greater than about $9g \approx 88\text{ m/s}^2$.)

Solution: Let's call the floor our $h = 0$ level. At the object's initial position, we have $h_i = 0$ (so $PE_i = 0$). At the shelf (the final position), we have $h_f = 2$ m. The question is to find the speed of the ball, v, at this point. Using Conservation of Total Mechanical Energy, we get

$$\begin{aligned}
KE_i + PE_i &= KE_f + PE_f \\
\tfrac{1}{2}mv_0^2 + 0 &= \tfrac{1}{2}mv^2 + mgh_f \\
\tfrac{1}{2}v_0^2 &= \tfrac{1}{2}v^2 + gh_f \\
v &= \sqrt{v_0^2 - 2gh_f} \\
&= \sqrt{(12 \text{ m/s})^2 - 2(10 \text{ m/s}^2)(2 \text{ m})} \\
\therefore v &\approx 10 \text{ m/s}
\end{aligned}$$

Notice that the direction of the initial velocity vector (given to be "at an angle of 85° with the horizontal") was irrelevant here. One of the most useful attributes of solving problems by Conservation of Total Mechanical Energy is that KE, PE, and E are all *scalars*. This makes it easier to solve questions because we don't have to worry about direction.

Using the Energy Method when There Is Friction

If friction acts during an object's motion, then total mechanical energy is no longer conserved. Consider this example: We give a block of mass 2 kg an initial speed of 6 m/s across a flat surface, where the coefficient of kinetic friction between the block and the surface is $\mu_k = 0.2$.

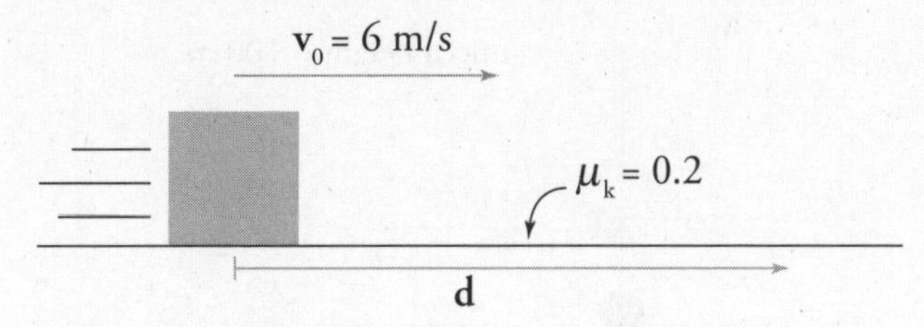

Kinetic friction will do work as the block slides. If d is the distance the block slides, then the work done by friction will be

$$W_{\text{by } F_f} = -F_f \cdot d = -\mu_k F_N d = -\mu_k mgd = -(0.2)(2 \text{ kg})(10 \text{ N/kg})d = -(4 \text{ N})d$$

In particular, when $d = 9$ m, the work done by friction will be

$$W_{\text{by } F_f} = -(4 \text{ N})d = -(4 \text{ N})(9 \text{ m}) = -36 \text{ J}$$

Since the initial kinetic energy of the block was

$$KE_i = \tfrac{1}{2}mv_0^2 = \tfrac{1}{2}(2 \text{ kg})(6 \text{ m/s})^2 = 36 \text{ J}$$

then the work-energy theorem tells us that the final kinetic energy of the block will be 0:

$$W = \Delta KE = KE_f - KE_i \rightarrow KE_f = KE_i + W = (36\text{ J}) + (-36\text{ J}) = 0\text{ J}$$

The block lost *KE* (and, therefore, *E*) as it moved because of friction. So, when friction acts, total mechanical energy is not a constant; in other words, it's not conserved.

Despite the fact that total mechanical energy is no longer conserved if friction acts, we can use a *modified* version of the Conservation of Total Mechanical Energy equation to handle questions with friction (or any force besides gravity). We can write this modified equation either in the form

$$\boxed{E_i + W_{\text{by F}} = E_f}$$

or as:

Conservation of Total Mechanical Energy (with outside forces)

$$KE_i + PE_i + W_{\text{by F}} = KE_f + PE_f$$

Since $W_{\text{by F}_f}$ is negative, E_f will be less than E_i, just as we expect, since friction takes away mechanical energy.

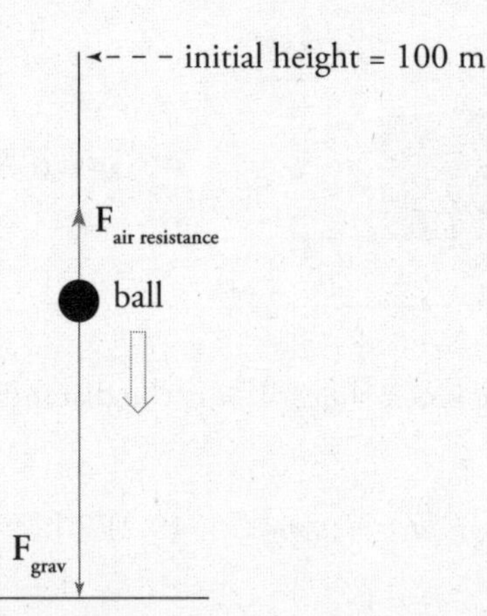

Example 6-24: A ball of mass 2 kg is dropped from a height of 100 m. As it falls, the ball feels an average force of air resistance of magnitude 4 N. What is the ball's speed as it strikes the ground?

Solution: Let's call the ground our $h = 0$ level. At the object's initial position, we have $h_i = 100$ m and $v_0 = 0$ (so $KE_i = 0$). As it hits the ground (the final position), we have $h_f = 0$ m (so $PE_f = 0$). The question is to find the speed of the ball, v, as it strikes the ground. Because the air resistance is given, and air resistance is friction exerted by the air on the moving object, we need to use the modified version of the energy equation, the one that includes the work done by friction.

Let's figure out the work done by the force of air resistance. Since the displacement of the ball is downward, the force of air resistance is upward; the opposite direction. This tells us that the work done by air resistance is negative, as we expect:

$$W_{\text{by } \mathbf{F}_f} = -F_f \cdot h = -(4\,\text{N})(100\,\text{m}) = -400\,\text{J}$$

Therefore, using the modified equation for Conservation of Total Mechanical Energy, we find that

$$\begin{aligned} KE_i + PE_i + W_{\text{by } \mathbf{F}_f} &= KE_f + PE_f \\ 0 + mgh + (-400\,\text{J}) &= \tfrac{1}{2}mv^2 + 0 \\ v &= \sqrt{2gh - \frac{800\,\text{J}}{m}} \\ &= \sqrt{2(10\text{ m/s}^2)(100\,\text{m}) - \frac{800\,\text{J}}{2\,\text{kg}}} \\ &= \sqrt{1600\text{ m}^2/\text{s}^2} \\ v &= 40\text{ m/s} \end{aligned}$$

Without air resistance, you can check that the ball's speed at impact would have been greater:

$$\sqrt{2000\text{ m}^2/\text{s}^2} \approx 45\text{ m/s}.$$

6.6 MOMENTUM

For an object of mass m moving with velocity **v**, we define the object's **momentum**, **p**, as the product of m and **v**. Notice that because **v** is a vector, momentum is a vector, too, pointing in the same direction as **v** (because m is always a *positive* scalar).

Momentum

$$\mathbf{p} = m\mathbf{v}$$

The SI unit of momentum is just the kg·m/s; there's no special name for it.

Example 6-25: A car whose mass is 2000 kg is traveling at a velocity of 15 m/s due east. What is its momentum? How does its momentum compare to that of a car whose mass is 2000 kg traveling at a velocity of 15 m/s due west?

Solution: Since **p** = m**v**, we have **p** = (2000 kg)(15 m/s, east) = 30,000 kg·m/s, east. If we call *east* the positive direction, then we can write **p** = +30,000 kg·m/s. For the car traveling west, the magnitude of its momentum will be the same, 30,000 kg·m/s, but the direction of its momentum will be to the west. So, if *east* is again the positive direction, then *west* is the negative direction, and we'd write **p** = –30,000 kg·m/s. Remember, momentum is a vector, and its direction must be taken into account.

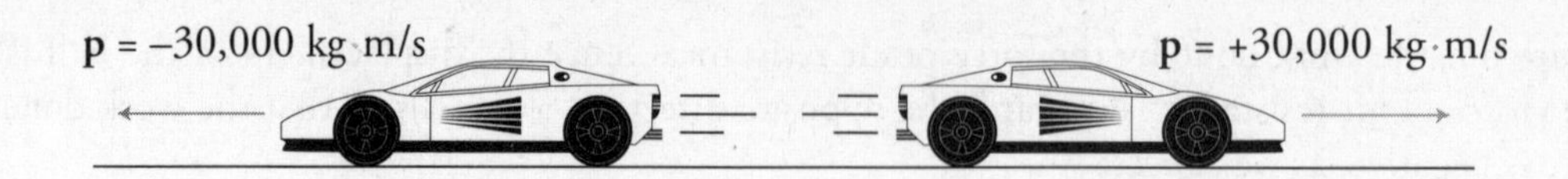

Example 6-26: An object of mass m is moving with velocity **v**. What will happen to its momentum if v doubles? What will happen to its kinetic energy?

Solution: Momentum has something in common with kinetic energy: namely, only moving objects have it. Also, the more massive an object, or the greater its velocity, the greater its momentum (and kinetic energy). However, there are two important differences. First, kinetic energy is a scalar, while momentum is a vector. Second, kinetic energy is proportional to v^2 whereas the magnitude of momentum is proportional only to v. So, if the object's speed doubles, then its momentum doubles while its kinetic energy increases by a factor of 4.

Now that we've defined momentum, let's see how it applies to the OAT.

Impulse

Let's say we exert a force **F** on an object of mass m over a time interval Δt. We can use Newton's second law, **F** = m**a**, to predict the effect of this force. Because **a** = Δ**v**/Δt, we can rewrite **F** = m**a** as

$$\mathbf{F} = m\frac{\Delta \mathbf{v}}{\Delta t}$$

Multiplying both sides by Δt gives

$$\mathbf{F}\Delta t = m\Delta \mathbf{v}$$

If the object's mass remains constant, then $m\Delta$**v** is the same as $\Delta(m$**v**$)$, so we get

$$\mathbf{F}\Delta t = \Delta(m\mathbf{v})$$

We now recognize the quantity on the right-hand side as Δ**p**, the change in momentum. The quantity on the left-hand side, force multiplied by time, is called **impulse**, denoted by **J**. (Don't confuse the variable for impulse, **J**, with the abbreviation for the joule, J.) So, this last equation can be written simply as **J** = Δ**p**. This alternative way of expressing Newton's second law is known as the

Impulse-Momentum Theorem

$$\mathbf{J} = \Delta\mathbf{p} = \Delta(m\mathbf{v}) = \mathbf{F}\Delta t$$

Example 6-27: A batter strikes a pitched baseball (mass = 0.15 kg) that was moving horizontally at 40 m/s, and it leaves his bat moving at speed of 50 m/s directly back toward the pitcher. The bat was in contact with the baseball for 15 ms.

a) What's the baseball's change in momentum?
b) What's the impulse of the force exerted by the batter?
c) What's the magnitude of the average force exerted by the bat on the ball?

Solution:

a) Since we're dealing with momentum, which is a vector, we need to define our positive direction. Let's choose *toward the pitcher* as the positive direction. This means that the initial momentum of the baseball (the momentum it had on its way from the pitcher to the batter) was negative, and the final momentum of the baseball (which is its momentum after the batter hits it) is positive. This gives

$$\mathbf{p}_\mathrm{i} = m\mathbf{v}_\mathrm{i} = (0.15\,\mathrm{kg})(-40\ \mathrm{m/s}) = -6\ \mathrm{kg \cdot m/s} \ \text{and} \ \mathbf{p}_\mathrm{f} = m\mathbf{v}_\mathrm{f} = (0.15\,\mathrm{kg})(+50\ \mathrm{m/s}) = 7.5\ \mathrm{kg \cdot m/s}$$

So the change in the baseball's momentum is

$$\Delta\mathbf{p} = \mathbf{p}_\mathrm{f} - \mathbf{p}_\mathrm{i} = (+7.5\ \mathrm{kg \cdot m/s}) - (-6\ \mathrm{kg \cdot m/s}) = +13.5\ \mathrm{kg \cdot m/s}$$

b) Impulse is equal to force multiplied by the time during which it acts. However, we are not told what the force is; in fact, we're asked that in part (c). So we need another way of figuring out the impulse. The impulse-momentum theorem tells us that the impulse is equal to the change in momentum, which we just computed in part (a). Since $\Delta\mathbf{p}$ = +13.5 kg·m/s, this is also the impulse of the force. (We can also write the unit as a newton-second, N·s, which is the most natural unit for impulse: $J = F\Delta t$ implies that $[J] = [F][\Delta t]$ = N·s. However, the unit of momentum, kg·m/s, is the same as the unit of impulse, N·s, so we could say that $\mathbf{J}$ = +13.5 N·s.)

c) Now that we know J, we can use the definition $J = F\Delta t$ to find F:

$$J = F\Delta t \rightarrow \quad F = \frac{J}{\Delta t} = \frac{13.5\,\mathrm{N \cdot s}}{0.015\,\mathrm{s}} = 900\,\mathrm{N}$$

Because F usually varies while it acts, this is actually the *average* force exerted by the bat. To be more precise, we should place a bar over the F and write the definition of impulse as $J = \overline{F}\Delta t$.

Example 6-28: The graph at the right shows how a force **F** acting on an object of mass m = 1 kg varies as a function of time.

a) What is the magnitude of the impulse of this force?
b) If the object's initial velocity is +2 m/s, what will be the object's velocity after this force acts?

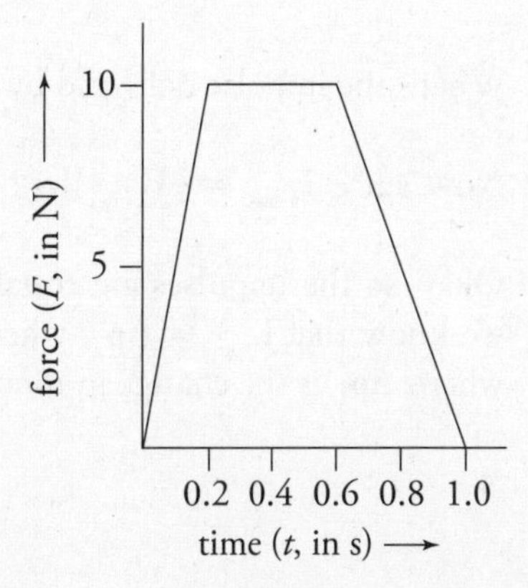

Solution:

a) Because impulse is equal to force × time, the area under a force vs. time graph gives the impulse. (Compare this to the statement from Chapter 1 that "The area under a velocity vs. time graph gives the displacement.") The area under the graph shown can be split into two right triangles and a rectangle, so the total area under the graph is

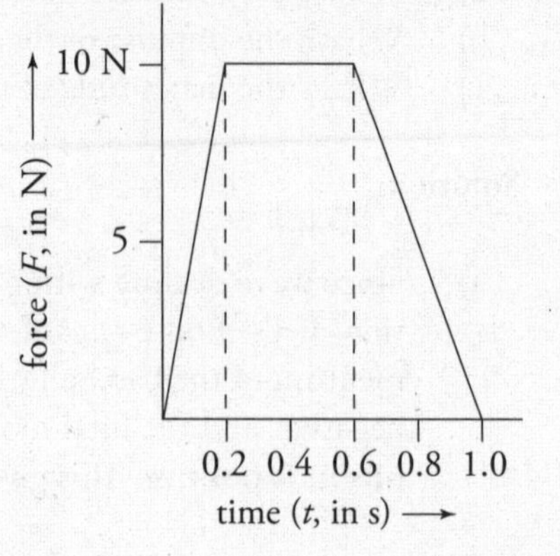

6.6

$$\begin{aligned}\text{area} &= (\text{first triangle}) + (\text{rectangle}) + (\text{second triangle})\\ &= \tfrac{1}{2}(0.2\,\text{s})(10\,\text{N}) + (0.6\,\text{s} - 0.2\,\text{s})(10\,\text{N}) + \tfrac{1}{2}(1\,\text{s} - 0.6\,\text{s})(10\,\text{N})\\ &= (1\,\text{N}\cdot\text{s}) + (4\,\text{N}\cdot\text{s}) + (2\,\text{N}\cdot\text{s})\\ \therefore J &= 7\,\text{N}\cdot\text{s}\end{aligned}$$

b) The impulse-momentum theorem says $\mathbf{J} = \Delta\mathbf{p} = \mathbf{p}_f - \mathbf{p}_i$, so

$$\mathbf{p}_f = \mathbf{p}_i + \mathbf{J} \rightarrow m\mathbf{v}_f = m\mathbf{v}_i + \mathbf{J}$$

$$\begin{aligned}\mathbf{v}_f &= \mathbf{v}_i + \frac{\mathbf{J}}{m}\\ &= (+2\text{ m/s}) + \frac{7\,\text{N}\cdot\text{s}}{1\text{ kg}}\\ &= (+2\text{ m/s}) + (7\text{ m/s})\end{aligned}$$

$$\therefore \mathbf{v}_f = +9\text{ m/s}$$

Conservation of Momentum

Consider a pair of objects, 1 and 2, that exert forces (an action/reaction pair) on each other. Let $\mathbf{F}_{1\text{-on-}2}$ be the force exerted by Object 1 on Object 2, let $\mathbf{F}_{2\text{-on-}1}$ be the force exerted by Object 2 on Object 1, and let Δt be the time during which these forces act.

What's the impulse delivered by $\mathbf{F}_{1\text{-on-}2}$? It's $\mathbf{J}_{1\text{-on-}2} = \mathbf{F}_{1\text{-on-}2}\Delta t$.

What's the impulse delivered by $\mathbf{F}_{2\text{-on-}1}$? It's $\mathbf{J}_{2\text{-on-}1} = \mathbf{F}_{2\text{-on-}1}\Delta t$.

Now, since $\mathbf{F}_{1\text{-on-}2} = -\mathbf{F}_{2\text{-on-}1}$ by Newton's third law, we'll automatically have $\mathbf{J}_{1\text{-on-}2} = -\mathbf{J}_{2\text{-on-}1}$.

Okay, so the impulses are equal but opposite. What will that do? By the impulse-momentum theorem, we know that $\mathbf{J}_{1\text{-on-}2} = \Delta\mathbf{p}_2$, where $\Delta\mathbf{p}_2$ is the change in momentum of Object 2, and that $\mathbf{J}_{2\text{-on-}1} = \Delta\mathbf{p}_1$, where $\Delta\mathbf{p}_1$ is the change in momentum of Object 1. So, because $\mathbf{J}_{1\text{-on-}2} = -\mathbf{J}_{2\text{-on-}1}$, we have

$$\Delta\mathbf{p}_2 = -\Delta\mathbf{p}_1$$

Therefore, the momentum changes if the two objects are equal but opposite too.

Now what if we ask, what's the change in momentum of both objects *together*? That is, what's $\Delta(\mathbf{p}_1 + \mathbf{p}_2)$? Well, if $\Delta\mathbf{p}_1$ and $\Delta\mathbf{p}_2$ are equal but opposite, then the total change in momentum is zero:

$$\Delta\mathbf{p}_2 + \Delta\mathbf{p}_1 \rightarrow \Delta\mathbf{p}_1 + \Delta\mathbf{p}_2 = 0 \rightarrow \Delta(\mathbf{p}_1 + \mathbf{p}_2) = 0$$

If the total momentum, $\mathbf{p}_1 + \mathbf{p}_2$, doesn't change, then it's a constant. We say that the total momentum is *conserved.*

In summary, what is shown above is simply that Newton's third law implies that when two objects interact only with each other, their total momentum doesn't change. That is, the total momentum *of the system* doesn't change. In fact, we could have any number of mutually interacting objects, not just two, and the result would be the same: The total momentum of the system will remain constant. This fact has the same stature as the Law of Conservation of Total Mechanical Energy, and it's called the Law of Conservation of Momentum:

Law of Conservation of Momentum

$$\Delta\mathbf{p}_{\text{system}} = 0$$

or

$$\text{total } \mathbf{p}_{\text{i}} = \text{total } \mathbf{p}_{\text{f}}$$

This law says that if a system of interacting objects feels no net external force (that is, if the forces the objects feel are only from other objects within the system) then the total momentum of the system will remain constant. The *individual* momenta of the objects in the system certainly can change, but always in such a way that their sum, the total momentum of all the objects, *doesn't* change. The second form of the law, total $\mathbf{p}_{\text{i}}$ = total $\mathbf{p}_{\text{f}}$, simply says that if we find the total momentum of an isolated system at one moment and then find the total momentum of the system at some later time, we'll get the same answer. We'll usually find it more convenient to use this second form when we solve problems, but of course, the two forms of the law say exactly the same thing.

Strictly speaking, the quantity $\mathbf{p} = m\mathbf{v}$ is known as **linear momentum**, so the law "$\Delta\mathbf{p}_{\text{system}} = 0$" or "total $\mathbf{p}_{\text{i}}$ = total $\mathbf{p}_{\text{f}}$" is known as the Law of Conservation of Linear Momentum. (There's another kind of momentum studied in physics: *angular momentum*. Since we rarely worry about this type of momentum for the OAT, we just use the word "momentum" for "linear momentum".)

Example 6-29: An astronaut (total mass, body + suit + equipment = 100 kg) is floating at rest in deep space near her ship, when she notices that the cord that's supposed to keep her connected to the ship has broken. She reaches into her pocket, finds a metal tool of mass 1 kg and throws it out into space with a velocity of 10 m/s, directly away from the ship. If she's 5 m away from the ship, how long will it take her to reach it?

Solution: Consider the astronaut and the metal tool as the system. Initially, both are at rest, so their total momentum is zero. Because of the Law of Conservation of Momentum, $\Delta\mathbf{p}_{\text{system}} = 0$, we know that after the astronaut throws the tool, the total momentum will still be zero:

$$m_{\text{astronaut}}\mathbf{v}'_{\text{astronaut}} + m_{\text{tool}}\mathbf{v}'_{\text{tool}} = 0$$

We can now solve for the astronaut's velocity after throwing the tool:

$$\begin{aligned} m_{\text{astronaut}}\mathbf{v}'_{\text{astronaut}} &= -m_{\text{tool}}\mathbf{v}'_{\text{tool}} \\ \mathbf{v}'_{\text{astronaut}} &= -\frac{m_{\text{tool}}\mathbf{v}'_{\text{tool}}}{m_{\text{astronaut}}} \\ &= -\frac{(1\text{ kg})(-10\text{ m/s})}{100\text{ kg}} \\ \therefore \mathbf{v}'_{\text{astronaut}} &= 0.1\text{ m/s} \end{aligned}$$

The minus sign on $\mathbf{v}'_{\text{tool}}$ simply indicates that we're calling *away from the ship* the negative direction; as a result, the astronaut's velocity is in the opposite direction, toward the ship and positive. Now, the question is, traveling at a rate of 0.1 m/s, how long will it take her to move the 5 m to the ship? Using distance = rate × time, we find that

$$t = \frac{d}{v} = \frac{5\text{m}}{0.1\text{ m/s}} = 50\text{s}$$

Example 6-30: A radioactive atom of polonium-204, initially at rest, undergoes alpha decay. Show that, as a result of ejecting the alpha particle, the daughter nucleus recoils with a speed equal to 2% of the speed of the alpha particle.

Solution: Initially, the parent nucleus is at rest, so its total momentum is zero. Because of the Law of Conservation of Momentum, $\Delta\mathbf{p}_{\text{system}} = 0$, we know that after the decay, the total momentum of the daughter atom (actually, ion, but we'll ignore the electrons because they're such a small portion of the mass) and the alpha particle will still be zero; that is, $m_D\mathbf{v}_D + m_\alpha\mathbf{v}_\alpha = 0$, where D represents the daughter. This gives

$$m_D\mathbf{v}_D = -m_\alpha\mathbf{v}_\alpha \rightarrow \mathbf{v}_D = -\frac{m_\alpha}{m_D}\mathbf{v}_\alpha \rightarrow v_D = -\frac{m_\alpha}{m_D}v_\alpha$$

Now, since the daughter atom has a mass number that's 4 less than that of the parent, we'll have m_D = 204 – 4 ≈ 200 u; and, since we know that $m_\alpha \approx 4$ u, we find that

$$v_D = -\frac{m_\alpha}{m_D}v_\alpha = -\frac{4\text{ u}}{200\text{ u}}v_\alpha = -\frac{1}{50}v_\alpha = -2\%v_\alpha$$

Collisions

Conservation of momentum is used to analyze collisions between objects. For example, consider this situation:

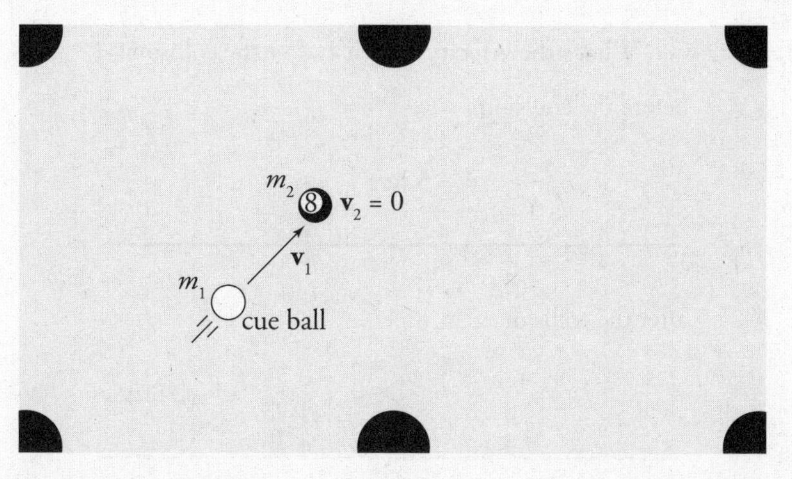

Let the cue ball and the 8-ball constitute our *system*, that is, the objects whose impending collision we're going to analyze. Before the collision, the cue ball is moving toward the 8-ball with a certain velocity, $\mathbf{v}_1$, and the 8-ball is at rest ($\mathbf{v}_2 = 0$). After the collision, the individual velocities of the objects change, to $\mathbf{v}_1'$ and $\mathbf{v}_2'$, respectively,

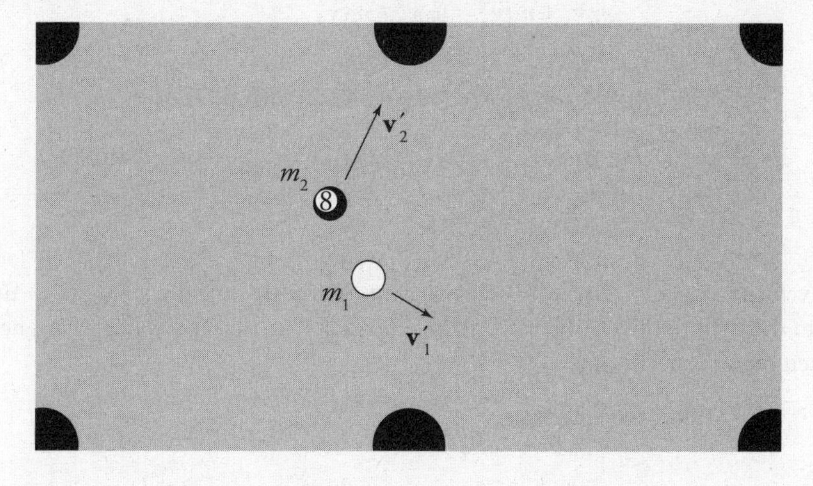

but in such a way that the *total* momentum *doesn't* change, because we must have $\Delta\mathbf{p}_{\text{system}} = 0$. Equivalently, we can say that $\mathbf{p}_{\text{total}}$ before the collision is equal to $\mathbf{p}_{\text{total}}$ after the collision:

$$\mathbf{p}_{\text{total before}} = \mathbf{p}_{\text{total after}}$$
$$m_1\mathbf{v}_1 + m_2\mathbf{v}_2 = m_1\mathbf{v}_1' + m_2\mathbf{v}_2'$$
$$m_1\mathbf{v}_1 = m_1\mathbf{v}_1' + m_2\mathbf{v}_2'$$

In this case, $\mathbf{v}_2 = 0$, which is why the term $m_2\mathbf{v}_2$ dropped out of the last equation.

Let's look at a simpler collision, one in which the motion of the objects is along a straight line.

Example 6-31: Ball 1 rolls with velocity $\mathbf{v}_1 = 5$ m/s toward Ball 2, which is initially at rest. Ball 1 has a mass of $m_1 = 1$ kg, and Ball 2 has a mass of $m_2 = 4$ kg. After the collision, Ball 2 is observed to move with a velocity of $\mathbf{v}_2' = 2$ m/s. What's the velocity of Ball 1 after the collision?

before the collision

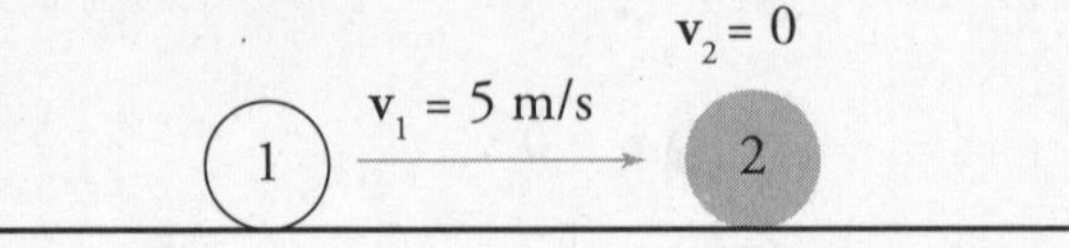

after the collision

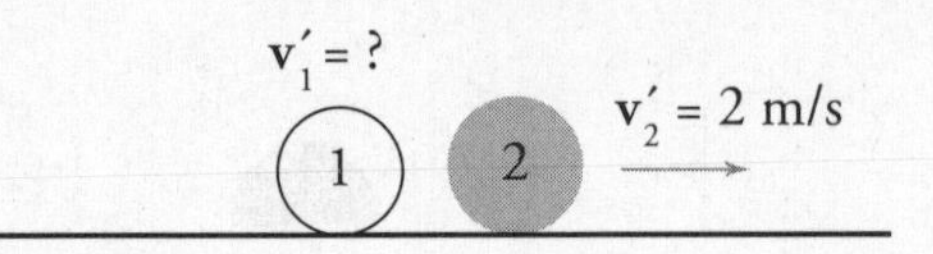

Solution: Using Conservation of Momentum, we get

$$\mathbf{p}_{\text{total before}} = \mathbf{p}_{\text{total after}}$$
$$m_1\mathbf{v}_1 + m_2\mathbf{v}_2 = m_1\mathbf{v}_1' + m_2\mathbf{v}_2'$$
$$m_1\mathbf{v}_1 = m_1\mathbf{v}_1' + m_2\mathbf{v}_2'$$
$$(1\text{ kg})(5\text{ m/s}) = (1\text{ kg})\mathbf{v}_1' + (4\text{ kg})(2\text{ m/s})$$
$$\therefore \mathbf{v}_1' = -3\text{ m/s}$$

Notice that the velocity of Ball 1 after the collision is negative; this means it points to the left (since we called velocities to the right positive). This isn't surprising. When an object collides with a heavier object, the lighter object often bounces backward.

after the collision

$\mathbf{v}'_1 = -3$ m/s (1) (2) $\mathbf{v}'_2 = 2$ m/s

Example 6-32: Ball 1 and Ball 2 are rolling toward each other at the same speed, 5 m/s. Ball 1 has a mass of $m_1 = 8$ kg, and Ball 2 has a mass of $m_2 = 2$ kg. After the collision, Ball 1 is observed to move with a velocity of 2 m/s in the same direction as $\mathbf{v}_1$. What's the velocity of Ball 2 after the collision?

before the collision

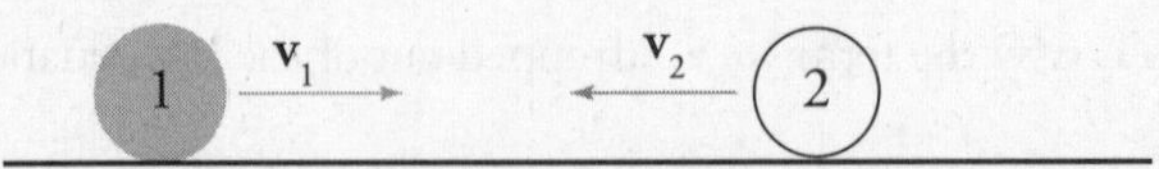

after the collision

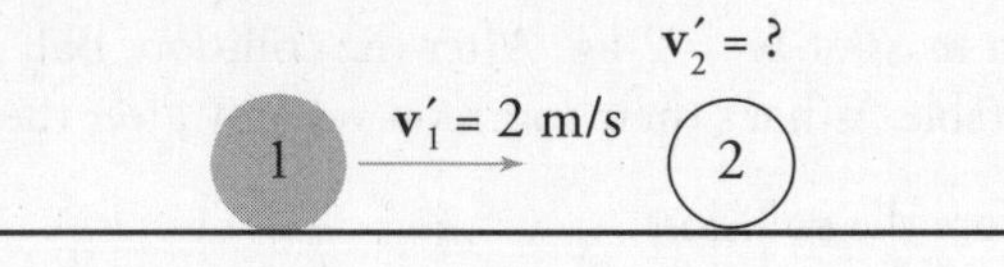

Solution: Since $\mathbf{v}_1$ and $\mathbf{v}_2$ point in opposite directions, we need to choose which direction to call positive. Let's choose *to the right* as our positive direction; then $\mathbf{v}_1 = +5$ m/s and $\mathbf{v}_2 = -5$ m/s. Now, using Conservation of Momentum, we get

$$\mathbf{p}_{\text{total before}} = \mathbf{p}_{\text{total after}}$$
$$m_1\mathbf{v}_1 + m_2\mathbf{v}_2 = m_1\mathbf{v}_1' + m_2\mathbf{v}_2'$$
$$(8\text{ kg})(+5\text{ m/s}) + (2\text{ kg})(-5\text{ m/s}) = (8\text{ kg})(+2\text{ m/s}) + (2\text{ kg})\mathbf{v}_2'$$
$$30\text{ kg}\cdot\text{m/s} = 16\text{ kg}\cdot\text{m/s} + (2\text{ kg})\mathbf{v}_2'$$
$$14\text{ kg}\cdot\text{m/s} = (2\text{ kg})\mathbf{v}_2'$$
$$\therefore \mathbf{v}_2' = +7\text{ m/s}$$

Notice that the velocity of Ball 2 after the collision is positive; this means it points to the right (since we called velocities to the right positive). This isn't surprising. When a heavy object collides with a lighter one, the lighter object often gets pushed forward.

after the collision

$\mathbf{v}'_1 = 2$ m/s $\mathbf{v}'_2 = 7$ m/s

Now that we've looked at some collisions, it's time to classify them. Collisions can be grouped into two major types: elastic and inelastic. A collision is said to be **elastic** if the total *kinetic* energy is conserved also. (Notice I say "also," because total *momentum* is already conserved.) A collision is said to be **inelastic** if total kinetic energy is *not* conserved. Further, as a subcategory of inelastic collisions, we have **perfectly** (or **completely**) **inelastic** collisions; on the OAT, these are collisions in which the objects stick together afterwards.[2] *Perfectly inelastic collisions are the OAT's favorite type.*

Elastic Collision: Total momentum *and* total kinetic energy are conserved.
Inelastic Collision: Total momentum is conserved but total kinetic energy is not.
Perfectly Inelastic: An inelastic collision in which the objects stick together afterwards.

[2] Technically, a perfectly inelastic collision is one in which the loss of kinetic energy is as great as possible (consistent with Conservation of Momentum). Luckily, we don't need to worry about this definition, because collisions in which the objects stick together are always perfectly inelastic.

6.6

Example 6-33: Ball 1 and Ball 2 are rolling toward each other at the same speed, 5 m/s. Ball 1 has a mass of $m_1 = 8$ kg, and Ball 2 has a mass of $m_2 = 2$ kg. After the collision, Ball 1 and Ball 2 stick together and slide frictionlessly across the table. What's their common velocity after the collision?

before the collision

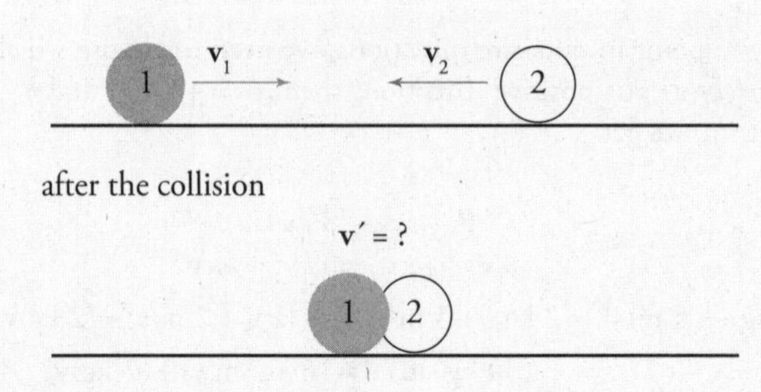

Solution: Choosing *to the right* as our positive direction, we have $\mathbf{v}_1 = +5$ m/s and $\mathbf{v}_2 = -5$ m/s. Now, using Conservation of Momentum, we get

$$\mathbf{p}_{\text{total before}} = \mathbf{p}_{\text{total after}}$$
$$m_1\mathbf{v}_1 + m_2\mathbf{v}_2 = (m_1 + m_2)\mathbf{v}'$$
$$(8\text{ kg})(+5\text{ m/s}) + (2\text{ kg})(-5\text{ m/s}) = (8\text{ kg} + 2\text{ kg})\mathbf{v}'$$
$$30\text{ kg}\cdot\text{m/s} = (10\text{ kg})\mathbf{v}'$$
$$\therefore \mathbf{v}' = +3\text{ m/s}$$

The OAT likes these collisions because the math is easier; after the collision, we have just one object, with a combined mass of $m_1 + m_2$, moving with a *single* velocity, $\mathbf{v}'$.

after the collision

$\mathbf{v}' = 3$ m/s

Example 6-34: Recall Example 6-31: Ball 1 rolled with velocity $\mathbf{v}_1 = 5$ m/s toward Ball 2, which was initially at rest. Ball 1's mass was $m_1 = 1$ kg, and Ball 2's mass was $m_2 = 4$ kg. After the collision, Ball 2 moved with a velocity of $\mathbf{v}_2' = 2$ m/s. We found that the velocity of Ball 1 after the collision was $\mathbf{v}_1' = -3$ m/s. Was this collision elastic or was it inelastic?

before the collision

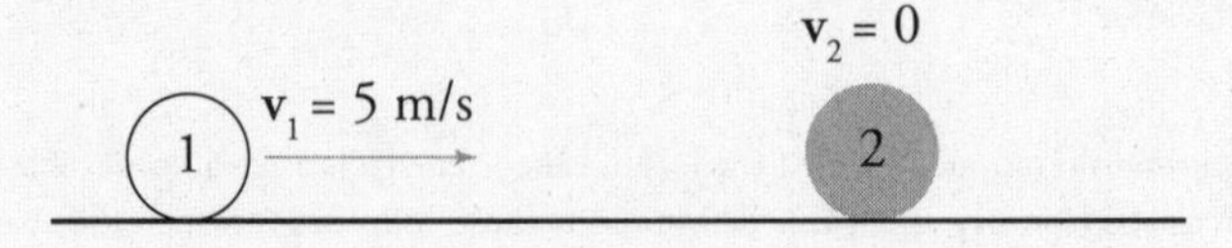

after the collision

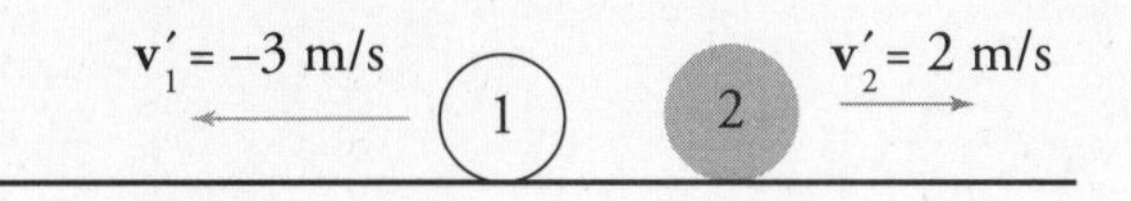

Solution: We need to decide whether total kinetic energy was conserved. Consider the following:

$$KE_{\text{before collision}} = \tfrac{1}{2}m_1v_1^2 + \tfrac{1}{2}m_2v_2^2 = \tfrac{1}{2}(1\text{ kg})(5\text{ m/s})^2 + 0 = \tfrac{25}{2}\text{ J}$$

and

$$KE_{\text{after collision}} = \tfrac{1}{2}m_1v_1'^2 + \tfrac{1}{2}m_2v_2'^2 = \tfrac{1}{2}(1\text{ kg})(3\text{ m/s})^2 + \tfrac{1}{2}(4\text{ kg})(2\text{ m/s})^2 = \tfrac{25}{2}\text{ J}$$

Since the kinetic energy was conserved in this case, we can conclude that this collision was elastic.

Example 6-35: Recall Example 6-32: Ball 1 and Ball 2 were rolling toward each other at the same speed, 5 m/s. Ball 1's mass was $m_1 = 8$ kg, and Ball 2's mass was $m_2 = 2$ kg. After the collision, Ball 1 moved with a velocity of 2 m/s in the same direction as $\mathbf{v}_1$. We found that the velocity of Ball 2 after the collision was 7 m/s. Was this collision elastic or was it inelastic?

Solution: We need to check whether total kinetic energy was conserved. Consider the following:

$$KE_{\text{before collision}} = \tfrac{1}{2}m_1v_1^2 + \tfrac{1}{2}m_2v_2^2 = \tfrac{1}{2}(8\text{ kg})(5\text{ m/s})^2 + \tfrac{1}{2}(2\text{ kg})(5\text{ m/s})^2 = 125\text{ J}$$

and

$$KE_{\text{after collision}} = \tfrac{1}{2}m_1v_1'^2 + \tfrac{1}{2}m_2v_2'^2 = \tfrac{1}{2}(8\text{ kg})(2\text{ m/s})^2 + \tfrac{1}{2}(2\text{ kg})(7\text{ m/s})^2 = 65\text{ J}$$

Since the kinetic energy was not conserved in this case, we can conclude that this collision was inelastic. This is what happens with macroscopic objects that collide. Some of the initial kinetic energy is converted to other forms: heat (mostly) and sound. The objects may also suffer some permanent deformation, which can also use up some of the pre-collision kinetic energy.

Example 6-36: Recall Example 6-33: Ball 1 and Ball 2 were rolling toward each other at the same speed, 5 m/s. Ball 1's mass was $m_1 = 8$ kg, and Ball 2's mass was $m_2 = 2$ kg. After the collision, Ball 1 and Ball 2 stuck together. We found that the common velocity of the combined object after the collision was $\mathbf{v}' = 3$ m/s. Was this collision elastic or inelastic?

Solution: Actually, there's no need for a calculation. If the objects stick together after the collision, then the collision is perfectly inelastic. That's certainly an inelastic collision.

Here's the proof, just to be sure you're convinced!

$$KE_{\text{before collision}} = \tfrac{1}{2}m_1v_1^2 + \tfrac{1}{2}m_2v_2^2 = \tfrac{1}{2}(8\text{ kg})(5\text{ m/s})^2 + \tfrac{1}{2}(2\text{ kg})(5\text{ m/s})^2 = 125\text{ J}$$

and

$$KE_{\text{after collision}} = \tfrac{1}{2}(m_1 + m_2)v' = \tfrac{1}{2}(8\text{ kg} + 2\text{ kg})(3\text{ m/s})^2 = 45\text{ J}$$

Notice that in the previous example (which described a generic inelastic collision), only 125 – 65 = 60 J (which is less than 50%) of the initial kinetic energy was lost as a result of the collision. In this case, however (a completely inelastic collision) we lost 125 – 45 = 80 J (or over 60%) of the initial kinetic energy. Completely inelastic collisions always result in the maximum possible loss of kinetic energy.

After our work on the Conservation of Total Mechanical Energy, you might be tempted to solve collision problems by Conservation of Energy. *Don't.* Total kinetic energy is conserved only for elastic collisions, and these are very special. In the everyday world of macroscopic-sized objects, collisions result in a loss of energy due to heat, sound, and deformation, so all such collisions are, by definition, *not* elastic. (In the subatomic domain, when particles such as neutrons and protons run into each other, elastic collisions are common.) So, the moral is: Unless the question specifically says, "Assume the collision is elastic," or "Assume that energy losses are negligible," then you should never assume that a collision between macroscopic-sized objects is elastic. And even if a collision is (or can be treated as) elastic, you can still use Conservation of Momentum, because total momentum is conserved in both types of collisions, elastic *and* inelastic.

Example 6-37: A fast-moving neutron collides with another neutron initially at rest. Could such a collision be elastic? If so, describe what would happen.

Solution: Yes, a collision between subatomic particles could be elastic. Assume that before the collision, the moving neutron had velocity **v** and the target neutron was at rest. If the resulting collision is elastic, the moving neutron hits the target and stops, and the target neutron moves away with the same velocity, **v**, that the first one had coming in to the collision. In other words, the moving neutron gives up all its momentum and kinetic energy to the target neutron. This conserves both total momentum and kinetic energy, and describes an elastic collision.

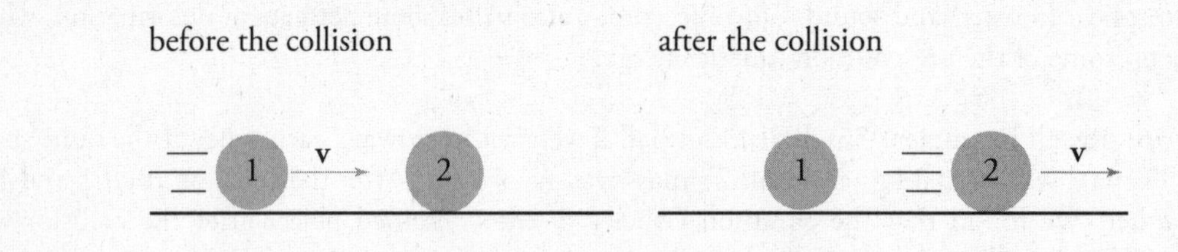

Summary of Formulas

Work: $W = Fd\cos\theta$ (θ = angle between **F** and **d**)

Power: $P = \frac{W}{t}$

$P = Fv$ if F is parallel to **v** and constant

Kinetic Energy: $KE = \frac{1}{2}mv^2$

Work-energy theorem: $W_{total} = \Delta KE$

Gravitational Potential Energy: $\Delta PE_{grav} = -W_{by\ F_{grav}} = -mg\Delta h$ (if g is constant)

Gravity is a conservative force (path independent)

Friction is NOT a conservative force (path dependent)

Total Mechanical Energy: $E = KE + PE$

Conservation of Total Mechanical Energy: $KE_i + PE_i = KE_f + PE_f$

If non-conservative forces (i.e., friction) act: $KE_i + PE_i + W_{other} = KE_f + PE_f$

Momentum: $\mathbf{p} = m\mathbf{v}$

Impulse-momentum theorem: $\mathbf{J} = \Delta\mathbf{p} = \mathbf{F}\Delta t$

Conservation of Total Momentum: total $\mathbf{p}_i$ = total $\mathbf{p}_f$

$m_1\mathbf{v}_1 + m_2\mathbf{v}_2 ... = m_1\mathbf{v}_1' + m_2\mathbf{v}_2' ...$

Collisions always conserve momentum

–Elastic collisions also conserve *KE*

–Inelastic collisions do NOT conserve *KE* (lose *KE*)

–Perfectly inelastic collisions lose the most *KE* (objects stick together after collision)

Chapter 7
Fluids and Elasticity of Solids

7.1 HYDROSTATICS: FLUIDS AT REST

In this section and the next, we'll discuss some of the fundamental concepts dealing with substances that can flow, which are known as **fluids**. *Both liquids and gases are fluids*, but there are distinctions between them. At the molecular level, a substance in the liquid phase is similar to one in the solid phase in that the molecules are close to, and interact with, one another. The molecules in a liquid are able to move around a little more freely than those in a solid, in which the molecules typically only vibrate around relatively fixed positions. By contrast, the molecules of a gas are not constrained and fly around in a chaotic swarm, with hardly any interaction. On a macroscopic level, there is another distinction between liquids and gases. If you pour a certain volume of a liquid into a container of a greater volume, the liquid will occupy its original volume, whatever the shape and size of the container. However, if you introduce a sample of gas into a container, the molecules will fly around and fill the *entire* container.

Density and Specific Gravity

The **density** of a substance is the amount of mass contained in a unit of volume. In SI units, density is usually expressed in kg/m^3 or g/cm^3.

$$\text{density} = \frac{\text{mass}}{\text{volume}}$$

$$\rho = \frac{m}{V}$$

There is one substance whose density you should memorize: The density of liquid water is taken to be 1000 kg/m^3 or 1 g/cm^3. (Another useful version of the same value: 1 kg/L, where L stands for a liter; a liter is 1000 cm^3.)

Sometimes the OAT mentions **specific gravity**. This (poorly named) unitless number tells us how dense something is compared to water:

$$\text{specific gravity} = \frac{\text{density of substance}}{\text{density of water}}$$

$$\text{sp. gr.} = \frac{\rho}{\rho_{H_2O}}$$

For solids, density doesn't change much with surrounding pressure or temperature. For example, the density of marble is pretty close to 2700 kg/m^3 under most conditions. Liquids behave the same way: the density of water is pretty close to 1000 kg/m^3 under all conditions at which it's a liquid. However, the density of a gas changes markedly with pressure and temperature. (The ideal gas law tells us that $PV = nRT$, so the density of a sample of an ideal gas is given by the equation $\rho_{gas} = m/V = mP/nRT$, which depends on P and T.)

Example 7-1: Turpentine has a specific gravity of 0.9. What is the density of this liquid?

Solution: By definition, we have

$$\rho_{turpentine} = (\text{sp. gr.}_{turpentine})(\rho_{H_2O}) = (0.9)(1000\ \text{kg/m}^3) = 900\ \text{kg/m}^3$$

Example 7-2: A 2 cm^3 sample of osmium, one of the densest substances on Earth, has a mass of 45 g. What's the specific gravity of this metal?

Solution: The density of osmium is

$$\rho = \frac{m}{V} = \frac{45\,\text{g}}{2\,\text{cm}^3} = 22.5\ \text{g/cm}^3$$

Since this is 22.5 times the density of water (which is 1 g/cm^3), the specific gravity of osmium is 22.5.

Example 7-3: A cork has volume of 4 cm^3 and weighs 0.01 N. What is its density? What is its specific gravity?

Solution: Because the cork weighs 10^{-2} N, its mass is

$$m = \frac{w}{g} = \frac{10^{-2}\ \text{N}}{10\ \text{N/kg}} = 10^{-3}\ \text{kg}$$

Therefore, its density is

$$\rho_{cork} = \frac{m}{V} = \frac{10^{-3}\ \text{kg}}{4\ \text{cm}^3} \times \left(\frac{10^2\ \text{cm}}{1\ \text{m}}\right)^3 = \tfrac{1}{4} \times 10^3\ \text{kg/m}^3 = 2.5 \times 10^2\ \text{kg/m}^3$$

and its specific gravity is

$$\text{sp. gr.}_{cork} = \frac{\rho_{cork}}{\rho_{H_2O}} = \frac{\frac{1}{4} \times 10^3\ \text{kg/m}^3}{10^3\ \text{kg/m}^3} = \tfrac{1}{4} = 0.25$$

Force of Gravity for Fluids

When solving questions involving fluids, it is often handy to know how to find the force of gravity acting on the fluid itself or objects that are immersed in the fluid. In previous chapters, we have used $F_{grav} = mg$ without too much difficulty. However, with fluids, it is more difficult to remove a portion of fluid from a tank, place it on a scale, and find its mass. Using the relationship between mass, volume, and density, we can redefine the magnitude of F_{grav} for fluids questions:

$$\rho = \frac{m}{V} \rightarrow \quad m = \rho V \quad \rightarrow \quad \therefore F_{grav} = mg = \rho V g$$

With this new formula $F_{grav} = \rho V g$, it is important to make sure that the density (ρ) and the volume (V) describe the properties of the correct object or fluid.

Pressure

If we place an object in a fluid, the fluid exerts a contact force on the object. If we look at how that force is *distributed* over any small area of the object's surface, we have the concept of **pressure**:

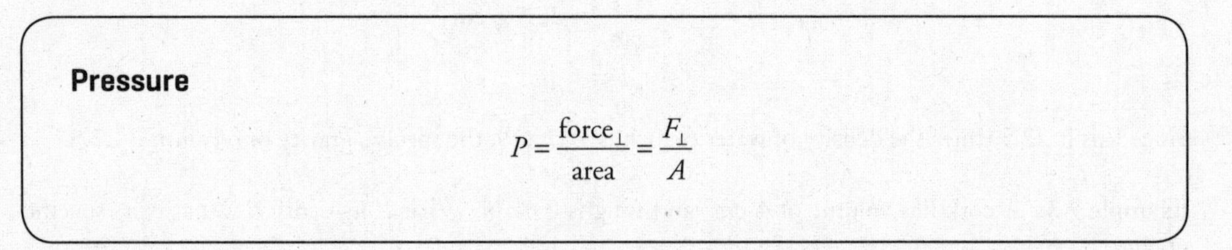

Pressure

$$P = \frac{\text{force}_\perp}{\text{area}} = \frac{F_\perp}{A}$$

The subscript $\perp$ (which means "perpendicular") indicates that pressure is defined as the magnitude of the force acting *perpendicular* to the surface, divided by the area. We don't need to worry very much about this, because (for OAT purposes) at any given point in a fluid the pressure is the same in all directions, which means that the force does not depend on the orientation of the force.

Although the formula for pressure involves "force," pressure is actually a *scalar* quantity, because the perpendicular force is the same for all orientations of surface. The unit of pressure is the N/m^2, which is called a **pascal** (abbreviated **Pa**). Because 1 N is a pretty small force and 1 m^2 is a pretty big area, 1 Pa is very small. Often, you'll see pressure expressed in kPa (or even in MPa). For example, at sea level, normal atmospheric pressure is about 100 kPa.

Let's imagine we have a tank of water with a lid on top. Suspended from the lid is a string attached to a thin metal sheet. The figures on the following page show you two views of this.

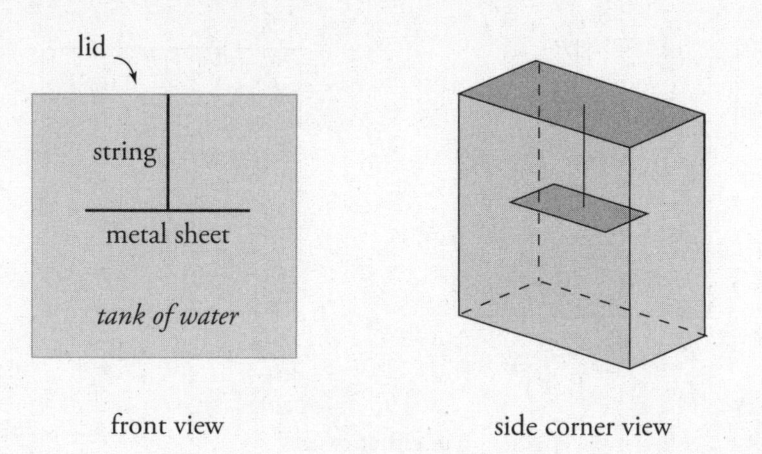

The weight of the water above the metal sheet produces a force that pushes down on the sheet. If we divide this force by the area of the sheet, w/A, we get the pressure, due to the water, on the sheet. The formula for calculating this pressure depends on the density of the fluid in the tank (ρ_{fluid}), the depth of the sheet (D), and the acceleration due to gravity (g).

$$P = \frac{w_{\text{fluid}}}{A} = \frac{m_{\text{fluid}}g}{A} = \frac{\rho_{\text{fluid}}V_{\text{fluid}}g}{A} = \frac{\rho_{\text{fluid}}ADg}{A} = \rho_{\text{fluid}}Dg$$

Hydrostatic Gauge Pressure

$$P_{\text{gauge}} = \rho_{\text{fluid}}gD$$

This formula gives the pressure due only to the fluid (in this case, the water) in the tank. This is called **hydrostatic gauge pressure**. It's called hydro*static*, because the fluid is at rest; and *gauge* pressure means that we don't take the pressure due to the atmosphere into account. If there were no lid on the water tank, then the water would be exposed to the atmosphere, and the *total* pressure at any point in the water would be equal to the atmospheric pressure pushing down on the surface *plus* the pressure due to the water (that is, the gauge pressure). So, below the surface, we'd have

$$P_{\text{total}} = P_{\text{atm}} + P_{\text{gauge}}$$

If the tank were closed to the atmosphere, but there were a layer of gas above the surface of the water, then the total pressure at a point below the surface would be the pressure of the gas pushing down at the surface plus the gauge pressure: $P_{\text{total}} = P_{\text{gas}} + P_{\text{gauge}}$. In general, we'll have

$$P_{\text{total}} = P_{\text{at surface}} + P_{\text{gauge}}$$

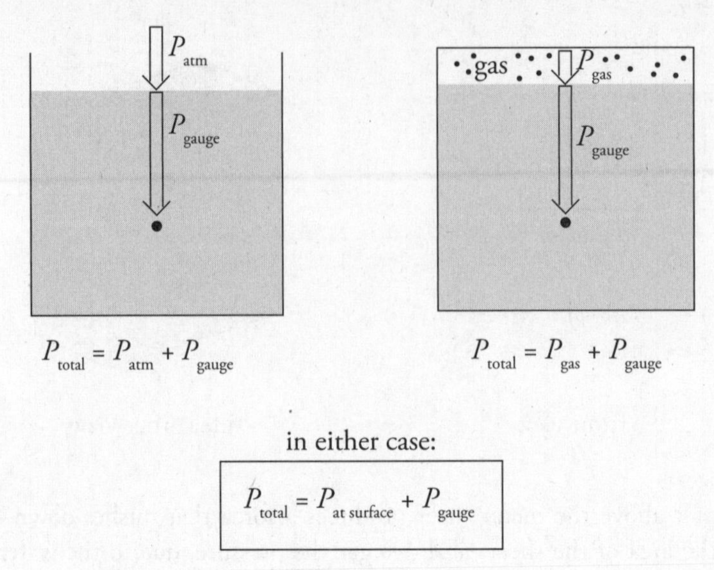

Notice that hydrostatic gauge pressure, $P_{gauge} = \rho_{fluid} gD$, is proportional to both the depth and the density of the fluid. *Total* pressure, however, is *not* proportional to either of these quantities if $P_{on\ surface}$ isn't zero.

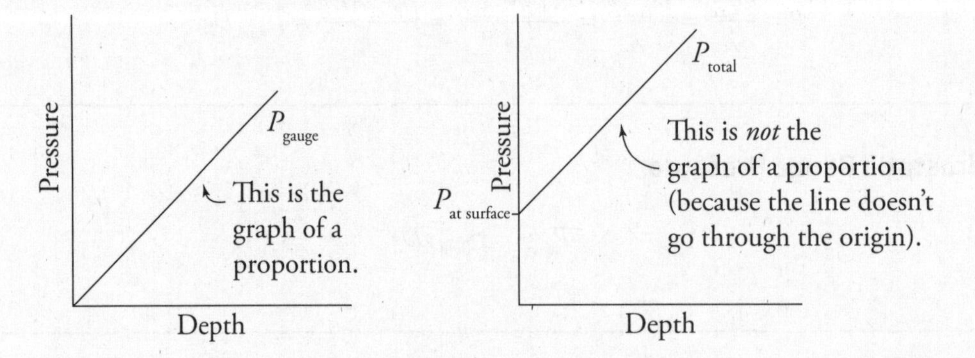

The lines in these graphs will be straight as long as the density of the liquid remains constant as the depth increases. Actually, ρ increases as the depth increases, but the effect is small enough that we generally consider liquids to be **incompressible**; that is, that the density of a liquid remains constant (so, in particular, the density doesn't increase with depth).

Example 7-4: The density of seawater is 1025 kg/m^3. Consider a point X that's 10 m below the surface of the ocean.

a) What's the gauge pressure at X?
b) If the atmospheric pressure is 1.015×10^5 Pa, what is the total pressure at X?
c) Consider a point Y that's 50 m below the surface. How does the gauge pressure at Y compare to the gauge pressure at X? How does the total pressure at Y compare to the total pressure at X?

Solution:

a) The gauge pressure at X is

$$P_{\text{gauge}} = \rho_{\text{fluid}} g D = (1025 \text{ kg/m}^3)(10 \text{ N/kg})(10 \text{ m}) = 1.025 \times 10^5 \text{ Pa}$$

b) The total pressure at X is the atmosphere pressure plus the gauge pressure:

$$P_{\text{total at X}} = P_{\text{atm}} + P_{\text{gauge}} = (1.015 \times 10^5 \text{ Pa}) + (1.025 \times 10^5 \text{ Pa}) = 2.04 \times 10^5 \text{ Pa}$$

c) Since P_{gauge} is proportional to D, an increase in D by a factor of 5 will mean the gauge pressure will also increase by a factor of 5. Therefore, the gauge pressure at Y will be $5\left(P_{\text{gauge at X}}\right) = 5.125 \times 10^5 \text{ Pa}$. The total pressure at Y is equal to the atmospheric pressure plus the gauge pressure at Y, so

$$P_{\text{total at Y}} = P_{\text{atm}} + P_{\text{gauge}} = (1.015 \times 10^5 \text{ Pa}) + (5.125 \times 10^5 \text{ Pa}) = 6.14 \times 10^5 \text{ Pa}$$

Notice that $P_{\text{total at Y}}$ is not 5 times $P_{\text{total at X}}$. *Total* pressure is *not* proportional to depth.

Example 7-5: A large storage tank fitted with a tight lid holds a liquid. The space between the surface of the liquid and the lid of the tank is filled with molecules of the stored liquid in the gaseous phase. At a depth of 40 m, the total pressure is 520 kPa, while at a depth of 50 m, the total pressure is 600 kPa. What's the pressure of the gas above the surface of the liquid?

Solution: Let P_{gas} be the pressure that the gas exerts on the surface of the liquid. Then we have

$$P_{\text{total at } D_1=40 \text{ m}} = P_{\text{gas}} + \rho_{\text{fluid}} g D_1 = P_{\text{gas}} + \rho_{\text{fluid}} g (40 \text{ m}) = 520 \text{ kPa}$$
$$P_{\text{total at } D_2=50 \text{ m}} = P_{\text{gas}} + \rho_{\text{fluid}} g D_2 = P_{\text{gas}} + \rho_{\text{fluid}} g (50 \text{ m}) = 600 \text{ kPa}$$

We have two equations and two unknowns (P_{gas} and ρ_{fluid}). If we subtract the first equation from the second, we get $\rho_{\text{fluid}} g (10 \text{ m}) = 80 \text{ kPa}$, which tells us that $\rho_{\text{fluid}} g = 8 \text{ kPa/m}$. Plugging this back into either one of the equations will give us P_{gas}. Choosing, say, the first one, we find that

$$P_{\text{gas}} + (8 \text{ kPa/m})(40 \text{ m}) = 520 \text{ kPa} \rightarrow P_{\text{gas}} = 200 \text{ kPa}$$

Example 7-6: The containers shown below are all filled with the same liquid. At which point (A, B, C, D, E, or F) is the gauge pressure the lowest?

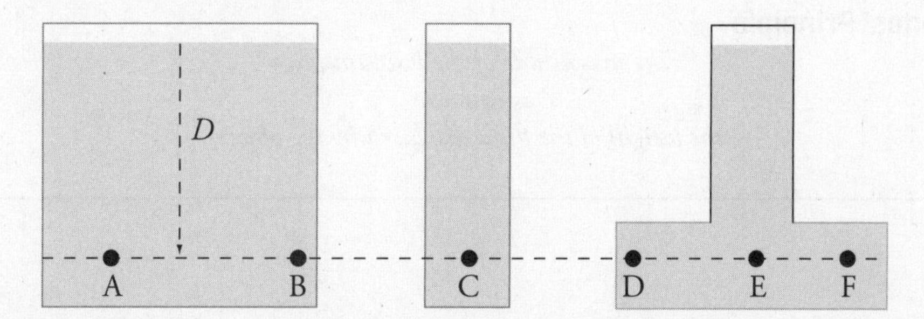

Solution: It's important to remember that the formula $P_{gauge} = \rho_{fluid} gD$ applies regardless of the shape of the container in which the fluid is held. If all the containers are filled with the same fluid, then the pressure is the *same* everywhere along the horizontal dashed line. This is because every point on this line (and within one of the containers) is at the same depth, D, below the surface of the fluid. The fact that the first container is wide, the second container is narrow, and the third container is wide at the base but has a narrow neck makes no difference. Even the fact that Points D and F (in the third container) aren't *directly* underneath a column of fluid of height D makes no difference either.

Pressure is the magnitude of the force per area, so pressure is a *scalar.* Pressure has no direction. The force *due to the pressure* is a vector, however, and the direction of this force on any small surface is always perpendicular to that surface. For example, in the figure below, the pressure at Point A is the same as the pressure at Point B, because they're at the same depth. But, as you can see, the direction of the force due to the pressure varies depending on the orientation of the surface (and even which side of the surface) the force is pushing on.

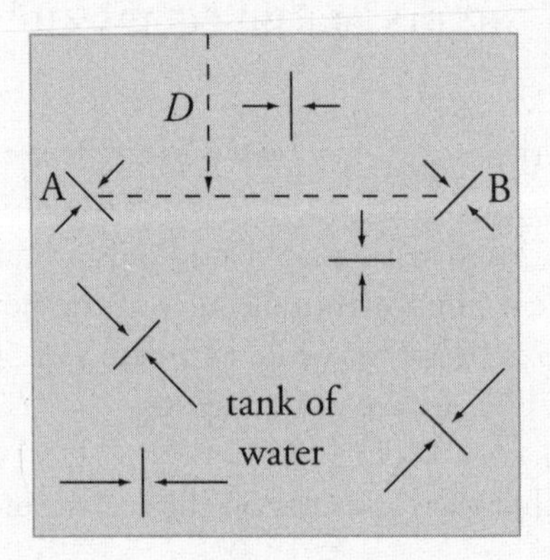

Buoyancy and Archimedes' Principle

Let's place a wooden block in our tank of water. Since the pressure on each side of the block depends on its average depth, we see that there's more pressure on the bottom of the block than there is on the top of it. Therefore, there's a greater force pushing up on the bottom of the block than there is pushing down on the top. The forces due to the pressure on the other four sides (left and right, front and back) cancel out, so the net fluid force on the block is upward. This net upward fluid force is called the **buoyant** force (or just **buoyancy** for short), which we'll denote by F_{Buoy} (or F_B).

We can calculate the magnitude of the buoyant force using Archimedes' principle:

Archimedes' Principle

The magnitude of the buoyant force
is equal to
the weight of the fluid displaced by the object.

When an object is partially or completely submerged in a fluid, the volume of the object that's submerged, which we call V_{sub}, is the volume of the fluid displaced.

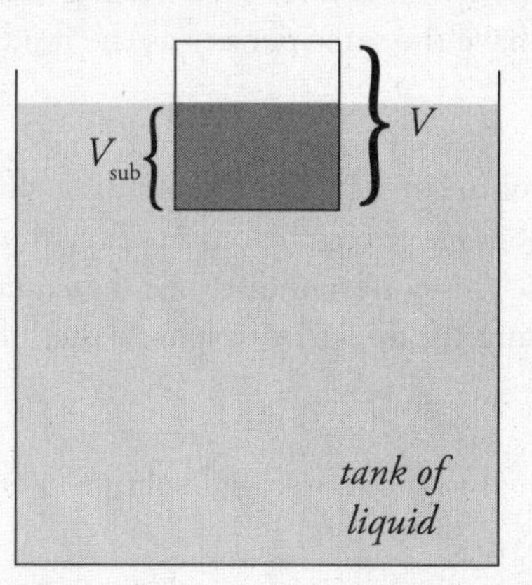

By multiplying V_{sub} by the density of the fluid, we get the *mass* of the fluid displaced; then, multiplying this mass by g gives us the weight of the fluid displaced. So, here's Archimedes' principle as a mathematical equation:

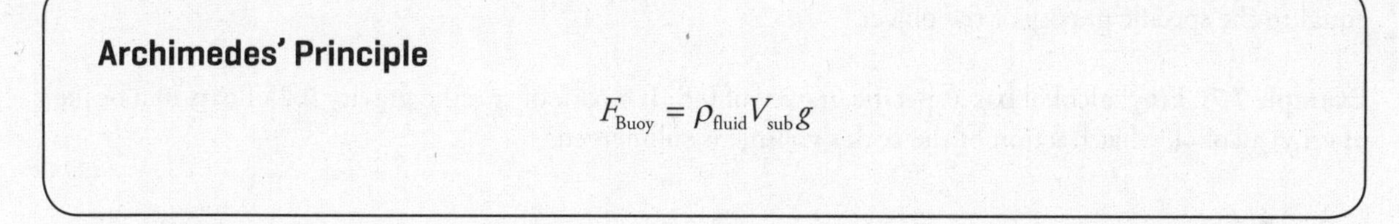

Archimedes' Principle

$$F_{Buoy} = \rho_{fluid} V_{sub} g$$

When an object floats, its submerged volume is just enough to make the buoyant force it feels balance its weight. That is, for a floating object, we always have $w_{object} = F_{Buoy}$. If an object's density is ρ_{object} and its volume is V, its weight will be $\rho_{object} V_{object} g$. The buoyant force it feels is $\rho_{fluid} V_{sub} g$. Setting these equal to each other, we find that

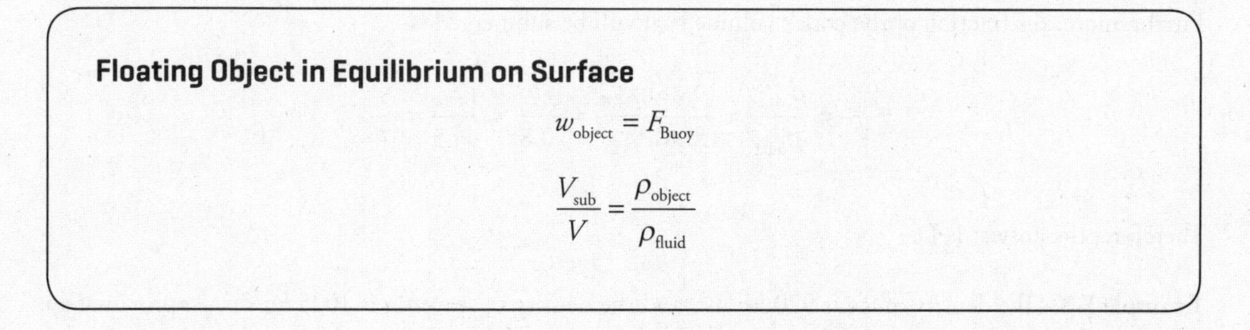

Floating Object in Equilibrium on Surface

$$w_{object} = F_{Buoy}$$

$$\frac{V_{sub}}{V} = \frac{\rho_{object}}{\rho_{fluid}}$$

So, if $\rho_{object} < \rho_{fluid}$, then the object will float; and the fraction of its volume that's submerged is the same as the ratio of its density to the fluid's density. *This is a very helpful fact to know for the OAT.* For example, if the object's density is 3/4 the density of the fluid, then 3/4 of the object will be submerged (and vice versa).

If an object is denser than the fluid, then the object will sink. In this case, even if the entire object is submerged (in an attempt to maximize the buoyant force), the object's weight is still greater than the buoyant force. This leaves a net force in the downwards direction, causing the object to sink by accelerating downwards. If an object just happens to have the same density as the fluid, it will be happy hovering (in static equilibrium) underneath the fluid.

For an object that is completely submerged in the surrounding fluid, the actual weight of the object ($w_{object} = \rho_{object}Vg$) remains unchanged. However, the object's "apparent" weight is less due to the buoyant force "buoying" the object upwards. This corresponds to the measurement of a scale placed at the bottom of a tank of liquid in order to measure the apparent weight of the submerged object, or the normal force acting on the object.

Since the volume of the object is equal to the submerged volume ($V = V_{sub}$), the buoyant force F_{Buoy} on the object is equal to $\rho_{fluid}Vg$. Therefore,

$$\frac{w_{object}}{F_{Buoy}} = \frac{\rho_{object}Vg}{\rho_{fluid}Vg} = \frac{\rho_{object}}{\rho_{fluid}}$$

If the fluid in which the object is submerged is water, the ratio of the object weight to the buoyant force is equal to the specific gravity of the object.

Example 7-7: Ethyl alcohol has a specific gravity of 0.8. If a cork of specific gravity 0.25 floats in a beaker of ethyl alcohol, what fraction of the cork's volume is submerged?

A. 4/25
B. 1/5
C. 1/4
D. 5/16

Solution: Because the cork has a lower density than the ethyl alcohol, we know that the cork will float. Furthermore, the fraction of the cork's volume that will be submerged is

$$\frac{V_{sub}}{V} = \frac{\rho_{object}}{\rho_{fluid}} = \frac{(0.25)\rho_{H_2O}}{(0.8)\rho_{H_2O}} = \frac{0.25}{0.8} = \frac{1/4}{4/5} = \frac{5}{16}$$

Therefore, the answer is D.

Example 7-8: The density of ice is 920 kg/m^3, and the density of seawater is 1025 kg/m^3. Approximately what percent of an iceberg floats above the surface of the ocean (in other words, how much is "the tip of the iceberg")?

A. 5%
B. 10%
C. 90%
D. 95%

Solution: Because the ice has a lower density than the seawater, we know that the iceberg will float. Furthermore, the fraction of the iceberg's volume that will be submerged is

$$\frac{V_{\text{sub}}}{V} = \frac{\rho_{\text{object}}}{\rho_{\text{fluid}}} = \frac{920\ \text{kg/m}^3}{1025\ \text{kg/m}^3} = \frac{900}{1000} = 90\%$$

However, the answer is not C. The question asked what percent of the iceberg floats *above* the surface. So, if 90% is submerged, then 10% is above the surface, and the answer is B. Watch for this kind of tricky wording; it is a common OAT tactic.

Example 7-9: A glass sphere of specific gravity 2.5 and volume 10^{-3} m^3 is completely submerged in a large container of water. What is the apparent weight of the sphere while immersed?

Solution: Because the buoyant force pushes up on the object, the object's *apparent weight*, $w_{\text{apparent}} = w - F_{\text{Buoy}}$, is less than its true weight, w. Because the sphere is completely submerged, we have $V_{\text{sub}} = V$, so the buoyant force on the sphere is

$$\begin{aligned} F_{\text{Buoy}} &= \rho_{\text{fluid}} V_{\text{sub}} g \\ &= \rho_{H_2O} V g \\ &= (1000\ \text{kg/m}^3)(10^{-3}\ \text{m}^3)(10\ \text{N/kg}) \\ &= 10\,\text{N} \end{aligned}$$

The true weight of the glass sphere is

$$\begin{aligned} w &= \rho_{\text{glass}} V g \\ &= (\text{sp. gr.}_{\text{glass}} \times \rho_{H_2O}) V g \\ &= (2.5 \times 1000\ \text{kg/m}^3)(10^{-3}\ \text{m}^3)(10\ \text{N/kg}) \\ &= 25\,\text{N} \end{aligned}$$

Therefore, the apparent weight of the sphere while immersed is

$$w_{\text{apparent}} = w - F_{\text{Buoy}} = 25\ \text{N} - 10\ \text{N} = 15\ \text{N}$$

Example 7-10: An object weighs 50 N, but weighs only 30 N when it's completely immersed in a liquid of specific gravity 0.8. What's the specific gravity of this object?

Solution: The weight of the object is $w_{\text{object}} = \rho_{\text{object}} Vg$, and the buoyant force it feels when completely immersed (that is, when $V_{\text{sub}} = V$) is $F_{\text{Buoy}} = \rho_{\text{fluid}} Vg$. Therefore,

$$\frac{w_{\text{object}}}{F_{\text{Buoy}}} = \frac{\rho_{\text{object}} Vg}{\rho_{\text{fluid}} Vg} = \frac{\rho_{\text{object}}}{\rho_{\text{fluid}}}$$

Now, since this 50 N object weighs only 30 N when immersed, the buoyant force must be 20 N. So, we can write

$$\frac{w_{\text{object}}}{F_{\text{Buoy}}} = \frac{50\text{N}}{20\text{N}} = \frac{5}{2}$$

We now have two expressions for the ratio $w_{\text{object}} / F_{\text{Buoy}}$. Therefore,

$$\frac{\rho_{\text{object}}}{\rho_{\text{fluid}}} = \frac{5}{2}$$

If the object's density is 5/2 times the fluid's density, then the object's specific gravity is 5/2 times the fluid's specific gravity; that is,

$$\text{sp. gr.}_{\text{object}} = \tfrac{5}{2}(\text{sp. gr.}_{\text{fluid}}) = \tfrac{5}{2}(0.8) = 2$$

Example 7-11: A balloon that weighs 0.18 N is then filled with helium so that its volume becomes 0.03 m^3. (Note: The density of helium is 0.2 kg/m^3.)

a) What is the net force on the balloon if it's surrounded by air? (Note: The density of air is 1.2 kg/m^3.)

b) What will be the initial upward acceleration of the balloon if it's released from rest?

Solution:

a) Remember that gases are fluids, so they also exert buoyant forces. If an object is immersed in a gas, the object experiences a buoyant force equal to the weight of the gas it displaces. In this case, the balloon is completely immersed in a "sea" of air (so $V_{\text{sub}} = V$), and Archimedes' principle tells us that the buoyant force on the balloon due to the surrounding air is

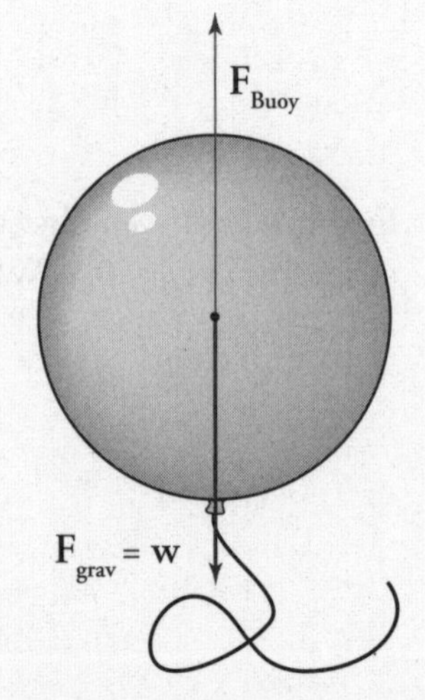

$$\begin{aligned} F_{\text{Buoy}} &= \rho_{\text{fluid}} V_{\text{sub}} g \\ &= \rho_{\text{air}} V g \\ &= (1.2 \text{ kg/m}^3)(0.03 \text{ m}^3)(10 \text{ N/kg}) \\ &= 0.36 \text{ N} \end{aligned}$$

The weight of the inflated balloon is equal to the weight of the balloon material (0.18 N) plus the weight of the helium:

$$\begin{aligned} w_{\text{total}} &= w_{\text{material}} + w_{\text{helium}} \\ &= w_{\text{material}} + \rho_{\text{helium}} V g \\ &= 0.18 \text{ N} + (0.2 \text{ kg/m}^3)(0.03 \text{ m}^3)(10 \text{ N/kg}) \\ &= 0.18 \text{ N} + 0.06 \text{ N} \\ &= 0.24 \text{ N} \end{aligned}$$

Because $F_{\text{Buoy}} > w_{\text{total}}$, the net force on the balloon is upward and has magnitude

$$F_{\text{net}} = F_{\text{Buoy}} - w_{\text{total}} = (0.36 \text{ N}) - (0.24 \text{ N}) = 0.12 \text{ N}$$

b) Using Newton's second law, $a = F_{\text{net}} / m$, we find that

$$a = \frac{F_{\text{net}}}{m} = \frac{F_{\text{net}}}{\frac{w}{g}} = \frac{0.12 \text{ N}}{\left(\frac{0.24 \text{ N}}{10 \text{ m/s}^2}\right)} = \frac{(0.12 \text{ N})(10 \text{ m/s}^2)}{0.24 \text{ N}} = \frac{10 \text{ m/s}^2}{2} = 5 \text{ m/s}^2$$

Pascal's Law

Pascal's law is a statement about fluid pressure. It says that a confined fluid will transmit an externally applied pressure change to all parts of the fluid and the walls of the container without loss of magnitude. In less formal language, if you squeeze a container of fluid, the fluid will transmit your squeeze perfectly throughout the container. The most important application of Pascal's law is to hydraulics.

Consider a simple hydraulic jack consisting of two pistons resting above two cylindrical vessels of fluid that are connected by a pipe. If you push down on one piston, the other one will rise. Let's make this more precise. Let F_1 be the magnitude of the force you exert down on one piston (whose cross-sectional area is A_1), and let F_2 be the magnitude of the force that the other piston (cross-sectional area A_2) exerts upward as a result.

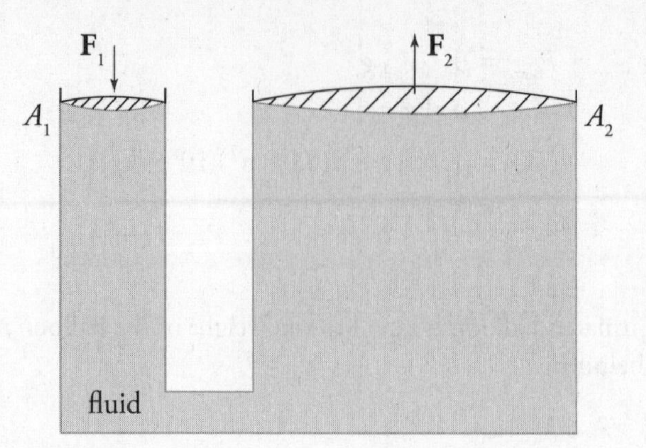

Pushing down on the left-hand piston with a force F_1 introduces a pressure increase of F_1/A_1. Pascal's law tells us that this pressure change is transmitted, without loss of magnitude, by the fluid to the other end. Since the pressure change at the other piston is F_1/A_1, we have, by Pascal's law,

$$\frac{F_1}{A_1} = \frac{F_2}{A_2}$$

Solving this equation for F_2, we get

$$F_2 = \frac{A_2}{A_1} F_1$$

So, if A_2 is greater than A_1 (as it is in the figure), then the ratio of the areas, A_2/A_1, will be greater than 1, so F_2 will be greater than F_1; that is, *the output force, F_2, is greater than your input force, F_1*. This is why hydraulic jacks are useful; we end up lifting something very heavy (a car, for example) by exerting a much smaller force (one that would be insufficient to lift the car if it were just applied directly to the car).

This seems too good to be true; doesn't this violate some conservation law? No, since there's no such thing as a "Conservation of Force" law. However, there *is* a price to be paid for the magnification of the force. Let's say you push the left-hand piston down by a distance d_1, and that the distance the right-hand piston moves upward is d_2. Assuming the fluid is incompressible, whatever fluid you push out of the left-hand cylinder must appear in the right-hand cylinder. Since volume is equal to cross-sectional area times distance, the volume of the fluid you push out of the left-hand cylinder is A_1d_1, and the extra volume of fluid that appears in the right-hand cylinder is A_2d_2.

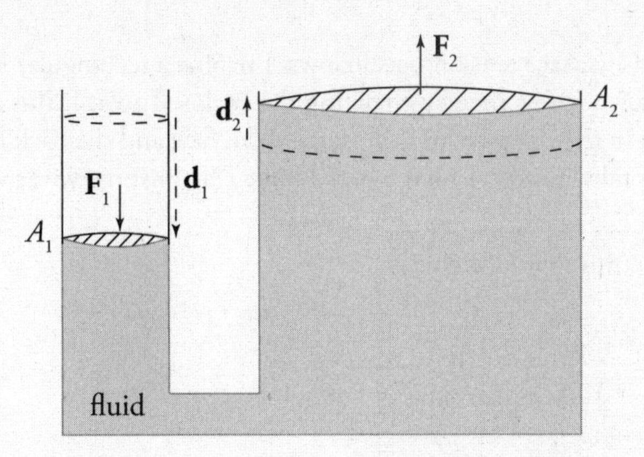

But these volumes have to be the same, so $A_1d_1 = A_2d_2$. Solving this equation for d_2, we get

$$d_2 = \frac{A_1}{A_2}d_1$$

If the area of the right-hand piston (A_2) is greater than the area of the left-hand piston (A_1), the ratio A_1/A_2 will be *less* than 1, so d_2 will be less than d_1. In fact, the decrease in d is the same as the increase in F. For example, if A_2 is five times larger than A_1, then F_2 will be five times greater than F_1, but d_2 will only be *one-fifth* of d_1. We can now see that the product of F and d will be the same for both pistons:

$$F_2d_2 = \left(\frac{A_2}{A_1}F_1\right)\cdot\left(\frac{A_1}{A_2}d_1\right) = F_1d_1$$

Recall that the product of F and d is the amount of work done. What we have shown is that the work you do pushing the left-hand piston down is equal to the work done by the right-hand piston as it pushes upward. Just as when we discussed simple machines in Chapter 4, we can't cheat when it comes to work. True, we can do the same job with less force, but we will always pay for that by having to exert that smaller force through a greater distance. This is the whole idea behind all simple machines, not just a hydraulic jack.

Surface Tension

To complete our section on fluids at rest, we introduce the phenomenon of **surface tension**. We have all seen long-legged bugs that can walk on the surface of a pond or have watched a slowly-leaking faucet form a drop of water that grows until it finally drops into the sink. Both of these are illustrations of surface tension. The surface of a fluid can behave like an elastic membrane or thin sheet of rubber. A liquid will form a drop because the surface tends to contract into a sphere (to minimize surface area); however, when you see a drop hanging precariously from a faucet, its spherical shape is distorted by the pull of gravity. In fact, the reason it eventually falls into the sink is that the force due to surface tension causing the drop to cling to the head of the faucet is overwhelmed by the increasing weight of the drop. It can't hang on, and away it goes.

A standard way to define the surface tension is as follows. Imagine a rectangular loop of thin wire with one side able to slide up and down freely, thereby changing the enclosed area. If this apparatus is dipped into a fluid, a thin film will form in the enclosed area. Both the front face and the back face of the film are pulling upward on the free horizontal wire with a total upward force F against the wire's weight.

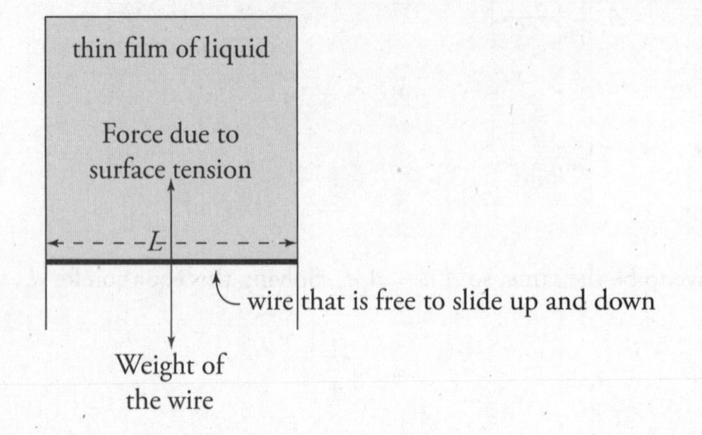

The strength of the surface tension force depends on the particular liquid and is determined by the *coefficient of surface tension*, γ, which is the force per unit length. Since there are *two* surfaces here (the front and the back), each of which acts along a length L, the force F due to surface tension acts along a total length of $2L$. The coefficient of surface tension is defined to be $\gamma = F/2L$, so $F_{\text{surf tension}} = 2\gamma L$. To give you an idea of the values of γ, the surface tension coefficient of water is 0.07 N/m at room temperature (and decreases as the temperature increases). A fluid with one of the highest surface tension coefficients is mercury. Its surface tension coefficient is nearly seven times greater than that of water: $\gamma_{\text{Hg}} = 0.46\,\text{N/m}$ at room temperature. Note that these values are really quite small. The surface of a pond of water can support the weight of a bug, but a frog isn't about to walk across the pond supported by surface tension.

Summary of Formulas

HYDROSTATICS

Assume liquids are incompressible unless otherwise stated

Standard atmospheric pressure = 1 atm = 760 mmHg = 760 torr ≈ 100 kPa

Density: $\rho = \frac{m}{V}$

Specific gravity: $\text{sp.gr.} = \frac{\rho}{\rho_{H_2O}}$

$$\left(\rho_{H_2O} = 1000 \text{ kg/m}^3 \text{ or } 1 \text{ g/cm}^3 \text{ or } 1 \text{ kg/L}\right)$$

Force of gravity: $mg = \rho V g$

Pressure: $P = \frac{F_\perp}{A}$

Hydrostatic gauge pressure: $P_{\text{gauge}} = \rho_{\text{fluid}} g D$

Hydrostatic gauge pressure is proportional to depth. Total hydrostatic pressure increases with increasing depth but is NOT proportional to depth.

Total hydrostatic pressure: $P_{\text{total}} = P_{\text{at surface}} + P_{\text{gauge}}$

Archimedes' principle: $F_{\text{Buoy}} = \rho_{\text{fluid}} V_{\text{sub}} g$

Buoyant force is equal to the weight of the displaced fluid.

Floating object: $\rho_{\text{object}} < \rho_{\text{fluid}} \rightarrow w_{\text{object}} = F_{\text{Buoy}}$

$$\frac{V_{\text{sub}}}{V} = \frac{\rho_{\text{object}}}{\rho_{\text{fluid}}}$$

Apparent weight of submerged object: $w_{\text{apparent}} = w_{\text{object}} - F_{\text{Buoy}}$

Pascal's law: $\frac{F_1}{A_1} = \frac{F_2}{A_2}$

Chapter 8
Electrostatics

8.1 ELECTRIC CHARGE

An atom is composed of a central nucleus (which is itself composed of protons and neutrons) surrounded by a cloud of one or more electrons. The fact that an atom is held together as a single unit is due to the fact that protons and electrons have a special property: They carry **electric charge**, which gives rise to an attractive force between them.

Electric charge exists in two varieties, which are called **positive** and **negative.** By convention, we say that protons carry positive charge and electrons carry negative charge. (Neutrons are well-named: They're neutral, because they have no electric charge.) The charge of a proton is $+e$, where e is called the **elementary charge**, and the charge of an electron is $-e$. Notice that the proton and the electron carry exactly the same amount of charge; the only difference in their charges is that one is positive and the other is negative.

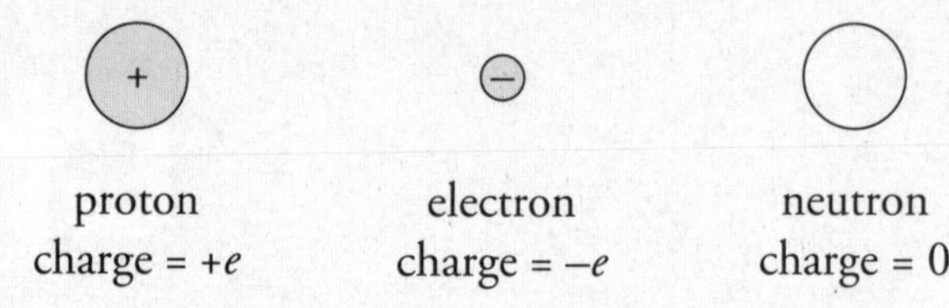

In SI units, electric charge is measured in **coulombs** (abbreviated **C**), and the value of the elementary charge, e, is 1.6×10^{-19} C.

Elementary Charge

$$e = 1.6 \times 10^{-19} \text{ C}$$

When an atom (or any other object) contains the same number of electrons as protons, its total charge is zero because the individual positive and negative charges add up and cancel. So, when the number of electrons (#e) equals the number of protons (#p), the object is *electrically neutral.* We say that an object is **charged** when there's an imbalance between the number of electrons and the number of protons. When an object has one or more extra electrons (#e > #p), the object is *negatively charged*, and when an object has a deficit of electrons (#e < #p), the object is *positively charged.* If a neutral atom has electrons removed or added, we say that it has been **ionized**, and the resulting electrically charged atom is called an **ion.** A positively charged ion is called a **cation**, and a negatively charged ion is called an **anion.** (An object can also become charged by gaining or losing protons, but these are usually locked up tight within the nuclei of the atoms. In virtually all cases, objects become charged by the transfer of *electrons.*)

Because an object can become charged only by losing or gaining electrons or protons, which can't be "sliced" into smaller pieces with fractional amounts of charge, the charge on an object can only be a whole number of $\pm e$'s; that is, charge is **quantized**. So, for any object, its charge is always equal to $n(\pm e)$, where n is a whole number. To remind us that charge is *q*uantized, electric charge is usually denoted by the letter q (or Q).

Charge is Quantized

$$q = n(\pm e)$$

where n = 0, 1, 2...

In chemistry, it's common to talk about the charge of an atom in terms of whole numbers like +1 or –2, etc. For example, we say that the charge of the fluoride ion, F^-, is –1, and the charge of the calcium ion, Ca^{+2}, is +2. This is just a convenient way of saying that the charge of the fluoride ion is –1 elementary unit (in other words, $-1e$), and the charge of the calcium ion is +2 elementary units, $+2e$. When we want to find the electric force between ions, we will express their charges in the proper unit (coulombs), and say, for example, that the charge of the fluoride ion is $-1e = -1.6 \times 10^{-19}$ C and the charge of the calcium ion is $+2e = +3.2 \times 10^{-19}$ C.

Finally, total electric charge is always conserved; that is, the total amount of charge before any process must always be equal to the total amount of charge afterward.[1]

Example 8-1: When you pet a cat, you rub electrons off the cat's fur, which are transferred to your hand. Assuming that you transfer 5×10^{10} electrons to your hand, what is the electric charge on your hand? What's the charge on the cat?

Solution: Because each electron carries a charge of $-e = -1.6 \times 10^{-19}$ C, and you've gained 5×10^{10} of them, the charge on your hand will be

$$(5\times10^{10})(-e) = (5\times10^{10})(-1.6\times10^{-19}) = -8\times10^{-9}\text{ C}$$

Since the cat has lost 5×10^{10} electrons, the charge on the cat will be

$$(5\times10^{10})(+e) = (5\times10^{10})(1.6\times10^{-19}) = +8\times10^{-9}\text{ C}$$

Notice that the *net* charge before and after petting the cat was zero; all you've done is transferred charge.

[1] This does not mean that electric charge cannot be created or destroyed, which happens all the time. For example, in the reaction $e^- + e^+ \rightarrow \gamma + \gamma$, an electron ($e^-$) and its antiparticle (the positron, e^+, which is, in effect, a positively charged electron) meet and annihilate each other, producing energy in the form of two gamma-ray photons (γ), which carry no charge. Charge has been destroyed, but the total charge (zero, in this case) has been conserved. Conversely, charge can be created in the opposite process, when energy is converted to mass and charge (but always with zero total charge).

Example 8-2: How much positive charge is contained in 1 mole of carbon atoms? How much negative charge? What is the total charge?

Solution: Every atom of carbon contains 6 protons, so the amount of positive charge in one carbon atom is $q_+ = +6e$. Therefore, if N_A denotes Avogadro's number, the total amount of positive charge in 1 mole of carbon atoms is

$$Q_+ = N_A \times q_+ = N_A \times (+6e) = (6.02 \times 10^{23}) \times (6)(+1.6 \times 10^{-19}\text{ C}) \approx +6 \times 10^5\text{ C}$$

Because every neutral carbon atom also contains 6 electrons, the amount of negative charge in a carbon atom is $q_- = 6(-e) = -6e = -q_+$, so the total amount of negative charge in 1 mole of carbon atoms is $Q_- = N_A \times q_- = -Q_+ \approx -6 \times 10^5\text{ C}$. The total charge on the carbon atoms, $Q_+ + Q_-$, is zero.

8.2 ELECTRIC FORCE AND COULOMB'S LAW

If two charged particles are a distance r apart,

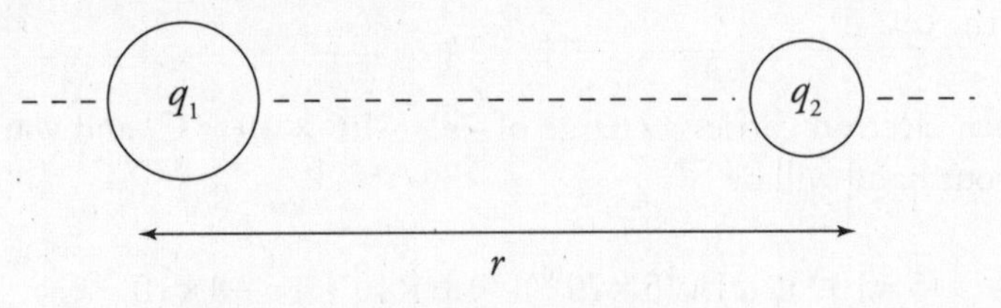

then the electric force between them, $\mathbf{F}_E$, is directed along the line joining them. The magnitude of this force is proportional to the charges (q_1 and q_2) and inversely proportional to r^2, as given by

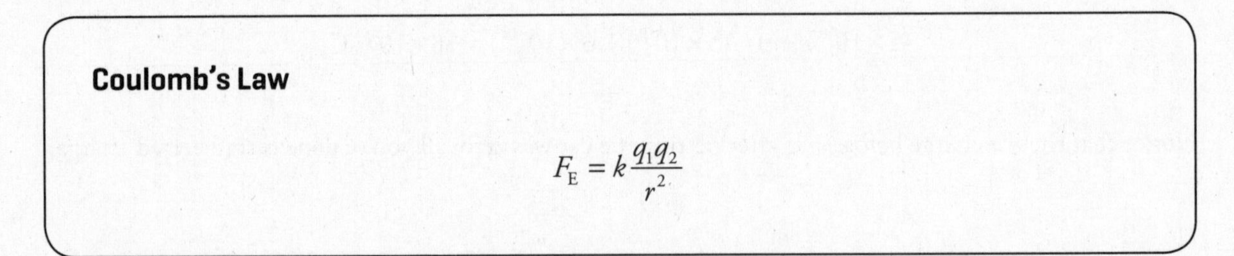

Coulomb's Law

$$F_E = k\frac{q_1 q_2}{r^2}$$

The proportionality constant is k, and in general, its value depends on the material between the particles. However, in the usual case where the particles are separated by empty space (or by air, for all practical purposes), the proportionality constant is denoted by k_0 and called **Coulomb's constant.** This is a fundamental constant of nature (equal in magnitude, by definition, to 10^{-7} times the speed of light squared), and its value is $k_0 = 9 \times 10^9\ \text{N} \cdot \text{m}^2/\text{C}^2$:[2]

Coulomb's Constant

$$k_0 = 9 \times 10^9 \text{ N} \cdot \text{m}^2 / \text{C}^2$$

This is the value of k you should use unless you're specifically given another value (which would happen only if the charges were embedded in some insulating material that weakens the electric force).

If we retain the signs of the charges q_1 and q_2 when we use the formula $F_E = kq_1q_2 / r^2$, then a positive F_E means that the particles repel each other; a negative F_E means they attract each other. This is consistent with the fact that like charges (two positives or two negatives) repel each other, and opposite charges (one positive and one negative) attract. Note that the two electric forces in each of the following diagrams form an action–reaction pair.

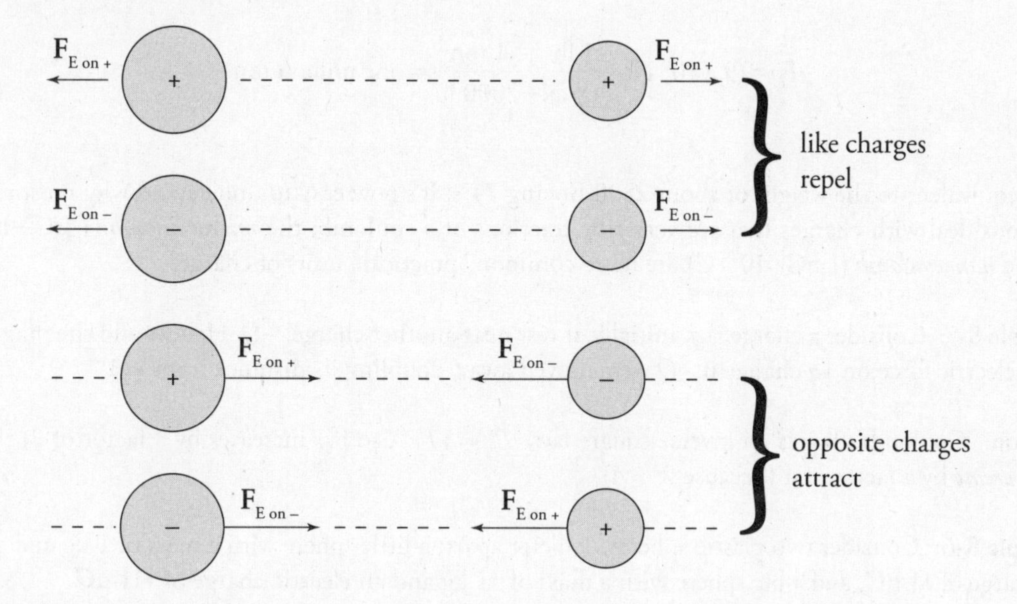

Example 8-3: Two charges, $q_1 = -2 \times 10^{-6}$ C and $q_2 = +5 \times 10^{-6}$ C, are separated by a distance of 10 cm. Describe the electric force between these particles.

Solution: Using Coulomb's law, we find that

$$F_E = k_0 \frac{q_1 q_2}{r^2} = (9 \times 10^9 \text{ N} \cdot \text{m}^2 / \text{C}^2) \frac{(-2 \times 10^{-6} \text{ C})(+5 \times 10^{-6} \text{ C})}{(10^{-1} \text{ m})^2} = -9 \text{N}$$

The minus sign on F_E tells us that the electric force between the charges is attractive, which we expected since q_1 is negative and q_2 is positive. Therefore, the electric force on q_1 is directed toward q_2, the electric force on q_2 is directed toward q_1, and the magnitude of the electric force that each charge feels due to the other is 9 N.

8.2

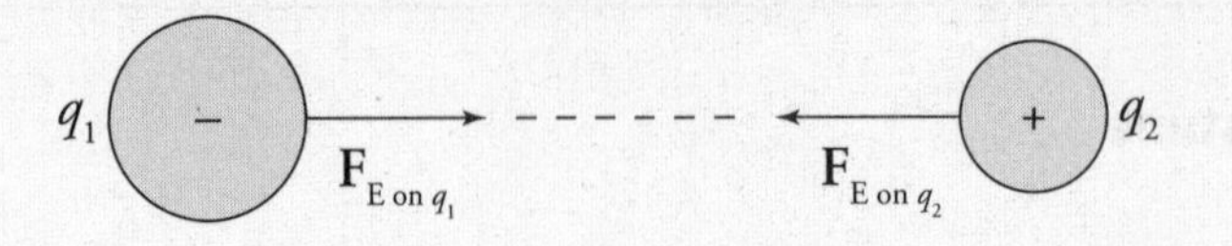

Example 8-4: A coulomb is a *lot* of charge. To get some idea just how much, imagine that we had two objects, each with a charge of 1 C, separated by a distance of 1 m. What would be the electric force between them?

Solution: Using Coulomb's law, we'd find that

$$F_E = k_0 \frac{q_1 q_2}{r^2} = (9\times10^9 \text{ N}\cdot\text{m}^2/\text{C}^2)\frac{(1\text{ C})(1\text{C})}{(1\text{ m})^2} = 9\times10^9 \text{ N}$$

To write this answer in terms of a more familiar unit, let's use the fact that 1 pound (1 lb) is about 4.5 N, and 1 ton is 2000 lb:

$$F_E = (9\times10^9 \text{ N})\cdot\frac{1\text{ lb}}{4.5\text{ N}}\cdot\frac{1\text{ ton}}{2000\text{ lb}} = \text{one million tons}$$

That's equivalent to the weight of about 2500 Boeing 747s! It's now easy to understand why most real-life situations deal with charges that are very tiny fractions of a coulomb; the *microcoulomb* (1 μC $=10^{-6}$ C) and the *nanocoulomb* (1 nC $=10^{-9}$ C) are more common "practical" units of charge.

Example 8-5: Consider a charge, $+q$, initially at rest near another charge, $-Q$. How would the magnitude of the electric force on $+q$ change if $-Q$ were moved away, doubling its distance from $+q$?

Solution: Coulomb's law is an inverse-square law, $F_E \propto 1/r^2$, so if r increases by a factor of 2, then F_E will *decrease* by a factor of 4 (because $2^2 = 4$).

Example 8-6: Consider two plastic spheres, 1 meter apart: a little sphere with a mass of 1 kg and an electric charge of +1 nC, and a big sphere with a mass of 11 kg and an electric charge of +11 μC.

a) Find the electric force and the gravitational force between these spheres. Which force is stronger?
b) If the big sphere is fixed in position, and the little sphere is free to move, describe the resulting motion of the little sphere if it's released from rest.

Solution:

a) Using Coulomb's law, we find that the electric force between the spheres is

$$F_E = k_0 \frac{Qq}{r^2} = (9 \times 10^9 \text{ N} \cdot \text{m}^2 / \text{C}^2) \frac{(11 \times 10^{-6} \text{ C})(1 \times 10^{-9} \text{ C})}{1 \text{m}^2} = 9.9 \times 10^{-5} \text{ N} \approx 10^{-4} \text{ N}$$

Using Newton's law of gravitation, the gravitational force between them is

$$F_G = G \frac{Mm}{r^2} = (6.7 \times 10^{-11} \text{ N} \cdot \text{m}^2 / \text{kg}^2) \frac{(1 \text{ kg})(11 \text{ kg})}{1 \text{ m}^2} \approx 7.4 \times 10^{-10} \text{ N}$$

Which force is stronger? It's no contest: The electric force is *much* stronger than the gravitational force. So, even though the spheres experience an attraction due to gravity, it is many orders of magnitude weaker than their electrical repulsion and can therefore be ignored.

b) The net force on the little sphere is essentially equal to the electrical repulsion it feels from the big sphere (since the gravitational force is *so* much smaller, it can be ignored). Therefore, the initial acceleration of the little sphere is

$$a = \frac{F_E}{m} = \frac{10^{-4} \text{ N}}{1 \text{ kg}} = 10^{-4} \text{ m/s}^2$$

directed away from the big sphere. Notice that as the little sphere moves away, its acceleration does not remain constant. Because the electric force is inversely proportional to the square of the distance between the charges, as the little sphere moves away, the repulsive force it feels weakens, so its acceleration decreases. Therefore, the little sphere moves directly away from the big sphere with decreasing acceleration.

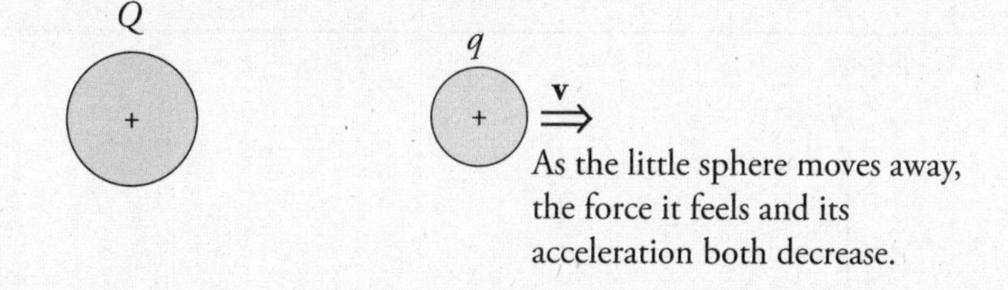

Nevertheless, because the acceleration of the little sphere always points in the same direction (namely, away from the big sphere), the speed of the little sphere is always increasing, although the rate of increase of speed gets smaller as the little sphere gets farther away.

The Principle of Superposition for Electric Forces

Coulomb's law tells us how to calculate the force that one charge exerts on another one. What if two (or more) charges affect a third one? For example, what is the electric force on q_3 in the following figure?

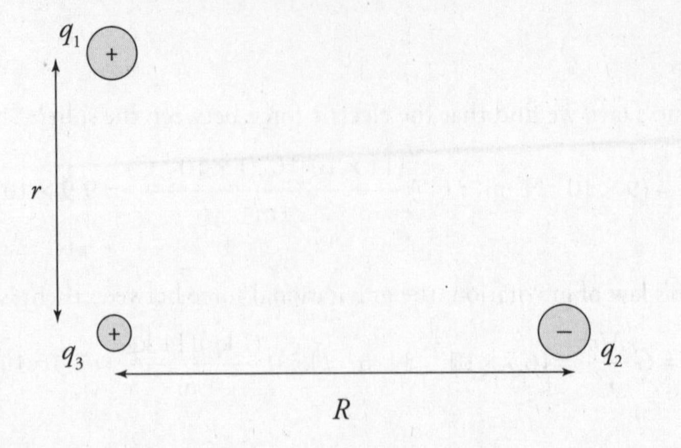

Here's the answer: If $\mathbf{F}_{1\text{-on-}3}$ is the force that q_1 *alone* exerts on q_3 (ignoring the presence of q_2) and if $\mathbf{F}_{2\text{-on-}3}$ is the force that q_2 *alone* exerts on q_3 (ignoring the presence of q_1), then the total force that q_3 feels is simply the vector sum $\mathbf{F}_{1\text{-on-}3} + \mathbf{F}_{2\text{-on-}3}$. The fact that we can calculate the effect of several charges by considering them individually and then just adding the resulting forces is known as the **principle of superposition.** (This important property will also be used when we study electric field vectors, electric potential, magnetic fields, and magnetic forces.)

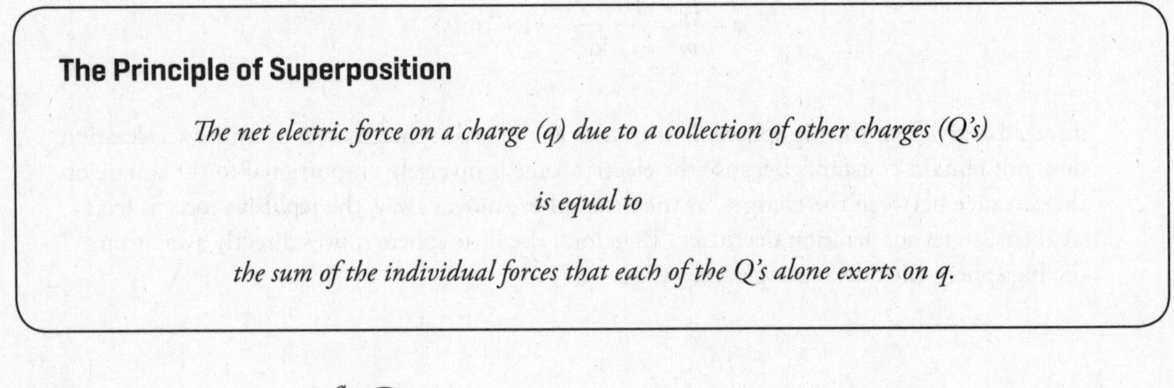

The Principle of Superposition

The net electric force on a charge (q) due to a collection of other charges (Q's)

is equal to

the sum of the individual forces that each of the Q's alone exerts on q.

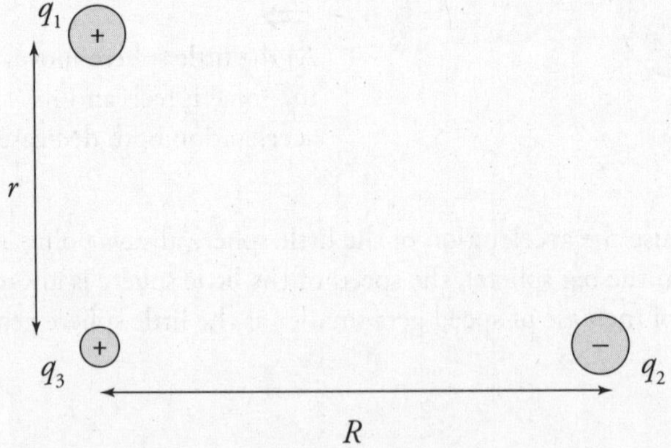

Example 8-7: In the figure above, assume that $q_1 = 2$ C, $q_2 = -8$ C, and $q_3 = 1$ nC. If $r = 1$ m and $R = 2$ m, which one of the following vectors best illustrates the direction of the net electric force on q_3?

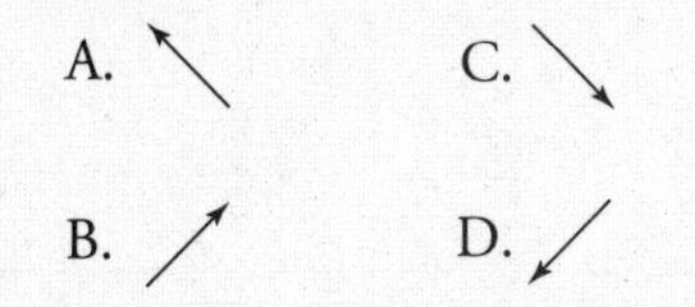

Solution: The individual forces $\mathbf{F}_{1\text{-on-}3}$ and $\mathbf{F}_{2\text{-on-}3}$ are shown in the figure below. Adding these vectors gives $\mathbf{F}_{\text{on }3}$, which points down to the right, so the answer is C.

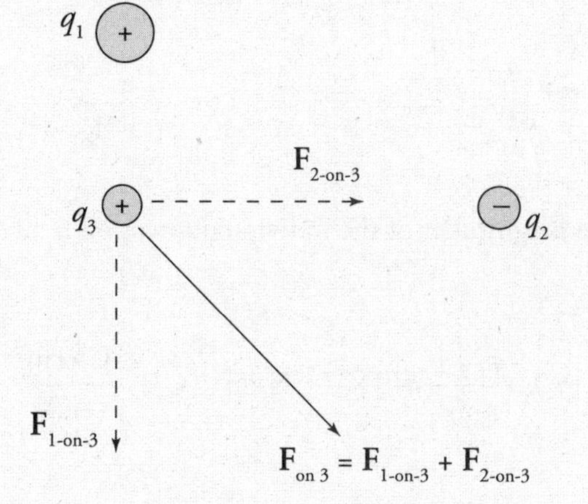

$$F_{1-\text{on}-3} = k_0 \frac{q_1 q_3}{r^2} = (9 \times 10^9 \text{ N} \cdot \text{m}^2 / \text{C}^2) \frac{(2\text{C})(1 \times 10^{-9} \text{ C})}{(1\text{m})^2} = 18\text{N}$$

(repulsive; away from q_1)

$$F_{2-\text{on}-3} = k_0 \frac{q_2 q_3}{R^2} = (9 \times 10^9 \text{ N} \cdot \text{m}^2 / \text{C}^2) \frac{(-8\text{C})(1 \times 10^{-9} \text{ C})}{(2 \text{ m})^2} = -18\text{N}$$

(attractive; toward q_2)

If the question had asked for the magnitude of the net electric force on q_3, then we'd use the Pythagorean theorem to find the length of the vector $\mathbf{F}_{\text{on }3}$. The vector $\mathbf{F}_{\text{on }3}$ is the hypotenuse of the right triangle whose legs are $\mathbf{F}_{1\text{-on-}3}$ and $\mathbf{F}_{2\text{-on-}3}$, so the magnitude of $\mathbf{F}_{\text{on }3}$ is found like this:

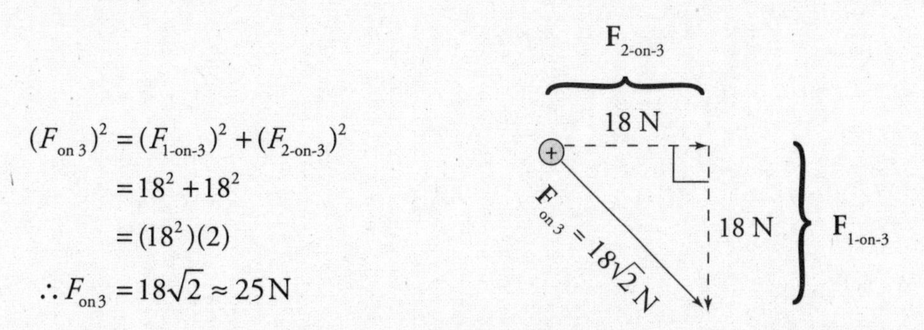

$$(F_{\text{on }3})^2 = (F_{1\text{-on-}3})^2 + (F_{2\text{-on-}3})^2$$
$$= 18^2 + 18^2$$
$$= (18^2)(2)$$
$$\therefore F_{\text{on}3} = 18\sqrt{2} \approx 25\text{N}$$

8.2

Example 8-8: In the figure below, assume that q_1 = 1 C, q_2 = –1 nC, and q_3 = 8 C. If q_4 is a negative charge, what must its value be in order for the net electric force on q_2 to be zero?

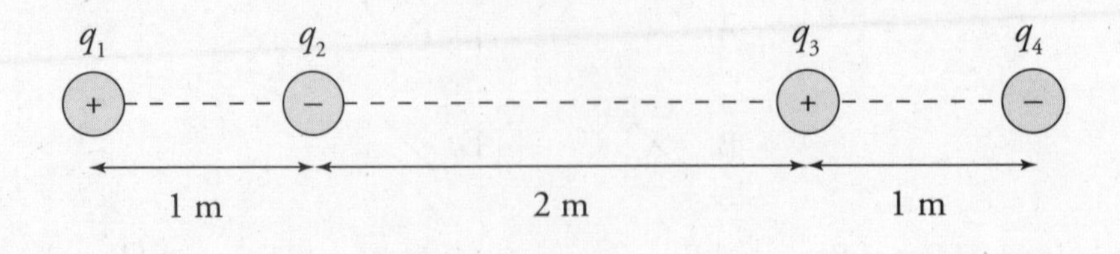

Solution: The individual forces $\mathbf{F}_{\text{1-on-2}}$, $\mathbf{F}_{\text{3-on-2}}$, and $\mathbf{F}_{\text{4-on-2}}$ are shown in the figure below. Notice that $\mathbf{F}_{\text{1-on-2}}$ and $\mathbf{F}_{\text{4-on-2}}$ point to the left, while $\mathbf{F}_{\text{3-on-2}}$ points to the right.

q_1 $\mathbf{F}_{\text{1-on-2}}$ q_2 $\mathbf{F}_{\text{3-on-2}}$ q_3 q_4

$\mathbf{F}_{\text{4-on-2}}$

If we let $q_4 = -x\text{ C}$, then the magnitudes of the individual forces on q_2 are

$$|F_{\text{1-on-2}}| = k_0\frac{q_1|q_2|}{(r_{1-2})^2} = (9\times10^9\ \text{N}\cdot\text{m}^2/\text{C}^2)\frac{(1\text{C})(1\text{nC})}{(1\text{m})^2} = 9\text{N}$$

$$|F_{\text{3-on-2}}| = k_0\frac{q_2|q_3|}{(r_{2-3})^2} = (9\times10^9\ \text{N}\cdot\text{m}^2/\text{C}^2)\frac{(1\text{nC})(8\text{C})}{(2\text{m})^2} = 18\text{N}$$

$$|F_{\text{4-on-2}}| = k_0\frac{q_2|q_4|}{(r_{2-4})^2} = (9\times10^9\ \text{N}\cdot\text{m}^2/\text{C}^2)\frac{(1\text{nC})(x\text{C})}{(3\text{m})^2} = x\text{N}$$

In order for the net electric force on q_2 to be zero, the sum of the magnitudes of $\mathbf{F}_{\text{1-on-2}}$ and $\mathbf{F}_{\text{4-on-2}}$ must be equal to the magnitude of $\mathbf{F}_{\text{3-on-2}}$. That is, 9 N + x N = 18 N so x = 9. Therefore, $q_4 = -x\text{ C} = -9\text{ C}$.

8.3 ELECTRIC FIELDS

There are several advantages to regarding electrical interactions in a slightly different way from the simple "charge Q exerts a force on charge q" mode of thinking. In this more sophisticated interpretation, the very existence of a charge (or a more general distribution of charge) alters the space around it, creating what we call an **electric field** in its vicinity. If a second charge happens to be there or to roam by, it will feel the effect of the field created by the original charge. That is, we think of the electric force on a second charge q as exerted *by the field*, rather than directly by the original charge(s). Qualitatively, we can represent electrical interactions as follows:

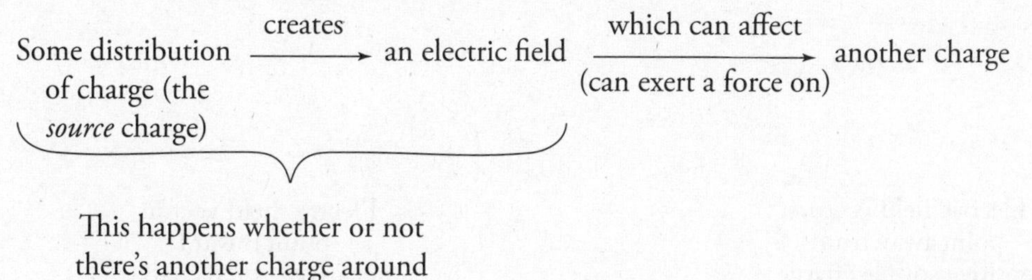

The charge(s) creating the electric field is/are called the **source charge(s)**; they're the source of the electric field. You may like to think of a source charge as a spider and its electric field as the spider's web. After a spider creates a web, when a small insect roams by, it is the web that ensnares the unfortunate bug, not the spider directly.

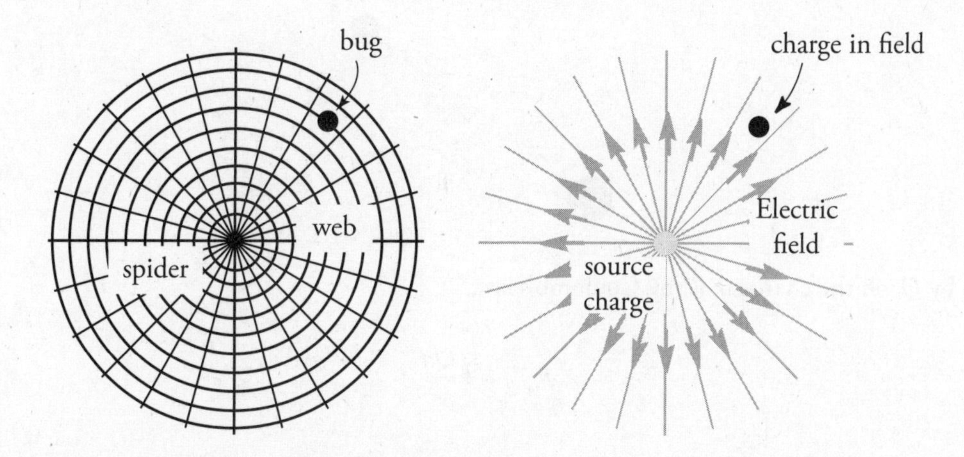

The figure on the right above illustrates one way to picture an electric field, but a few words of explanation are needed. First: An electric field is a **vector field**, which means that at each point in space surrounding the source charge, we associate a specific vector. The length of this vector will tell us the magnitude, or strength, of the field at that point, and the direction of the vector will tell us the direction of the resulting electric force that a *positive* test charge would feel if it were placed at that point. That's the convention: Although the charge that finds itself in an electric field can of course be positive or negative, for purposes of *illustrating* the field, we always think of a *positive* test charge. Because of this convention, *electric field vectors always point away from positive source charges and toward negative ones*. Also, the closer we are to the source charge, the stronger the resulting electric force a test charge would feel (because Coulomb's law is an *inverse*-square law). So, we expect the electric field vectors to be long at points close to the source

8.3

charge and shorter at points farther away. The following figures illustrate the electric field due to a positive source charge and the electric field due to a negative source charge.

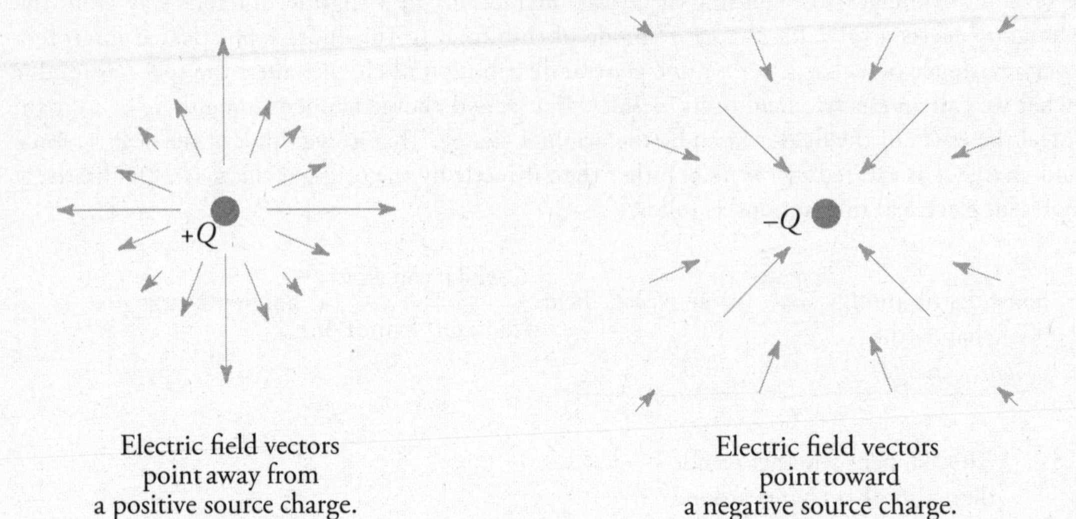

Electric field vectors point away from a positive source charge.

Electric field vectors point toward a negative source charge.

We can use Coulomb's law to find a formula for the strength of the electric field. Remember that a source charge creates an electric field whether or not there's another charge in the field to feel it. It takes *two* charges to create an electric *force*, but it takes only *one* (the source charge) to create an electric *field*. So, let's imagine we have a single source charge, Q, and another charge, q, at a distance r from Q.

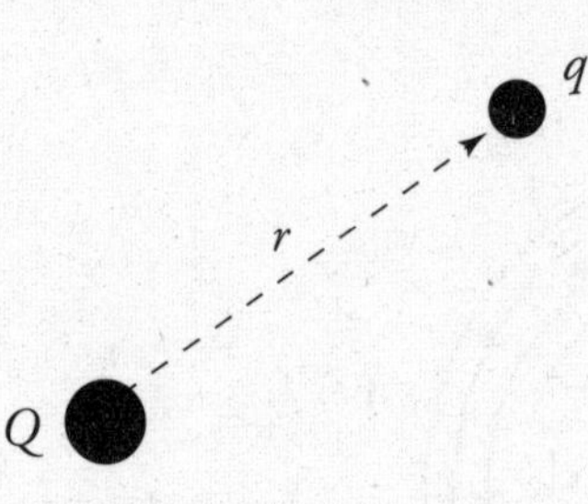

The force by Q, on the charge q, is, by Coulomb's law,

$$F_{\text{by } Q} = k\frac{Qq}{r^2}$$

Now we ask, "What if q weren't there? Do we still have something?" The answer is *yes*, we have the electric field created by the source charge, Q. "So, if q weren't there, what if we removed q from the formula for the force exerted on it by Q? Would we still have something?" The answer is *yes*, we'd have the formula for the electric field, **E**, created by the single source charge Q.

Electric Field

$$E_{\text{by } Q} = k\frac{Q}{r^2}$$

In the formula for the force by Q on q, the variable r represents the distance from Q to q. However, if q is not there, what does r mean now? Answer: It's simply the distance from Q to the point in space where we want to know the electric field vector.

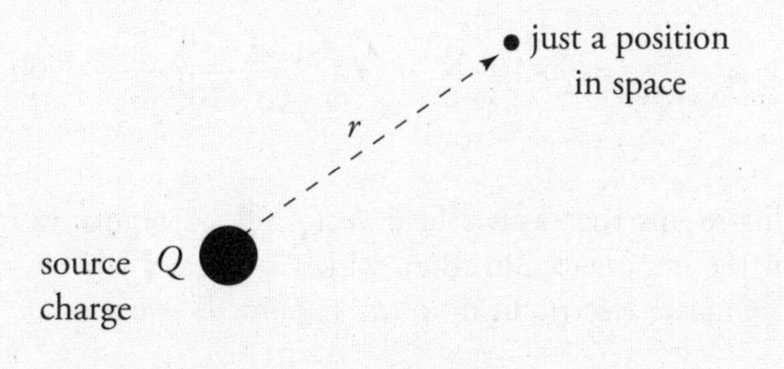

A final note: If we retain the sign of the source charge Q when we use the formula $E = kQ / r^2$, then a positive value for E means that the source charge Q is positive and the electric field vector at that point in space points away from Q; a negative value for E means that the source charge Q is negative and the electric field vector at that point in space points toward Q. (This makes the formula conform to the convention that electric field vectors are always pictured from the point of view of the force that a *positive* test charge would feel.)

Example 8-9: Let $Q = +4$ nC be a charge that is fixed in position at the origin of an x-y coordinate system. What is the magnitude and direction of the electric field at the point (10 cm,0)? At the point (–20 cm,0)?

Solution: In the figure below, the point A is (10 cm,0), which is 10 cm directly to the right of Q, and B is the point (–20 cm,0), which is 20 cm directly to the left of Q.

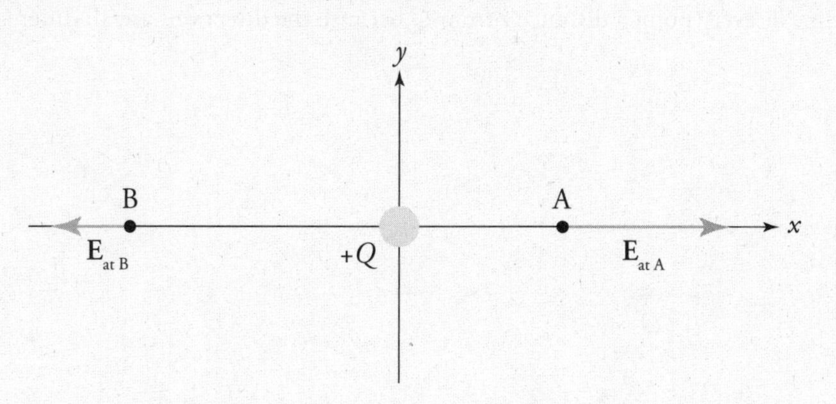

The electric field at point A is

$$E_{\text{at A}} = k_0 \frac{Q}{(r_{\text{to A}})^2} = (9\times10^9\ \text{N}\cdot\text{m}^2/\text{C}^2)\frac{(4\times10^{-9}\ \text{C})}{(10^{-1}\ \text{m})^2} = 3600\ \text{N/C}$$

Since $E_{\text{at A}}$ is positive, this means the electric field vector, $\mathbf{E}_{\text{at A}}$, points away from the source charge. Therefore, $\mathbf{E}_{\text{at A}}$ points in the positive *x* direction, which is usually written as the direction **i**. So, if we wanted to write the complete electric field vector at point A, we'd write $\mathbf{E}_{\text{at A}} = (3600\,\text{N/C})\mathbf{i}$.

The electric field at point B is

$$E_{\text{at B}} = k_0 \frac{Q}{(r_{\text{to B}})^2} = (9\times10^9\ \text{N}\cdot\text{m}^2/\text{C}^2)\frac{(4\times10^{-9}\ \text{C})}{(2\times10^{-1}\ \text{m})^2} = 900\ \text{N/C}$$

Since $E_{\text{at B}}$ is negative, this means the electric field vector, $\mathbf{E}_{\text{at B}}$, points away from the source charge. Therefore, $\mathbf{E}_{\text{at B}}$ points in the negative *x* direction, which is usually written as the direction $-\mathbf{i}$. So, if we wanted to write the complete electric field vector at point B, we'd write $\mathbf{E}_{\text{at B}} = (900\,\text{N/C})(-\mathbf{i})$ or $-(900\,\text{N/C})\mathbf{i}$.

Notice from the formula $E = kQ/r^2$ that the electric field obeys an inverse-square law, like the electric force. So the strength of an electric field from a single source charge decreases as we get farther from the source; in particular, $E \propto 1/r^2$. Also, for a given source charge *Q*, the electric field strength depends only on *r*, the distance from *Q*. So at every point on a circle (or more generally a sphere) of radius *r* centered on the source charge, the electric field strength is the same. In the electric field vector diagram below on the left, all the field vectors at the points on the smaller dashed circle have the same length, indicating that the electric field magnitude is the same at all points on this circle. Similarly, all the field vectors at the points on the larger dashed circle have the same length, indicating that the electric field magnitude is the same at all points on *this* circle. (Note that the field vectors at the points on the larger circle are shorter than those at the points on the smaller circle.) However, notice that the magnitude may be the same at every point on each circle (because they're all the same distance *r* from the source charge) but the directions of the electric field vectors are all different on each circle. Therefore, we're forced to say that the electric field isn't the same at every point a distance *r* from *Q* because the directions are all different.

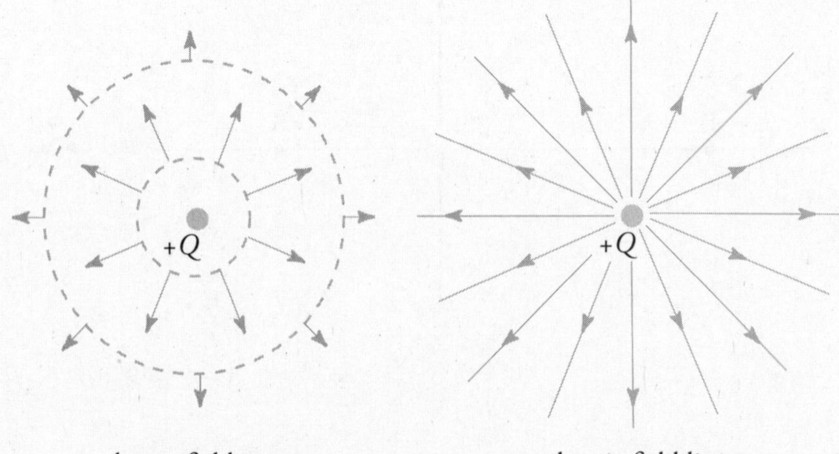

electric field vectors

electric field lines

The diagram on the left above and the two given earlier for the electric field produced by a positive source charge and by a negative source charge show the field represented by individual vectors. However, this is not the easiest way to draw an electric field.

Instead of drawing a bunch of separate vectors, we instead draw *lines* through them, like in the diagram on the right above. This drawing depicts the electric field using **field lines**. The direction of the field is indicated as usual; remember that, by convention, the electric field points away from positive source charges and toward negative ones and indicates the direction of the electric force that a positive test charge would feel if it were placed in the field.

Now that we've eliminated the separate vectors, it seems as though we've lost some information, namely, where the field is strong and where it's weak because we got this information from the lengths of the individual vectors. (Where the vectors were long, the field was strong, and where the vectors were shorter, the field was weaker.) However, we can still get a general idea of where the field is strong and where it's weak by looking at the *density* of the field lines: Where the field lines are cramped close together, the field is stronger; where the field lines are more spread out, the field is weaker.

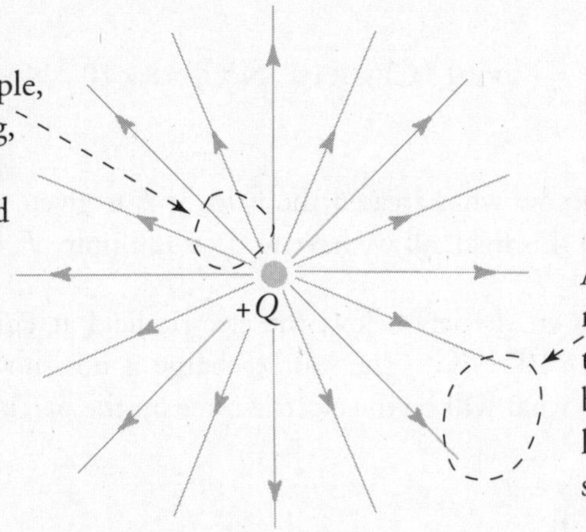

At points in this region, for example, the field is strong, because the field lines are cramped together.

+Q

At points in this region, for example, the field is weaker, becauses the field lines are more spread out.

Now, let's imagine that we have a source charge Q creating an electric field, and another charge, q, roams in to the field. What force will q feel? We want to find an equation for the force on q due to the electric field. Recall the formulas above: $F_{\text{on } q} = kQq / r^2$ and $E_{\text{by } Q} = kQ / r^2$. What would we need to do to E to get F? Just multiply it by q! That is, $F_{\text{on } q} = qE_{\text{by Q}}$. It turns out that this very important formula works not just for the electric field created by a single source charge; it works for *any* electric field:

Electric Force and Field

$$\mathbf{F}_{\text{on } q} = q\mathbf{E}$$

Notice also from this formula that $E = F / q$, so the units of E are N/C, which you saw in Example 8-9. The equation $\mathbf{E} = \mathbf{F} / q$ also gives us the definition of the electric field: It's the force per unit charge.

8.3

Finally, before we get to some more examples, realize that we've had two important (boxed) formulas in this section on the electric field: $E = kQ / r^2$ and $\mathbf{F} = q\mathbf{E}$. In the first formula, Q is the charge that *makes* the field, while in the second formula, q is the charge that *feels* the field.

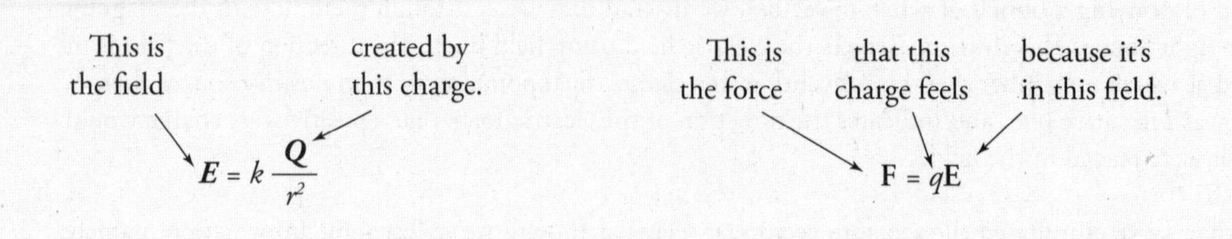

Example 8-10: A particle with charge $q = 2\ \mu\text{C}$ is placed at a point where the electric field has magnitude 4×10^4 N/C. What will be the strength of the electric force on the particle?

Solution: From the equation $F_{\text{on } q} = qE$, we find that

$$F = (2\times10^{-6}\ \text{C})(4\times10^{4}\ \text{N/C}) = 8\times10^{-2}\ \text{N}$$

Notice that we didn't need to know what created the field. If E is given, and the question asks for the force that some charge q feels in this field, all we have to do is multiply, $F = qE$, and we're done.

Example 8-11: In the diagram on the left below, the electric field at Point A points in the positive y direction and has magnitude 5×10^6 N/C. (The source charge is not shown.) If a particle with charge $q = -3\,\text{nC}$ is placed at point A, what will be the electric force on the particle?

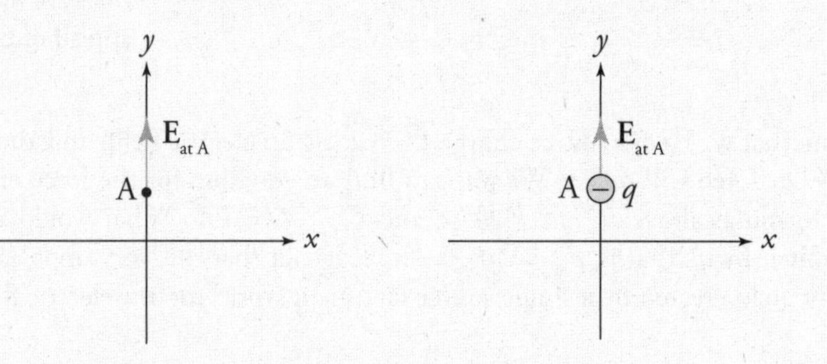

Solution: $\mathbf{E}_{\text{at A}}$ points in the positive y direction, which is usually written as the direction $\mathbf{j}$, so $\mathbf{E}_{\text{at A}} = (5\times10^6\ \text{N/C})\mathbf{j}$. The equation $\mathbf{F}_{\text{on g}} = q\mathbf{E}$ then gives us

$$\mathbf{F} = (-3\times10^{-9}\ \text{C})(5\times10^{6}\ \tfrac{\text{N}}{\text{C}})\text{j} = (1.5\times10^{-2}\ \text{N})(-\text{j})$$

That is, the force will have magnitude 1.5×10^{-2} N and point in the negative y direction ($-\mathbf{j}$). Notice that whenever q is negative, the force $F_{\text{on } q}$ will always point in the direction *opposite* to the electric field.

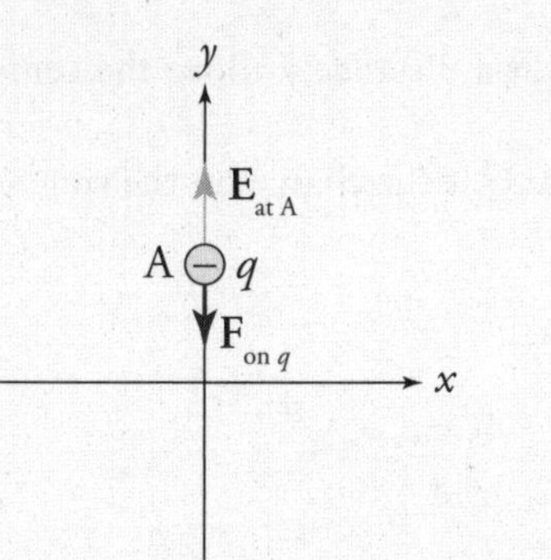

Example 8-12: A particle of mass m and charge q is placed at a point where the electric field is **E**. If the particle is released from rest, find its initial acceleration, **a**.

Solution: The acceleration of the particle is the force it feels divided by its mass: **a** = **F**/m. Because **F** = q**E**, we get

$$\mathbf{a} = \frac{\mathbf{F}}{m} = \frac{q\mathbf{E}}{m}$$

Notice that if q is negative, then **F** (and, consequently, **a**) will be directed *opposite* to the electric field **E**. Also, the question asked only for the *initial* acceleration, because once the particle starts moving, it will most likely move through locations where the electric field is different (in magnitude or direction or both), so the force on the particle will change; and if the force on the particle changes, so will the acceleration.

Example 8-13: The magnitude of the electric field at a distance r from a source charge $+Q$ is equal to E. What will be the magnitude of the electric field at a distance $4r$ from a source charge $+2Q$?

Solution: The first sentence tells us that $kQ/r^2 = E$. Now, if we change Q to $2Q$ and r to $4r$, we find that E decreases by a factor of 8, because

$$E' = k\frac{Q'}{(r')^2} = k\frac{2Q}{(4r)^2} = \frac{2}{16}\cdot k\frac{Q}{r^2} = \frac{1}{8}E$$

Example 8-14: The electric field at a distance y above the center of a ring of charge is given by the formula $E = k_0 Qy / (y^2 + R^2)^{\frac{3}{2}}$, where Q is the charge on the ring and R is its radius.

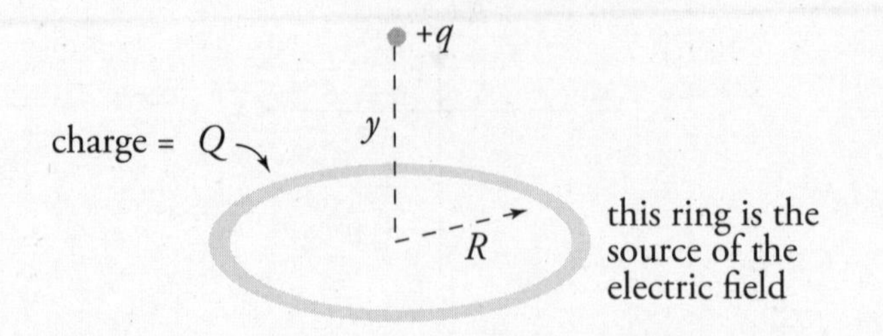

If Q = +25 mC and R = 3 m, find the force that a charge q = +25/9 nC would feel if it were placed at y = 4 m.

Solution: Even though the source of the electric field is not a point charge, we can still use the formula $F = qE$:

$$
\begin{aligned}
F &= q \cdot E \\
&= q \cdot k_0 \frac{Qy}{(y^2 + R^2)^{\frac{3}{2}}} \\
&= (\tfrac{25}{9} \times 10^{-9}\ \text{C}) \cdot (9 \times 10^9\ \text{N} \cdot \text{m}^2/\text{C}^2) \frac{(25 \times 10^{-3}\ \text{C})(4\ \text{m})}{[(4\ \text{m})^2 + (3\ \text{m})^2]^{\frac{3}{2}}} \\
&= (25\ \text{N} \cdot \text{m}^2/\text{C}) \frac{(10^{-1})\ \text{C} \cdot \text{m}}{(5^3)\ \text{m}^3} \\
&= 2 \times 10^{-2}\ \text{N}
\end{aligned}
$$

The Principle of Superposition for Electric Fields

The pictures we've drawn so far have been of electric fields created by a single source charge. However, we can also have two or more charges whose electric fields overlap, creating one combined field. For example, let's consider an **electric dipole**, which, by definition, is a pair of equal but opposite charges:

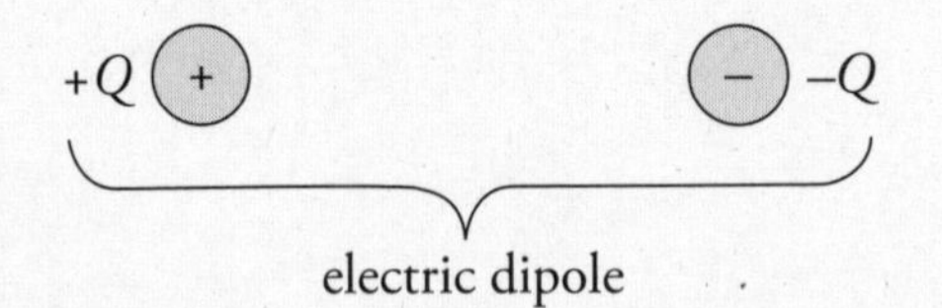

What if we regarded *both* of them as source charges; how would we find the electric field that they create together? By using the principle of superposition. If we wanted to find the electric field vector at, say, the point P in the diagram below,

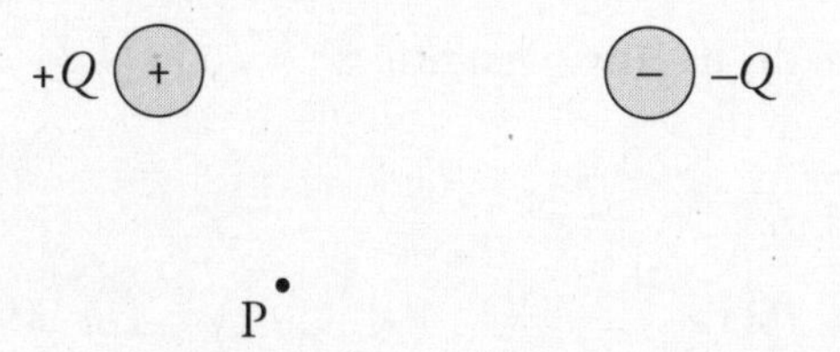

we'd first find the electric field vector, $\mathbf{E}_+$, at P due to the $+Q$ charge alone (ignoring the presence of the $-Q$ charge) and then we'd find the electric field vector, $\mathbf{E}_-$, at P due to the $-Q$ charge alone (ignoring the presence of the $+Q$ charge). The net electric field vector at P will then be the vector sum, $\mathbf{E}_+ + \mathbf{E}_-$.

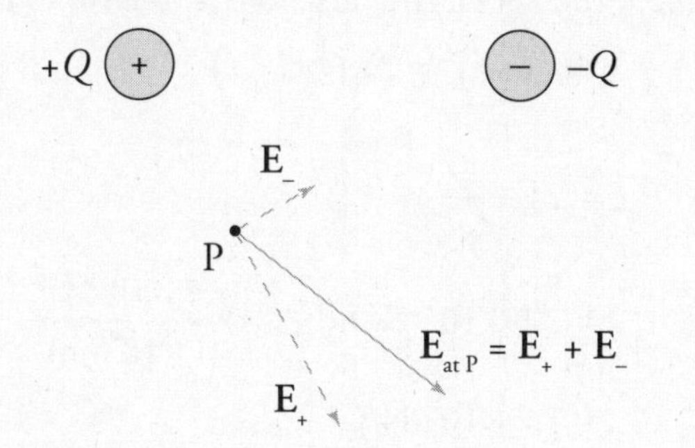

We can do this for as many points as we like and obtain a diagram of the electric field as a collection of vectors. The diagram in terms of electric field lines would look like this:

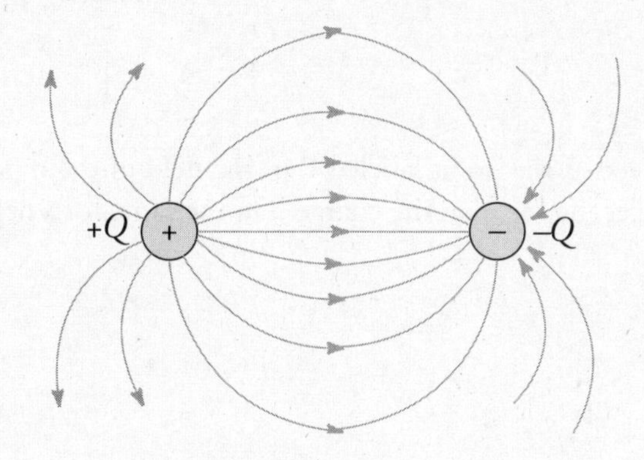

Notice that between the charges, where the field lines are dense, the field is strong; and as we move away from the charges, the field lines get more spread out, indicating that the field gets weaker.

Example 8-15: An electric dipole consists of two charges, $+Q$ and $-Q$, where $Q = 4\ \mu\text{C}$, separated by a distance of $d = 20$ cm. Find the electric field at the point midway between the charges.

Solution: The electric field at P due to the positive charge is $E_+ = k_0 Q / \left(\frac{1}{2}d\right)^2$, pointing away from $+Q$, and the electric field at P due to the negative charge is $E_- = k_0 Q / \left(\frac{1}{2}d\right)^2$, pointing toward $-Q$ (which is in the same direction as $\mathbf{E}_+$).

By the principle of superposition, the net electric field at P is the sum: $\mathbf{E} = \mathbf{E}_+ + \mathbf{E}_-$. The magnitude of $E_{\text{at P}}$ is $E_+ + E_- = k_0 Q / \left(\frac{1}{2}d\right)^2 + k_0 Q / \left(\frac{1}{2}d\right)^2 = 2k_0 Q / \left(\frac{1}{2}d\right)^2$:

$$
\begin{aligned}
E &= 2k_0 \frac{Q}{\left(\frac{1}{2}d\right)^2} \\
&= 2(9\times10^9\ \text{N}\cdot\text{m}^2/\text{C}^2)\frac{4\times10^{-6}\ \text{C}}{(1\times10^{-1}\ \text{m})^2} \\
&= 7.2\times10^6\ \text{N/C}
\end{aligned}
$$

The direction of $\mathbf{E}_{\text{at P}}$ is away from $+Q$ and toward $-Q$:

Example 8-16: A positive charge, $+q$, is placed at the point labeled P in the field of the dipole shown below. Describe the direction of the resulting electric force on the charge. Do the same for a negative charge, $-q$, placed at the point labeled N.

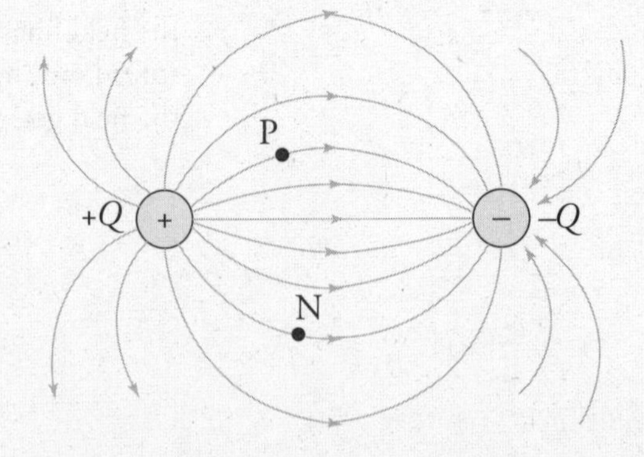

Solution: The electric field vector at any point is always *tangent* to the field line passing through that point and its direction is the same as that of the field line. Since $\mathbf{F} = q\mathbf{E}$, the force on a positive charge is in the same direction as $\mathbf{E}$ and the force on a negative charge is in the opposite direction from $\mathbf{E}$. The directions of $\mathbf{F}_{\text{on }+q}$ and $\mathbf{F}_{\text{on }-q}$ are shown in the figure below.

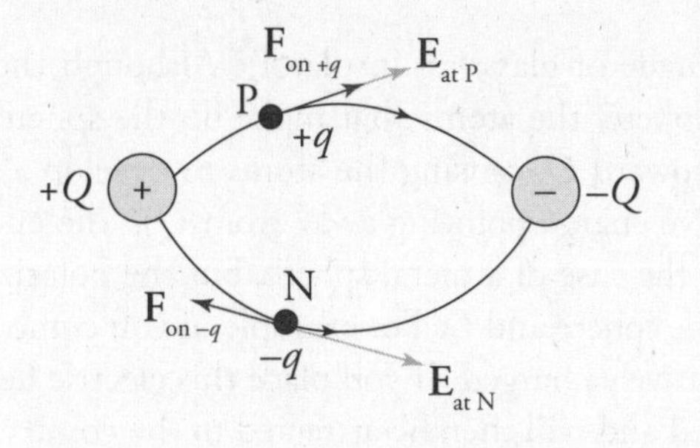

Conductors, Insulators, and Polarization

Most everyday materials can be classified into one of two major categories: *conductors* or *insulators* (also known as *dielectrics*). A material is a **conductor** if it contains charges that are free to roam throughout the material. Metals are the classic and most important conductors. In a metal, one or more valence electrons per atom are not strongly bound to any particular atom and are thus free to roam. If a metal is placed in an electric field, these free charges (called **conduction electrons**) will move in response to the field. Another example of a conductor would be a solution that contains lots of dissolved ions (such as saltwater).

Here's an interesting property of conductors: Imagine that we place a whole bunch of electrons on a piece of metal. It's now negatively charged. Since electrons repel each other, they'll want to get as far away from each other as possible. As a result, all this excess charge moves (rapidly) to the surface. Any net charge on a conductor resides on its surface. Since there's no excess charge within the body of the conductor, there cannot be an electrostatic field inside a conductor. You can block out external electric fields simply by surrounding yourself with metal; the free charges in the metal will move to the surface to shield the interior and keep **E** = 0 inside.

By contrast, an **insulator** (**dielectric**) is a material that doesn't have free charges. Electrons are tightly bound to their atoms and thus are not free to roam throughout the material. Common insulators include rubber, glass, wood, paper, and plastic.

Now, let's study this situation: Start with a neutral metal sphere and bring a charge (a positive charge) Q nearby without touching the original metal sphere. What will happen? The positive charge will attract free electrons in the metal, leaving the far side of the sphere positively charged. Since the negative charge is closer to Q than the positive charge, there'll be a net attraction between Q and the sphere. So, even though the sphere as a whole is electrically neutral, the separation of charge induced by the presence of Q will create a force of electrical attraction between them.

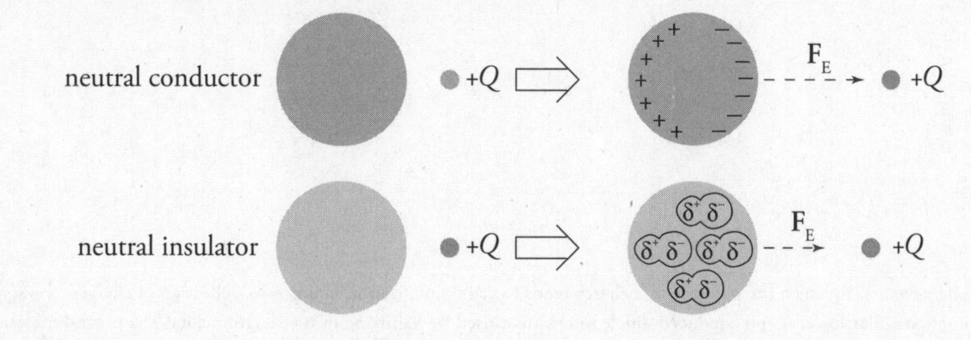

Now what if the sphere was made of glass (an insulator)? Although there aren't free electrons that can move to the near side of the sphere, the atoms that make up the sphere will become **polarized**. That is, their electrons will feel a tug toward *Q*, causing the atoms to develop a partial negative charge pointing toward *Q* (and a partial positive charge pointing away from *Q*). The effect isn't as dramatic as the mass movement of free electrons in the case of a metal sphere, but the polarization is still enough to cause an electrical attraction between the sphere and *Q*. For example, if you comb your hair, the comb will pick up extra electrons, making it negatively charged. If you place this electric field source near little bits of paper, the paper will become polarized and will then be attracted to the comb.[2]

8.4 ELECTRIC POTENTIAL

So far, we have viewed the electric field due to a source charge (or a more general charge distribution, such as a pair of charges, a ring, or a plate) as a collection of vectors. This point of view allowed us to answer questions about other *vector* quantities, like force and acceleration. The basic equations for finding these quantities were $\mathbf{F} = q\mathbf{E}$ and $\mathbf{a} = \mathbf{F}/m = q\mathbf{E}/m$.

What if we wanted to answer questions about *scalar* quantities, like energy, work, or speed? It turns out that the easiest way to answer these questions is to view the electric field in a different way, in terms of a scalar field. That is, instead of thinking of a vector at each point in the space around a source charge, we'll think of a scalar (just a *number*) at each point in space around a source charge. This scalar has a name: it's called **electric potential** (or just **potential** for short).

Let *Q* be a point source charge. At any point P that's a distance *r* from *Q*, we say that the electric potential at P is the scalar given by this formula:

Electric Potential

$$\phi = k\frac{Q}{r}$$

---

[2] The same phenomenon, in which the presence of a charge tends to cause polarization in a nearby collection of charges, is responsible for a kind of intermolecular force: Dipole-induced dipole forces are caused by a shifting of the electron cloud of a neutral molecule toward positively charged ions or away from a negatively charged ion; in each case, the resulting force between the ion and the atom is attractive.

The **London dispersion force**, in which electrically neutral molecules temporarily induce polarization in each other, is a much weaker version of the same phenomenon—again, electron clouds shift a little bit to create dipoles.

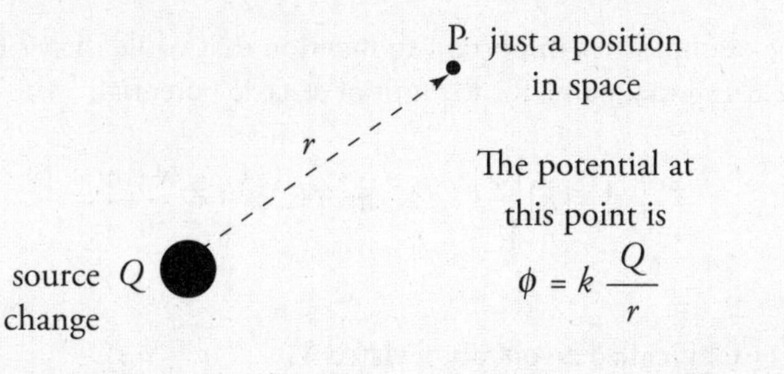

Notice the differences between this formula and the one for the electric field. First, the potential is kQ divided by r, while the electric field is kQ divided by r^2. Second, the electric field has a specific direction at each point (because it's a vector quantity); the potential, on the other hand, is not a vector, so it has no direction. While the electric field has the same magnitude at every point a distance r from Q, the field has a different direction at every point on the circle (or, more generally, the sphere) of radius r centered on Q. Therefore, we're forced to say that the electric field isn't the same at every point a distance r from Q because the directions are all different. The potential, however, is easier because it has no direction: The potential *is* the same at every point that's a distance r from Q.

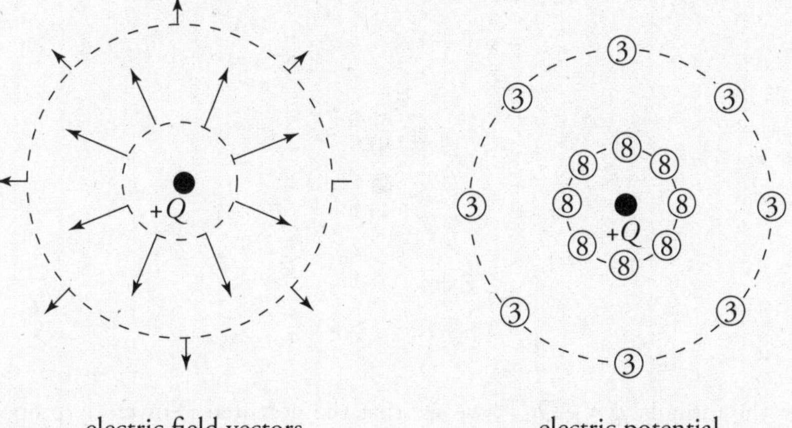

electric field vectors   electric potential

The dashed circles shown in the figure on the right above are called **equipotentials** ("equal potentials"), because the potential is the same at every point on them. For example, the potential is equal to 8 units everywhere on the inner dashed circle, and equal to 3 units everywhere on the outer dashed circle. As we move around on either dashed circle, the electric field changes (because the direction of **E** changes), but the potential doesn't change.

The formula given above for the potential, $\phi = kQ/r$, assumes that the potential decreases to 0 as we move far away from the source charges (that is, as $r \to \infty$); this is the standard, conventional assumption. With this formula, you can see that if Q is a positive charge, then the values of the potential due to this source charge are also positive (if Q is positive, then kQ/r is positive); on the other hand, the values of the potential due to a negative source charge are negative (if Q is negative, then kQ/r is negative). The sign of the potential (that is, whether it's positive or negative) is not an indication of a direction; remember, potential is a scalar, so it has no direction.

Before we get to some examples, it's important to mention that while there's no special name for the unit of electric field, there *is* a special name for the unit of electric potential:

$$[\phi]=[k]\frac{[Q]}{[r]}=(\text{N}\cdot\text{m}^2/\text{C}^2)\frac{\text{C}}{\text{m}}=\frac{\text{N}\cdot\text{m}}{\text{C}}=\frac{\text{J}}{\text{C}}$$

A joule per coulomb (J/C) is called a **volt**, abbreviated V.

Example 8-17: What is the electric potential at a distance of $r = 30$ cm from a source charge $Q = -20$ nC ?

Solution: Using the formula $\phi = k_0 Q / r$, we find that

$$\phi = k_0\frac{Q}{r}=(9\times10^9\ \text{N}\cdot\text{m}^2/\text{C}^2)\frac{-20\times10^{-9}\ \text{C}}{30\times10^{-2}\ \text{m}}=-600\ \text{V}$$

Example 8-18: In the figure below, the potential at Point A is 1,000 V. What's the potential at Point B ?

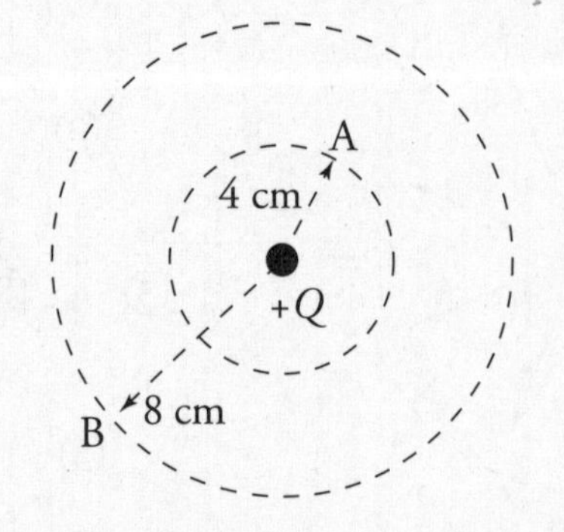

Solution: From the formula $\phi = k_0 Q / r$, we see that the potential is inversely proportional to *r*: Thus, $\phi \propto 1/r$. Because the distance from *Q* to B is twice the distance from *Q* to A, the potential at B should be half the potential at A. Therefore, $\phi_{\text{at B}} = 500\ \text{V}$. (Notice that because the potential at A is 1,000 V, the potential at *every* point on the inner circle is 1,000 V; and since the potential at B is 500 V, the potential at *every* point on the outer circle is 500 V.)

Now that we know how to calculate electric potential, how do we use it to answer questions about the scalar quantities energy, work, and speed? The applications of electric potential all follow from this one fundamental equation:

Change in Electrical Potential Energy

$$\Delta PE = q\Delta\phi = qV$$

That is, the change in potential energy of a charge *q* that moves between two points whose potential difference is $\Delta\phi$ is just given by the product, $q\Delta\phi$; it also can be expressed as *qV*, where *V* is defined in the change in potential and is known as the *voltage*. For example, let's say a charge $q = +0.03\text{C}$ moves from a point on the inner circle to a point on the outer circle in the figure accompanying the preceding example:

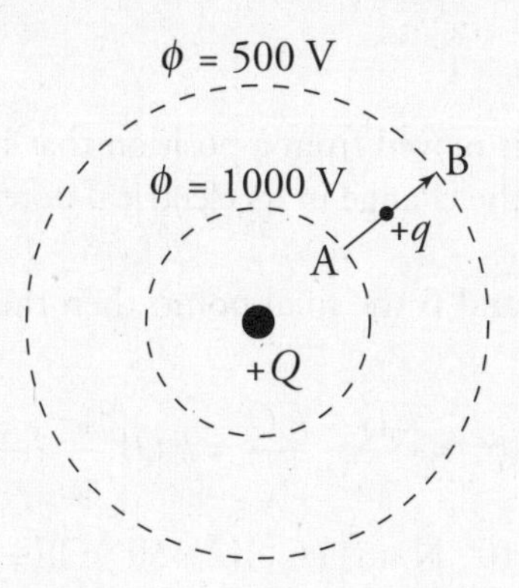

Then the change in the electrical potential energy of the charge q is

$$\Delta PE_{\text{A}\to\text{B}} = q\Delta\phi_{\text{A}\to\text{B}} = q(\phi_{\text{B}} - \phi_{\text{A}}) = (+0.03\text{C})(500\,\text{V} - 1000\,\text{V}) = -15\,\text{J}$$

We expected that the change in potential energy would be negative (that is, the potential energy would decrease), because the positive charge is moving farther from the positive source charge; because q moves in a way it naturally "wants" to move (since the positive charge q is naturally repelled by the positive charge Q), its potential energy should decrease.

If the charge q were instead pushed (by some outside force) from Point B to Point A, then its potential energy would increase:

$$\Delta PE_{\text{B}\to\text{A}} = q\Delta\phi_{\text{B}\to\text{A}} = q(\phi_{\text{A}} - \phi_{\text{B}}) = (+0.03\text{C})(1000\,\text{V} - 500\,\text{V}) = +15\,\text{J}$$

What if the charge q were moved from one point on the outer circle (Point B, say) to another point on the outer circle, B′?

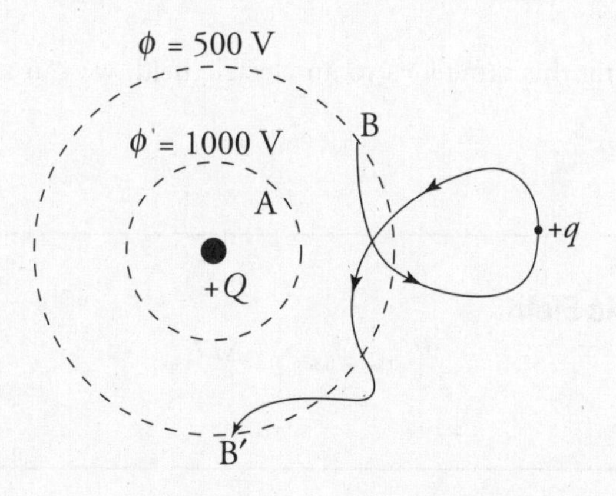

Its potential energy would not change. Because the potential is the same everywhere on the outer circle, the potential at B is the same as the potential at B′, so the potential *difference* between Points B and B′ is zero; and if $\Delta\phi = 0$, then $\Delta PE = 0$ as well. *A charge experiences no change in potential energy when its initial and final positions are at the same potential.*

The figure above also illustrates that the path taken by the charge is irrelevant. Like the gravitational force, the electric force is conservative; all that matters is where the charge began and where it ended; the specific path it takes doesn't matter.

Example 8-19: A charge $q = -8$ nC is moved from a position that's 10 cm from a charge $Q = +2$ μC to a position that's 20 cm away. What is the change in its electrical potential energy?

Solution: Let A be the initial point and B the final point; then the change in potential from Point A to Point B is

$$\Delta\phi = \phi_B - \phi_A = \frac{k_0 Q}{r_B} - \frac{k_0 Q}{r_A} = k_0 Q\left(\frac{1}{r_B} - \frac{1}{r_A}\right)$$
$$= (9\times10^9\ \text{N}\cdot\text{m}^2/\text{C}^2)(2\times10^{-6}\ \text{C})\left(\frac{1}{0.2\ \text{m}} - \frac{1}{0.1\ \text{m}}\right)$$
$$= -9\times10^4\ \text{V}$$

Therefore, the change in potential energy of the charge q is

$$\Delta PE = q\Delta\phi = (-8\times10^{-9}\ \text{C})(-9\times10^4\ \text{V}) = 7.2\times10^{-4}\ \text{J}$$

Now that we've seen examples of how to calculate changes in potential energy in an electric field by using the concept of electric potential, how do we answer questions about work or kinetic energy? By using equations we already know from mechanics.

What if we want to find the work done by the electric field as a charge moves? If we move objects around in a *gravitational* field, we remember that the change in gravitational potential energy is equal to the opposite of the work done by the gravitational field. That is, $\Delta PE_{\text{grav}} = -W_{\text{by gravity}}$, which is the same as $W_{\text{by gravity}} = -\Delta PE_{\text{grav}}$. Applying this same idea to an electric field, we can say that the work done by the electric field is equal to $-\Delta PE_{\text{elec}}$:

Work Done by Electric Field

$$W_{\text{by electric field}} = -\Delta PE_{\text{elec}}$$

Now what about kinetic energy? Well, if there's no friction (which will be the case for charges moving around in empty space) or other forces doing work as a charge moves, then mechanical energy is conserved; that is, $KE + PE$ will remain constant. And if $KE + PE$ is constant, then $\Delta(KE + PE)$ will be zero.

That is, ΔKE will be equal to $-\Delta PE$. Since we know how to calculate ΔPE, we can calculate ΔKE by just changing the sign of ΔPE:

$$\Delta KE = -\Delta PE$$

So, as long as you remember the fundamental formula for potential energy changes in an electric field, $\Delta PE = q\Delta\phi$, you can answer questions about work or kinetic energy in an electric field by just using the formulas above.

Example 8-20: In the figure below, a particle whose charge q is +4 nC moves in the electric field created by a negative source charge, $-Q$.

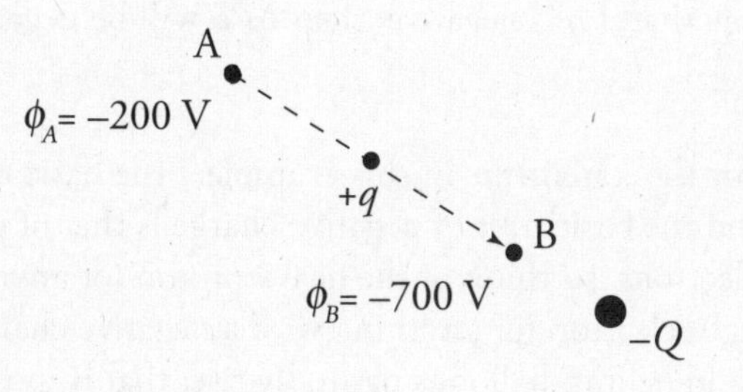

Find:

a) the change in potential energy,
b) the work done by the electric field, and
c) the change in kinetic energy of the particle as it moves from position A to position B.
d) If the mass of the particle is 10^{-8} kg and it started from rest at Point A, what will be its speed as it passes through Point B?

Solution:

a) $\Delta PE = q\Delta\phi = q(\phi_B - \phi_A) = (4\times10^{-9}\text{ C})[(-700\text{ V})-(-200\text{ V})]$
$= -2\times10^{-6}\text{ J}$

b) $W_{\text{by electric field}} = -\Delta PE_{\text{elec}} = -(-2\times10^{-6}\text{ J}) = 2\times10^{-6}\text{ J}$

c) $\Delta KE = -\Delta PE_{\text{elec}} = -(-2\times10^{-6}\text{ J}) = +2\times10^{-6}\text{ J}$

d) If the particle started from rest at Point A, then $KE_{\text{at B}} = \Delta KE = +2\times10^{-6}\text{ J}$, so

$$\frac{1}{2}mv_B^2 = 2\times10^{-6}\text{ J} \rightarrow v_B^2 = \frac{2(2\times10^{-6}\text{ J})}{m} \rightarrow v_B = \sqrt{\frac{4\times10^{-6}\text{ J}}{10^{-8}\text{ kg}}} = \sqrt{400\text{ m}^2/\text{s}^2} = 20\text{ m/s}$$

Example 8-21: Verify these statements:

a) Positive charges spontaneously accelerate (increase in kinetic energy) when they move toward a point of lower potential.
b) Negative charges spontaneously accelerate (increase in kinetic energy) when they move toward a point of higher potential.

Solution:

a) A charge will acquire more kinetic energy if it loses potential energy; that is, ΔKE will be positive if ΔPE is negative. So statement (a) is equivalent to this one: "A positive charge loses potential energy when it moves to a point of lower potential." To see that this is correct, notice first that if the charge moves to a point of lower potential, then the potential decreases, so $\Delta\phi$ is negative. It's now easy to see that if q is positive, then ΔPE will indeed be negative here, since $\Delta PE = q\Delta\phi = (+)(-) = (-)$.
b) Here, we want to show that if q is negative, then ΔPE will be negative if $\Delta\phi$ is positive. Thus, $\Delta PE = q\Delta\phi = (-)(+) = (-)$.

Here's a mnemonic for the statements in this example: The basic unit of positive charge is that of the proton, and the basic unit of negative charge is that of the electron. Protons are much heavier than electrons, so think of the heavy proton (or anything with a positive charge) like a rock and the light electron (or anything with a negative charge) like a helium balloon. Rocks naturally fall and helium balloons naturally rise; that is, positive charges naturally fall (to points at lower potential), while negative charges naturally rise (to points at higher potential).

Example 8-22: An electric field pulls an electron from one position to another such that the change in potential is +1 V. By how much does the electron's kinetic energy change?

Solution: The change in potential energy is

$$\Delta PE = q\Delta\phi = (-1.6\times10^{-19}\text{ C})(+1\text{ V}) = -1.6\times10^{-19}\text{ J}$$

so the change in kinetic energy is the opposite of this, $+1.6\times10^{-19}$ J. This amount of energy is known as 1 **electron volt** (eV). In fact, the abbreviation for this unit makes the definition easy to remember: An electron (e^-) moving through a potential difference of 1 V experiences a kinetic energy change of $-q\Delta\phi = (e)(1\text{ V}) = 1.6\times10^{-19}\text{ J} = 1\text{ eV}$. While the joule is the SI unit for energy, it's too big to be convenient when discussing atomic-sized systems. The electron volt is commonly used instead.

Example 8-23: An electric field pushes a proton from one position to another such that the change in potential is –500 V. By how much does the kinetic energy of the proton increase, in electron volts?

Solution: The change in potential energy is

$$\Delta PE = q\Delta\phi = (+e)(-500\text{ V}) = -500\text{ eV}$$

so the change in kinetic energy, ΔKE, is $-\Delta PE = -(-500\text{ eV}) = +500\text{ eV}$.

The Principle of Superposition for Electric Potential

The formula $\phi = kQ/r$ tells us how to find the potential due to a single point source charge, Q. To find the potential in an electric field that's created by more than one charge, we use the principle of superposition. In fact, applying this principle is even easier here than for electric forces and fields because potential is a scalar. When we add up individual potentials, we're simply adding numbers; we're not adding vectors.

Let's illustrate with an example. In the figure below, the source charges Q_1 = +10 nC and Q_2 = –5 nC are fixed in the positions shown; the charges and the two points, A and B, form the vertices of a rectangle. What is the potential at Point A? At Point B?

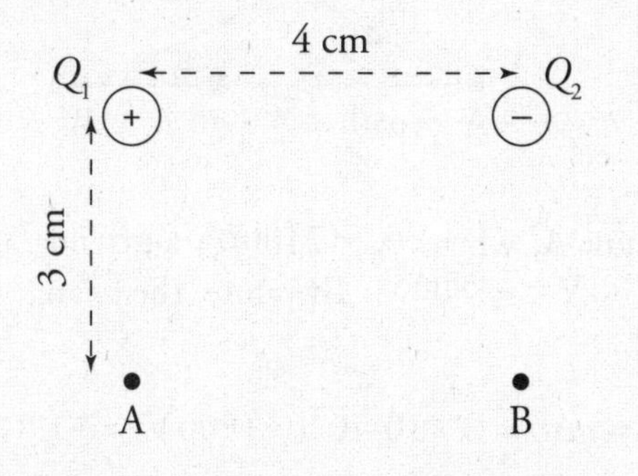

The potential at Point A due to Q_1 alone (ignoring the presence of Q_2) is

$$\phi_{A1} = k_0 \frac{Q_1}{r_{A1}} = (9 \times 10^9\ \text{N} \cdot \text{m}^2/\text{C}^2)\frac{+10 \times 10^{-9}\ \text{C}}{3 \times 10^{-2}\ \text{m}} = 3000\ \text{V}$$

Since Point A is 5 cm from Q_2 (it's the hypotenuse of a 3-4-5 right triangle), the potential at Point A due to Q_2 alone (ignoring the presence of Q_1) is

$$\phi_{A2} = k_0 \frac{Q_2}{r_{A2}} = (9 \times 10^9\ \text{N} \cdot \text{m}^2/\text{C}^2)\frac{-5 \times 10^{-9}\ \text{C}}{5 \times 10^{-2}\ \text{m}} = -900\ \text{V}$$

Therefore, the total electric potential at Point A, due to both source charges, is

$$\phi_A = \phi_{A1} + \phi_{A2} = (3000\ \text{V}) + (-900\ \text{V}) = 2100\ \text{V}$$

Similarly, the total electric potential at Point B is

$$\begin{aligned}
\phi_B = \phi_{B1} + \phi_{B2} &= k_0 \frac{Q_1}{r_{B1}} + k_0 \frac{Q_2}{r_{B2}} \\
&= (9 \times 10^9\ \text{N} \cdot \text{m}^2/\text{C}^2)\frac{+10 \times 10^{-9}\ \text{C}}{5 \times 10^{-2}\ \text{m}} + (9 \times 10^9\ \text{N} \cdot \text{m}^2/\text{C}^2)\frac{-5 \times 10^{-9}\ \text{C}}{3 \times 10^{-2}\ \text{m}} \\
&= (1800\ \text{V}) + (-1500\ \text{V}) \\
&= 300\ \text{V}
\end{aligned}$$

Example 8-24: A charge $q = 1$ nC is moved from position A to position B, along the path labeled *a* in the figure below. Find the work done by the electric field. How would your answer change if *q* had been moved from position A to position B, along the path labeled *b*?

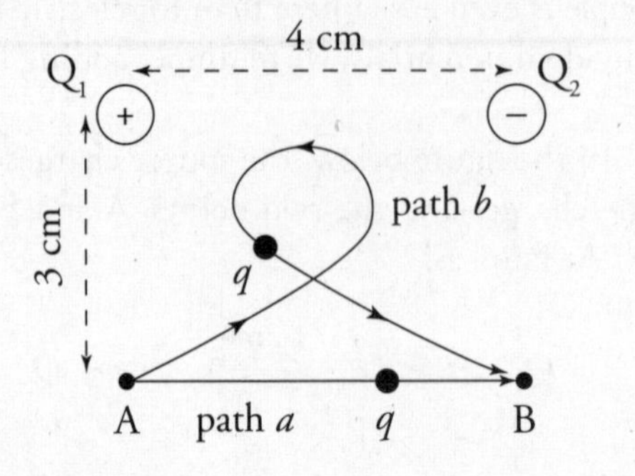

Solution: Path *a* begins at Point A, where $\phi_A = 2100\,\text{V}$, and ends at Point B, where $\phi_B = 300\,\text{V}$, so $\Delta\phi_{A\to B} = \phi_B - \phi_A = 300\,\text{V} - 2100\,\text{V} = -1800\,\text{V}$. Therefore, the change in potential energy of the charge *q* is

$$\Delta PE = q\Delta\phi = (1\times10^{-9}\,\text{C})(-1800\,\text{V}) = -1.8\times10^{-6}\,\text{J}$$

This means that the work done by the electric field, $W_{\text{by E}}$, is equal to $-\Delta PE = 1.8\times10^{-6}\,\text{J}$. If *q* had followed path *b*, the change in potential energy and the work done by the electric field would have been the same as for path *a*. The shape or length of the path is irrelevant; all that matters is the initial point and the ending point, and both paths begin at Point A and end at Point B.

We can't use the formula "work = force × distance" here, because the force is not constant during the object's displacement. To calculate work in an electric field, we use electric potential and the formula $W_{\text{by E}} = -\Delta PE_{\text{elec}}$.

Example 8-25: The figure below shows two source charges, $+2Q$ and $-Q$. What is the minimum amount of work that must be done by some outside force against the electric field to move a negative charge, $-q$, from position A to position B along the semicircular path shown?

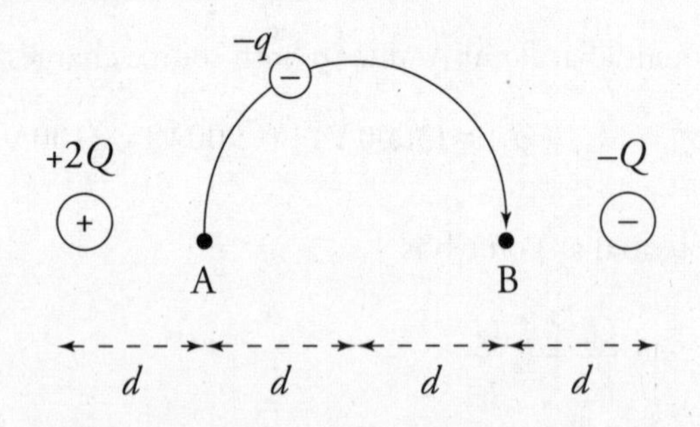

Solution: First, remember that neither the shape nor the length of the path matters; the fact that the path is a semicircle is irrelevant. All that matters is the initial point and the ending point of the path. Using the principle of superposition, the potentials at Points A and B are

$$\phi_A = \frac{k(+2Q)}{d} + \frac{k(-Q)}{3d} = \frac{5kQ}{3d} \quad \text{and} \quad \phi_B = \frac{k(+2Q)}{3d} + \frac{k(-Q)}{d} = -\frac{kQ}{3d}$$

Therefore, the change in potential energy of the charge $-q$ as it's moved from A to B is

$$\Delta PE = (-q)(\phi_B - \phi_A) = (-q)\left(\frac{-kQ}{3d} - \frac{5kQ}{3d}\right) = \frac{2kQq}{d}$$

Since the change in *PE* is positive, we know that the charge $-q$ is not moving as it would naturally on its own (after all, we can see from the figure that it's being moved from a point near a positive source charge, to which it's attracted, to a point near a negative charge, from which it's repelled). Therefore, some outside force is pushing this charge, doing work against the electric field. Since the work done *by* the electric field is $-\Delta PE = -2kQq / d$, the work done *against* the electric field by some outside force must be the opposite of this: $2kQq / d$.

Example 8-26: An electric dipole consists of a pair of equal but opposite charges, $+Q$ and $-Q$, separated by a distance *d*. What is the electric potential at the point (call it P) that's midway between these source charges?

Solution: The potential at P due to the positive charge alone is $k(+Q)/(\frac{1}{2}d)$, and the potential at P due to the negative charge alone is $k(-Q)/(\frac{1}{2}d)$. Adding these, we get zero, which is the potential at P due to both charges. (Notice that although the potential at P is zero, the electric field at P is *not* zero. We can have the "opposite" situation as well; that is, it's possible to have a point where the electric field is zero, but the potential is not. For example, if we had two equal source charges of the *same* sign, say $+Q$ and $+Q$, separated by a distance *d*, then the potential at the point that's midway between them would not be zero [it would be $2k(+Q)/(\frac{1}{2}d)$] but the electric field there *would* be zero.)

Example 8-27: An electric dipole consists of a pair of equal but opposite charges, $+Q$ and $-Q$, separated by a distance *d*. The dashed curves in the figure below are equipotentials. (Notice that the equipotentials are always perpendicular to the electric field lines, wherever they intersect. This is true for *any* electrostatic field, not just for the field created by a dipole.)

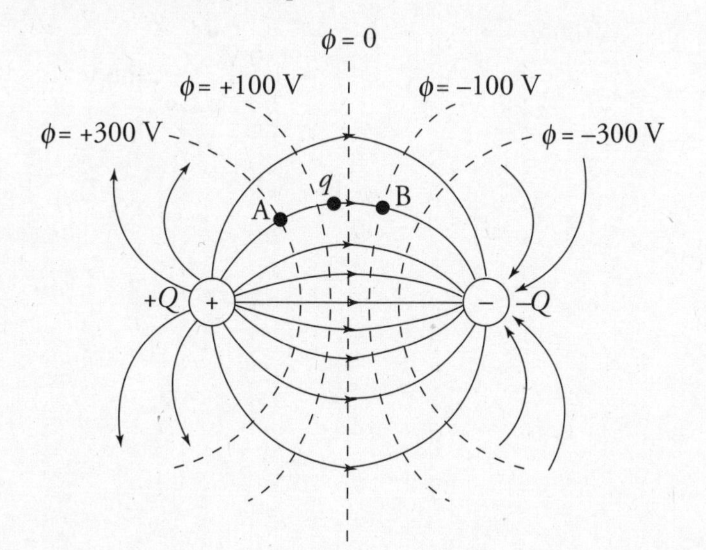

If a particle of mass $m = 1 \times 10^{-6}$ kg and charge q = 5 nC starts from rest at Point A and moves to Point B,

a) How much work is done by the electric field?
b) What is the speed of the particle when it reaches Point B?

Solution:

a) The work done by the electric field is equal to the opposite of the change in the particle's electrical potential energy $W_{\text{by E}} = -\Delta PE_{\text{elec}}$. Since the potential at Point A is $\phi_A = +300\text{ V}$ (because A lies on the $\phi = +300\text{ V}$ equipotential) and the potential at Point B is $\phi_B = -100\text{ V}$ (because B lies on the $\phi = -100\text{ V}$ equipotential), the change in potential from A to B is $\phi_B - \phi_A = (-100\text{ V}) - (300\text{ V}) = -400\text{ V}$. Therefore,

$$W_{\text{by E}} = -\Delta PE_{\text{elec}} = -q\Delta\phi = -(5\times10^{-9}\text{ C})(-400\text{ V}) = 2\times10^{-6}\text{ J}$$

b) Since the total work done on the particle is equal to its change in kinetic energy (the work-energy theorem), we have $\Delta KE = 2\times10^{-6}\text{ J}$. Because the particle started from rest at Point A, we have $KE_{\text{at B}} = \Delta KE_{A\to B} = 2\times10^{-6}\text{ J}$, so

$$\frac{1}{2}mv_B^2 = 2\times10^{-6}\text{ J} \rightarrow v_B = \sqrt{\frac{2(2\times10^{-6}\text{ J})}{1\times10^{-6}\text{ kg}}} = 2\text{ m/s}$$

Example 8-28: The figure below shows several point source charges, $+Q_1$, $+Q_2$, $-Q_3$, and $-Q_4$, and the electric potential at various points (A, B, C, Z, Y, and Z) in the electric field they produce:

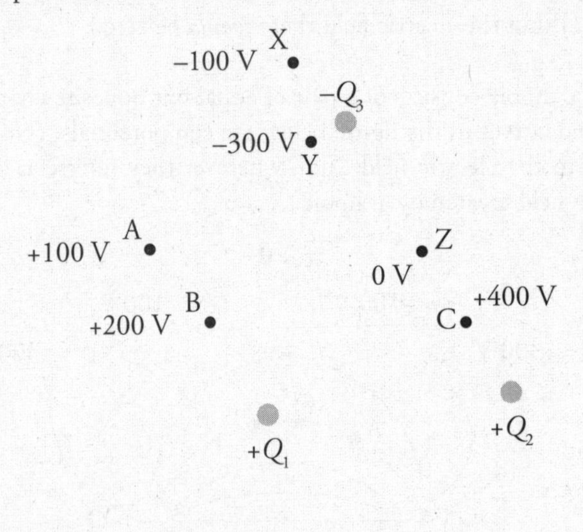

The difference in electric potential between two points is called the **voltage**, *V*. That is, $V = \Delta\phi$. For example, the voltage from Point A to Point B is $\phi_B - \phi_A = (+200\text{ V}) - (+100\text{ V}) = +100\text{ V}$, and the voltage from X to Y is $V = (-300\text{ V}) - (-100\text{ V}) = -200\text{ V}$.

a) How much work does the electric field do on a charge q = +2 μC as q is moved from Point X to Point C?

b) True or false? If the charge q is placed at Point Z, it will remain at this point because the electric potential is 0 V.

Solution:

a) The work done by the electric field is equal to the opposite of the change in the electrical potential energy $W_{\text{by E}} = -\Delta PE_{\text{elec}}$. Since $\Delta\phi = V$, the fundamental equation $\Delta PE = q\Delta\phi$ becomes simply

$$\Delta PE = qV$$

Since $V_{X\to C} = \phi_C - \phi_X = (+400\text{ V}) - (-100\text{ V}) = +500\text{ V}$, we have

$$\Delta PE = qV = (2\times10^{-6}\text{ C})(5\times10^{2}\text{ V}) = 1\times10^{-3}\text{ J}$$

Therefore, $W_{\text{by E}} = -1\times10^{-3}\text{ J}$. (Does it make sense that ΔPE is positive and $W_{\text{by E}}$ is negative? *Yes,* because a positive charge q would have to be pushed by some outside force from Point X (which is near a negative charge) to Point C (which is near a positive charge). When an external force has to do positive work against the electric field, the electrical potential energy increases and the work done by the electric field is negative.)

b) False. If q were placed at a point where the *electric field* was zero, *then* it would feel no force and remain there. However, if q is placed at a point where the electric potential is zero, it will be accelerated toward a point where the potential is lower (because q is positive; recall Example 8-21). In this case, q would be accelerated by the electric field toward the negative source charge $-Q_3$.

Summary of Formulas

Elementary charge: $e = 1.6\times10^{-19}$ C

charge of proton = $+e$; charge of electron = $-e$

Charge is quantized: $e = 1.6\times10^{-19}$ C

Coulomb's law: $F_{\text{elec}} = k\dfrac{Qq}{r^2}$

Opposite charges attract, like charges repel.

Coulomb's constant: $k_0 = 9\times10^{9}\ \text{N}\cdot\text{m}^2/\text{C}^2$

Principle of Superposition:

The net force, electric field, or electric potential on a charge q (for force) or point P (for electric field or electric potential) due to a collection of other charges (Qs) is equal to the sum of individual effects of each Q.

Electric field due to point charge Q: $E = k\dfrac{Q}{r^2}$

Direction of electric field:

Positive charges want to move in the direction of the electric field (**E**).

Negative charges want to move opposite the direction of the electric field (**E**).

Electric force and field: $\mathbf{F} = q\mathbf{E}$

Electric potential: $\phi = k\dfrac{Q}{r}$

(a scalar, not a vector)

Positive charges want to move to regions of lower potential.

Negative charges want to move to regions of higher potential.

Change in electrical *PE*: $\Delta PE_{\text{elec}} = q\Delta\phi = qV$

Work done by electric field: $W_{\text{by E}} = -\Delta PE_{\text{elec}}$

Change in *KE*: $\Delta KE = -\Delta PE$

For conductors, charge rests on the outer surface and the electric field inside is zero.

Chapter 9 Electricity and Magnetism

9.1 ELECTRIC CIRCUITS

An electric circuit is a pathway for the movement of electric charge, consisting of a voltage source, connecting wires, and other components.

Current

Current can be defined as the movement of charge, but for the purposes of analyzing an electric circuit, we need a more precise definition. For example, imagine picking up a metal paper clip and untwisting it to make it relatively straight. If we could look inside this piece of metal wire at the individual atoms, we would see a lattice with about one electron per atom free to roam freely, unbound to any particular atom. These free electrons are known as **conduction electrons**. (Recall the discussion of metallic bonding in OAT General Chemistry.) The conduction electrons in a metal are zooming around throughout the lattice at very high speeds. However, we only have a current when there is a *net* movement of charge. Let's look at this a little more closely.

The figure below shows an imagined magnified view inside a metal wire. The conduction electrons move at an average speed on the order of a million meters per second ($v \sim 10^6$ m/s). If we chose any cross-sectional slice of the wire, we would see that these conduction electrons cross from left to right as often as they cross from right to left. So, while there is movement of charge, there's no *net* movement of charge; that is, there's no current.

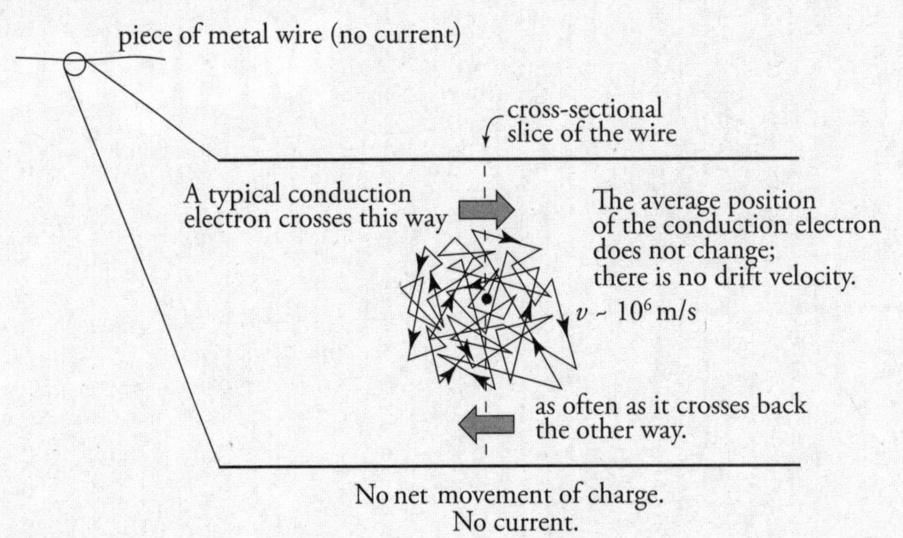

So how would this same piece of wire look if there *were* current in it? Superimposed on the conduction electrons' going-nowhere-fast zooming, we would see that there's a slight drift in one particular direction. This is known as the electrons' **drift velocity** (v_d). If we chose any cross-sectional slice of the wire, we'd see that these conduction electrons move across it from, say, left to right more often than they cross back. Thus, the average positions of the conduction electrons do change and there is a *net* movement of charge (in the case pictured below, negative charge to the right). This is **current**.

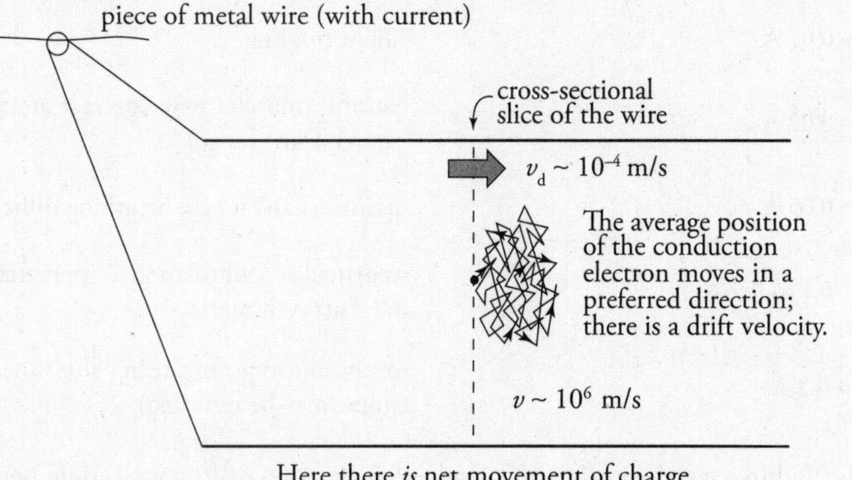

Here there *is* net movement of charge.
This is current.

In the first figure, there was no drift velocity and, therefore, no preferred direction for the movement of charge and no current. In the figure above, however, there is a drift velocity, so there is a flow of charge: a current.

Now, how do we measure current? Since current is the flow of charge, it makes sense to measure current as the amount of charge that moves past a certain point per unit time. Current is denoted by the letter I, and is equal to charge (Q) divided by time (t):

Current

$$I = \frac{Q}{t}$$

The unit of current is the coulomb per second (C/s), which has its own special name: the **ampère** (or just **amp**, for short), abbreviated A. Thus, 1 A = 1 C/s.[1] Since we know that one coulomb is a lot of charge (recall Example 8-4 in the preceding chapter), we would expect that one amp is a lot of current. The following table shows that even a small fraction of a coulomb is enough to kill you.

Current	Physiological Effect
~ 0.01 A	slight tingling
~ 0.02 A	painful; muscles may contract around source (can't let go)
~ 0.05 A	painful; can't let go; breathing difficult
~ 0.1 to 0.2 A	ventricular fibrillation (potentially fatal arrhythmia)
> 0.2 A	severe burning; breathing stops; heart stops (may be restarted)

Example 9-1: Within a metal wire, 5×10^{17} conduction electrons drift past a certain point in 4 seconds. What is the magnitude of the current?

Solution: The magnitude of charge that passes the point in $t = 4$ seconds is

$$Q = ne = (5\times10^{17})(1.6\times10^{-19}\text{ C}) = 8\times10^{-2}\text{ C}$$

Therefore, the value of the current is

$$I = \frac{Q}{t} = \frac{8\times10^{-2}\text{ C}}{4\text{ s}} = 0.02\text{ A}$$

[1] Notice that current is defined in about the same way that we defined *flow rate* in Chapter 5: amount of stuff per unit time. You can think of current as the flow rate of charge.

Voltage

Now that we know how to measure current, the next question is, *What causes it?* Look back at the picture of the wire in which there was a current. What would make an electron drift to the right? One answer is to say that there's an electric field inside the wire, and since negative charges move in the direction opposite to the electric field lines, electrons would be induced to drift to the right if the electric field pointed to the left:

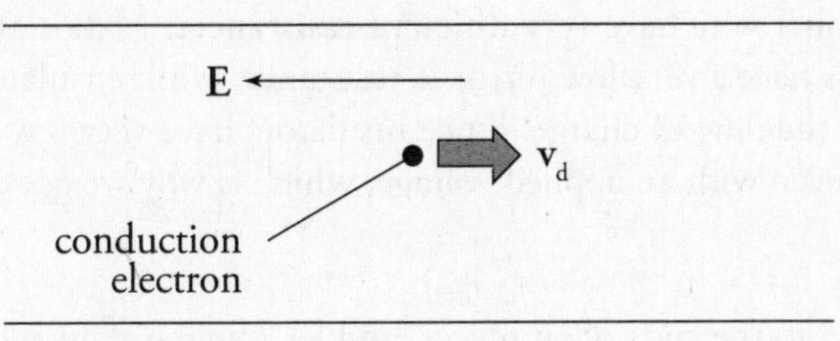

Another (equivalent) answer to the question, "What would make an electron drift to the right?" is that there's a potential difference (a voltage) between the ends of the wire. Because we know that negative charges naturally move toward regions of higher electric potential, electrons would be induced to drift to the right if the right end of the wire were maintained at a higher potential than the left end.

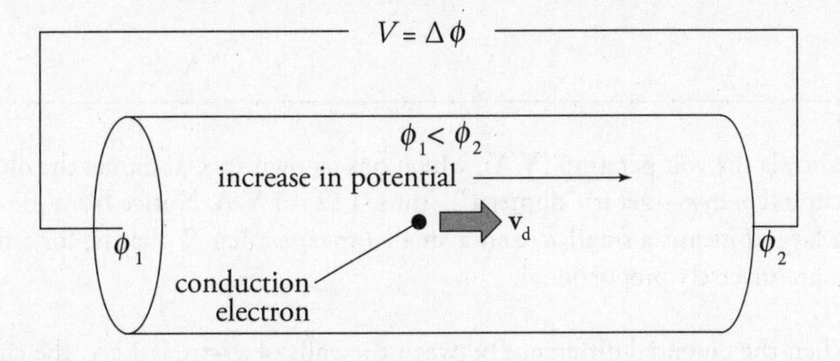

For our purposes in analyzing circuits, this second interpretation of the answer will be the one we use: that is, *it is a voltage that creates a current.* If there's no voltage (no potential difference) then the conduction electrons will just zoom around their original positions, going essentially nowhere; without a potential difference, they'd have no reason to do anything differently.

It is not uncommon to see the voltage that creates a current referred to as **electromotive force (emf)**, since it is the cause that sets the charges into motion in a preferred direction. Notice, however, that calling it a "force" really isn't correct; it's a voltage.

Resistance

Now that we know what current is, how to measure it, and what causes it, the next question is, *How much do we get?* The answer is, *It depends.* If we took a paper-clip wire and touched its two ends to the terminals of a battery, we'd get a measurable current. Now imagine picking up a rubber band and cutting it, so that it becomes essentially a straightened out "wire" of rubber. If we took this rubber wire and touched its two ends to the terminals of the same battery, we'd get essentially zero current. What's the difference? The metal wire and the rubber wire have very different **resistances**. Metals are conductors and rubber is an insulator. That is, metals have a very low intrinsic resistance, while insulators (like rubber) have a very high intrinsic resistance to the flow of charge. Since insulators have very few free electrons, there's going to be virtually no current, even with an applied voltage, which is why we got essentially zero current with our rubber wire.

Let V be the voltage applied to the ends of an object, and let I be the resulting current. By definition, the resistance of the object, R, is given by this equation:

Resistance

$$R = \frac{V}{I}$$

The unit of resistance is the volt per amp (V/A), which has its own special name: the **ohm**, abbreviated Ω (the Greek letter capital *omega*—get it? "ohmega"). Thus, 1 Ω = 1 V/A. Notice from the definition that for a given voltage, a large I means a small R, and a small I means a big R; that is, for a fixed voltage, resistance and current are inversely proportional.

Example 9-2: When the potential difference between the ends of a wire is 12 V, the current is measured to be 0.06 A. What's the resistance of the wire?

Solution: Using the definition of resistance, we find that

$$R = \frac{V}{I} = \frac{12\text{ V}}{0.06\text{ A}} = 200\ \Omega$$

There's another way to calculate the resistance, using a formula that does not depend on V or I. Instead, it expresses the resistance in terms of the material's *intrinsic* resistance, which is known as its **resistivity** (and denoted by ρ, not to be confused with the material's density):

Resistance and Resistivity

$$R = \rho\frac{L}{A}$$

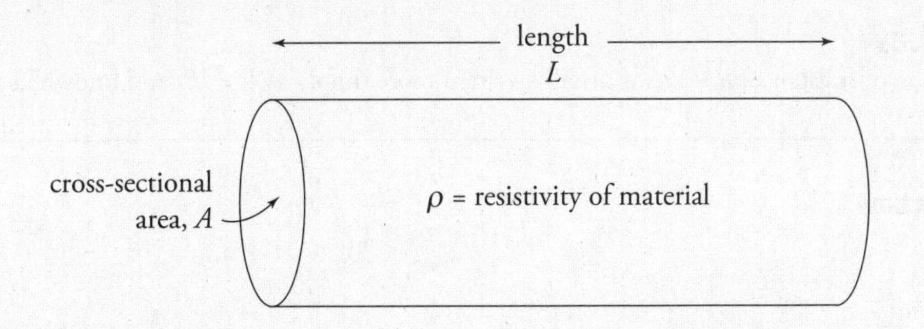

Notice that resistance and resistivity are not the same thing. Each material has its own resistivity; its *intrinsic* resistance. However, the resistance R depends on how we shape the material. For example, if we had two aluminum wires, one that was long and thin and another that was short and thick, both would have the same resistivity (because they're both made of the same material, aluminum), but the wires would have different resistances. The long, thin wire would have the greater resistance because R is proportional to L and inversely proportional to A.

Example 9-3: Consider two copper wires. Wire #1 has three times the length and twice the diameter of Wire #2. If R_1 is the resistance of Wire #1 and R_2 is the resistance of Wire #2, then which of the following is true?

A. $R_2 = (2/3)R_1$
B. $R_2 = (4/3)R_1$
C. $R_2 = 6R_1$
D. $R_2 = 12R_1$

Solution: We're told that $L_1 = 3L_2$, and since $d_1 = 2d_2$, we know that $A_1 = 4A_2$ (because area is proportional to the *square* of the diameter). Since both wires have the same resistivity (because they're both made of the same material), we find that

$$\frac{R_2}{R_1} = \frac{\rho L_2 / A_2}{\rho L_1 / A_1} = \frac{L_2}{L_1} \cdot \frac{A_1}{A_2} = \frac{1}{3} \cdot 4 = \frac{4}{3} \rightarrow R_2 = \frac{4}{3} R_1$$

Thus, the answer is B.

Example 9-4: The wire used for lighting systems is usually No. 12 wire, in the American Wire Gauge (AWG) system. The diameter of No. 12 wire is just over 2 mm (which means a cross-sectional area of 3.3×10^{-6} m^2). What would be the resistance of half a mile (800 m) of No. 12 copper wire, given that the resistivity of copper is 1.7×10^{-8} Ω·m?

Solution: Using the equation $R = \rho L / A$, we get

$$R = \rho \frac{L}{A} = (1.7 \times 10^{-8}\ \Omega\ \text{m}) \frac{8 \times 10^2\ \text{m}}{3.3 \times 10^{-6}\ \text{m}^2} \approx 4\Omega$$

If we wanted to give a more precise formula for the resistance in terms of resistivity, we would have to include the temperature dependence. The resistivity of conductors generally increases slightly with temperature. However, unless specifically mentioned otherwise, assume that the OAT will treat resistivity as a constant.

Ohm's Law

The definition of resistance, $R = V/I$, is usually written more simply as $V = IR$, and known as **Ohm's law.**

Ohm's Law

$$V = IR$$

However, the actual statement of Ohm's law isn't $V = IR$; rather, it's a statement about the behavior of certain conductors, and it isn't true for all materials. A material is said to obey Ohm's law if its resistance, R, remains constant as the voltage is varied; another requirement is that the current must reverse direction if the polarity of the voltage is reversed.[2] On the OAT, you can assume that materials are "ohmic" unless you are specifically told otherwise.

Resistors

A resistor is a component in an electric circuit that has a specific (and usually known) resistance. When we analyze a circuit, we generally ignore the resistance of the connecting metal wires and think of the resistance as being concentrated solely in the resistors placed in the circuit. We can do this because metal wires are such good conductors, i.e., their resistance is very low. Recall that in Example 9-4, we calculated that even half a mile of household wire has a resistance of only 4 Ω.

In the real world, a resistor is typically a little cylinder filled with an alloy (of carbon or of nickel and copper) and often encircled by colored bands to indicate the numerical value of its resistance, like this:

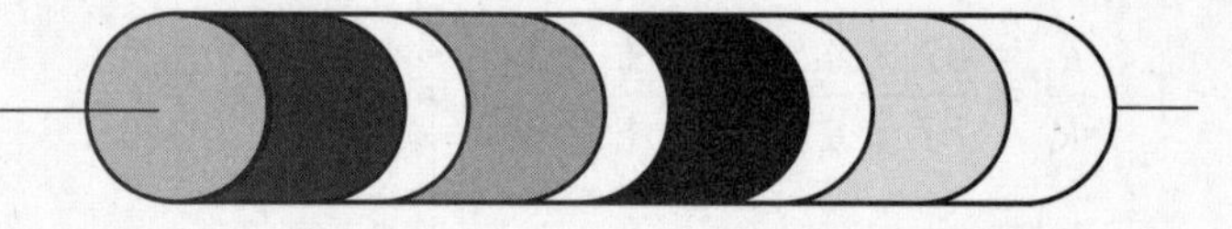

In circuit diagrams, however, a resistor is denoted by the following symbol:

Electric circuits on the OAT may contain just one resistor, but it's more likely that they'll have two or more. There are two ways the OAT will combine resistors: in series or in parallel. Two or more resistors are said to be in **series** if each follows the others along a single connection in a circuit. For example, these two resistors are in series, because R_2 directly follows R_1 along a single path.

[2] Some materials don't behave this way, and the relationship between voltage and current is more complex; on the OAT, however, it's safe to assume that $V = IR$ applies unless you're told otherwise.

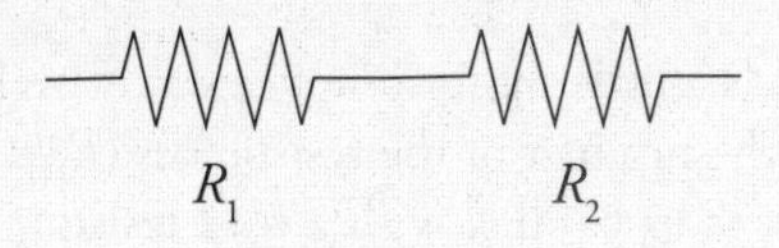

Resistors in Series

On the other hand, two or more resistors are said to be in **parallel** if they provide alternate routes from one point in a circuit to another. For example, the following two resistors are in parallel, because we get from Point P to Point Q in the circuit *either* by traveling through R_1 *or* by traveling through R_2; we don't go through both resistors like we would if they were in series.

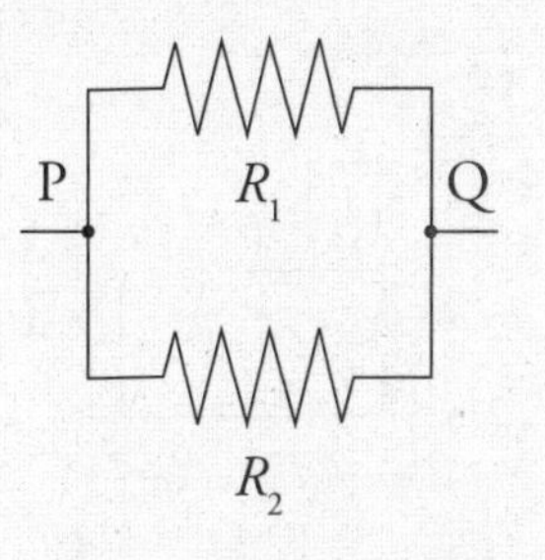

Resistors in Parallel

Typically, we analyze a circuit by first transforming it into a simpler one, one that contains just a single resistor. Therefore, we need a way to turn combinations of resistors (series combinations and parallel combinations) into a single, equivalent resistor; that is, one resistor that provides the same overall resistance as the combination. Here are the formulas:

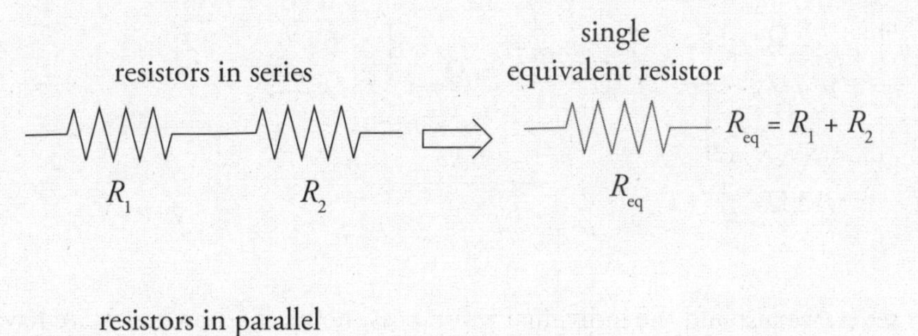

resistors in parallel

P R_1 Q

R_2

R_{eq}

$$R_{eq} = \frac{R_1 R_2}{R_1 + R_2}$$

So, for resistors in series, we simply add the resistances. For example, if a 20 Ω resistor is in series with a 30 Ω resistor, this combination is equivalent to a single 50 Ω resistor, because 20 + 30 = 50. Notice that for a series combination, the equivalent resistance is always greater than the largest resistance in the combination; that's why the "R" is bigger in the figure above for the series combination.

For resistors in parallel, the formula is a little more complicated. If we have two resistors in parallel, we get the equivalent resistance by taking the product of the resistances (R_1R_2) and dividing this by their sum ($R_1 + R_2$). For example, if a 3 Ω resistor is in parallel with a 6 Ω resistor, this combination is equivalent to a single 2 Ω resistor, because (3 × 6) divided by (3 + 6) is equal to 2. For a parallel combination, the equivalent resistance is always less than the smallest resistance in the combination; that's why the "R_{eq}" is smaller in the figure above for the parallel combination.

The "product over sum" formula for parallel resistors only works for *two* resistors. If you have three or more resistors in parallel, do them two at a time. Here's an example:

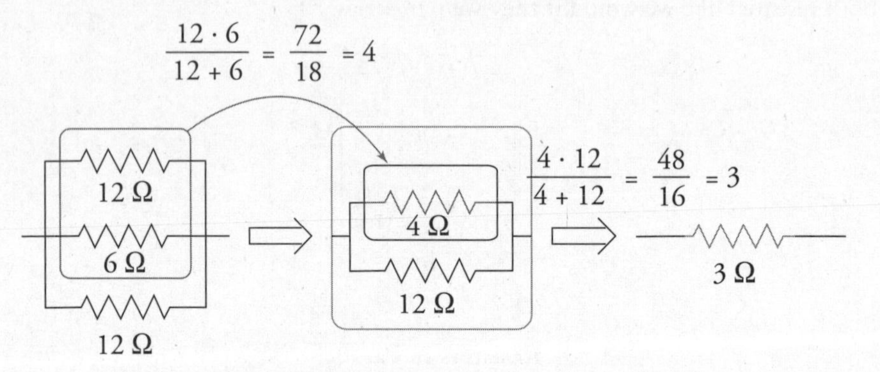

We could have also found the same answer this way:

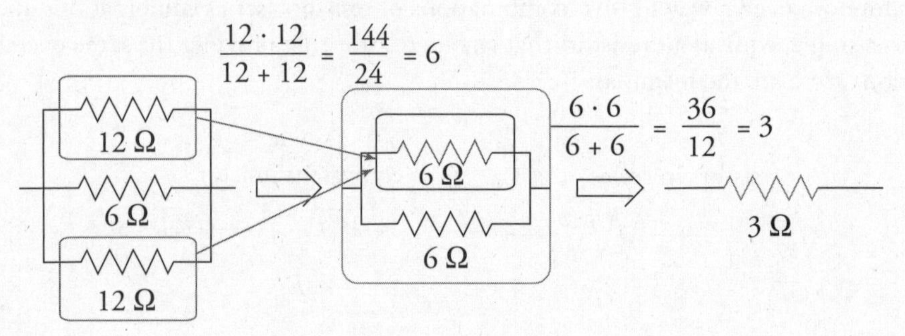

For resistors in series, we just add the individual resistances, no matter how many we have in a row. For example, if we have the following four resistors in series: 10 Ω, 20 Ω, 30 Ω, and 40 Ω, then we can reduce this combination of four series resistors to a single equivalent resistance of 100 Ω, because 10 + 20 + 30 + 40 = 100.

The formula for calculating the equivalent resistance, R, for a parallel combination of resistors R_1, R_2, ... is usually given as:

$$\frac{1}{R_{eq}} = \frac{1}{R_1} + \frac{1}{R_2} + \ldots$$

This formula works for any number of resistors in parallel, not just two. If you prefer this formula, that's perfectly okay. However, you may find adding the fractions to be messier than the "product over sum" rule above. Also, be sure to avoid the common error of forgetting to take the reciprocal of the left-hand side to get your final answer.

Example 9-5: Show that the equivalent resistance of two identical resistors in series is twice the resistance of either resistor, but the equivalent resistance of two identical resistors in parallel is half the resistance of either resistor.

Solution: Let the resistance of each resistor be R. Then, if two such resistors are in series, the equivalent resistance is $R_{eq} = R + R = 2R$. However, if two such resistors are in parallel, then their equivalent resistance is

$$R_{eq} = \frac{R \cdot R}{R + R} = \frac{R^2}{2R} = \frac{R}{2}$$

Example 9-6: What is the equivalent or total resistance of the following combination of resistors?

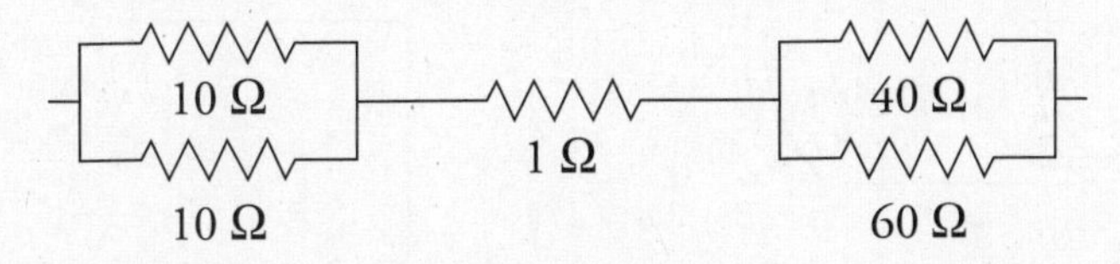

Solution: Here we have a mixture of parallel *and* series combinations. There's a parallel combination (the pair of 10 Ω resistors) that's in series with both a 1 Ω resistor and another parallel combination (the 40 Ω and 60 Ω resistors). To simplify this, we work in steps:

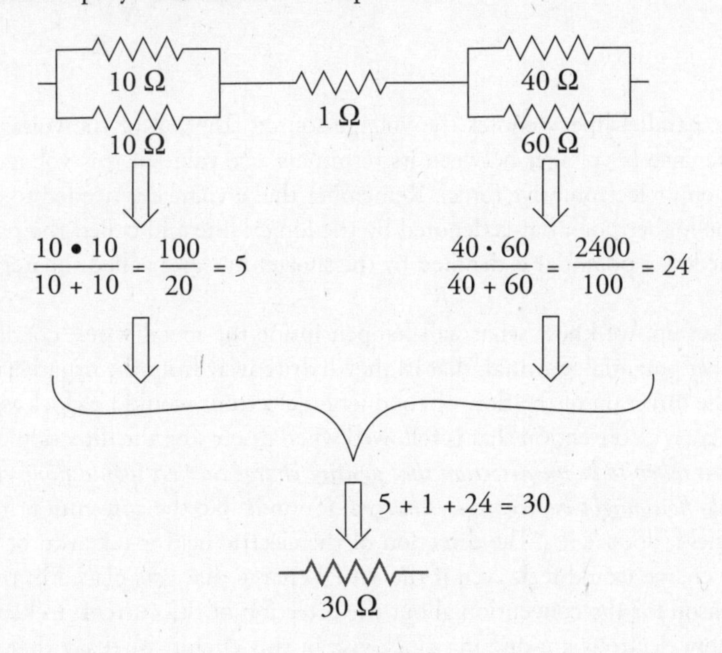

Therefore, the given combination of resistors is equivalent to a single 30 Ω resistor.

DC Circuits

Now that we know how to simplify series and parallel combinations of resistors, we're ready to analyze circuits. The simplest circuit consists of a voltage source (most commonly, it's a battery), a connecting wire between the terminals of the voltage source, and a resistor. As an example, imagine hooking up a light bulb to a typical flashlight battery; one wire connects the positive terminal of the battery to one of the "leads" on the light bulb, and another wire connects the other lead on the bulb to the negative terminal of the battery. This completes the circuit. The diagram on the right below shows the way this real-life circuit would be drawn schematically.

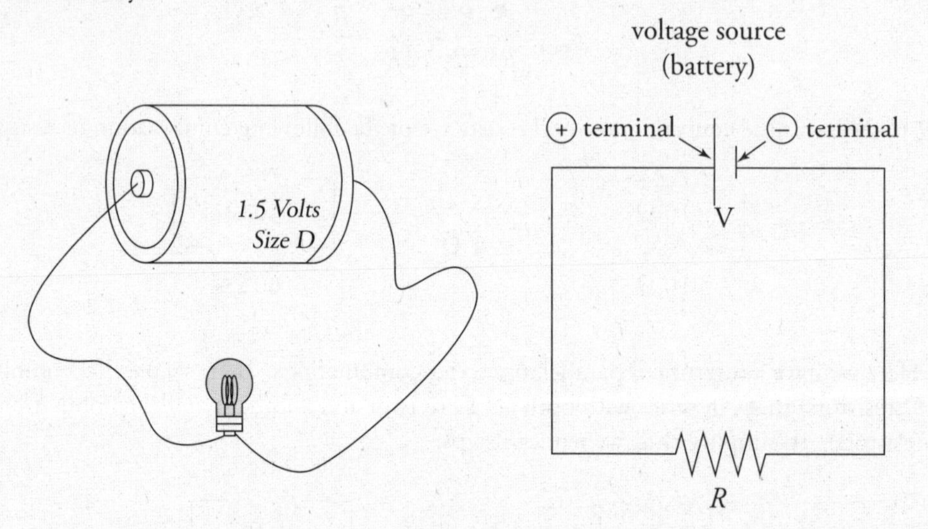

The pair of adjacent parallel lines denotes the voltage source. The job of the voltage source is to maintain a potential difference (a voltage) between its terminals; the value of this voltage is denoted by V or sometimes by ε, for emf (electromotive force). Remember that a voltage is needed to create a current. The terminal that's at the higher potential is denoted by the longer line and called the **positive terminal**; the terminal that's at the lower potential is denoted by the shorter line and called the **negative terminal**.

Once the circuit is set up, we know what will happen inside the metal wires: conduction electrons will drift toward the higher potential terminal; that is, they'll drift away from the negative terminal, toward the positive terminal. The direction of the flow of conduction electrons would be clockwise in the diagram as drawn. However, there is a convention that is followed when discussing the direction of the current. *The direction of the current is taken to be the direction that positive charge carriers would flow, even though the actual charge carriers that do flow might be negatively charged.* (Sounds like the convention for defining the direction of the electric field, doesn't it? "The direction of the electric field is taken to be the direction of the force that a positive charge would feel, even if the actual charge that gets placed in the field isn't positive." In fact, that's the reason for the convention about the direction of the current; to keep things consistent.) Even though we know electrons are drifting clockwise in this circuit, we'd say that the current, I, flows counterclockwise from the positive terminal around to the negative terminal.

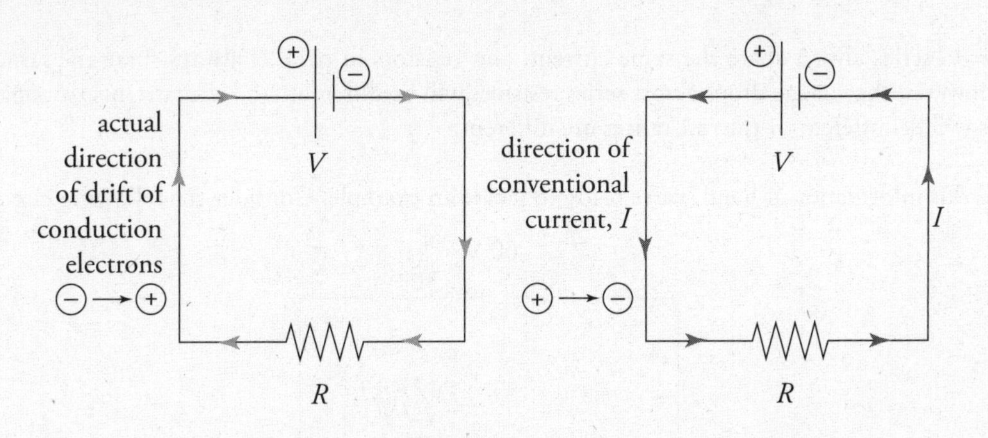

If we were asked for the value of the current in this circuit, this question would be easy to answer. We know V and R, and we want I. Using the equation $V = IR$, we'd say that

$$I = \frac{V}{R}$$

For example, if $V = 1.5$ V and $R = 150\ \Omega$, then $I = 0.01$ A. So, what made this problem so easy? The answer: There was only one resistor. This will usually be our goal: to simplify a circuit with multiple resistors into a circuit with just a single equivalent resistor. (We say "usually" because there are some question types that can be answered without changing the circuit into one with just a single resistor; we'll show you some examples of those, too.)

In order to simplify a circuit with multiple resistors, we first need a way to turn resistors in series and resistors in parallel into a single equivalent resistor; this we already know how to do. However, there are two other important quantities in circuits besides R; namely, I and V. We also need to know what happens to these other quantities when we convert a series or parallel combination of resistors into a single resistor. The following figure contains this needed information:

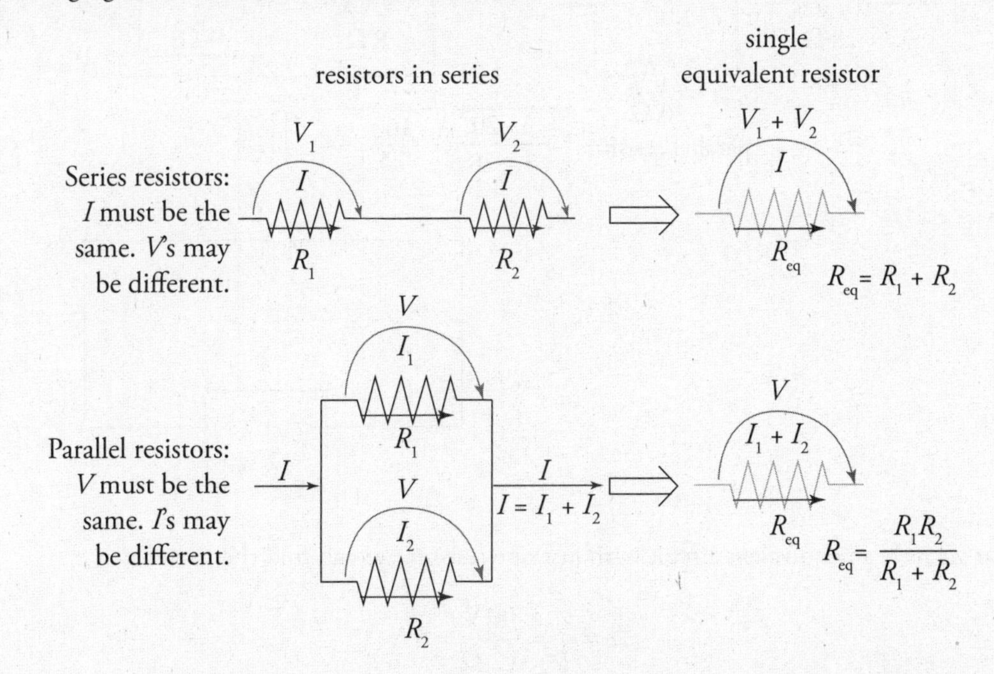

Resistors in series always share the same current, and resistors in parallel always share the same voltage drop. However, the voltage drops across series resistors will be different (and the currents through parallel resistors will be different) if the resistances are different.

With all this information at hand, we're ready to tackle an example. Consider the following circuit:

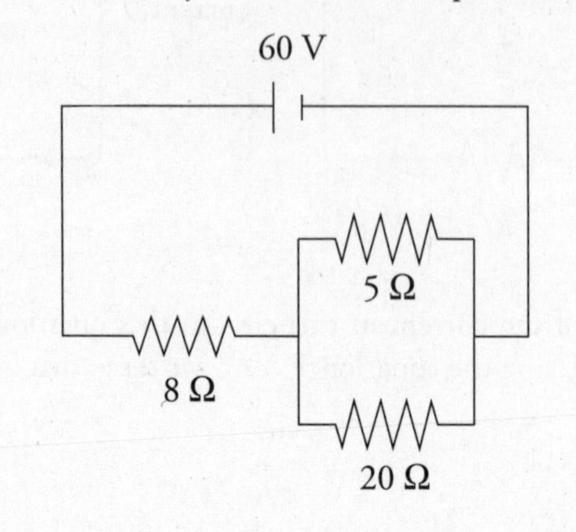

We'll find the current in the circuit, the current through each resistor, and the voltage across each resistor. The first stage of the solution involves simplifying this multiple-resistor circuit into a circuit with just a single equivalent resistor, like this:

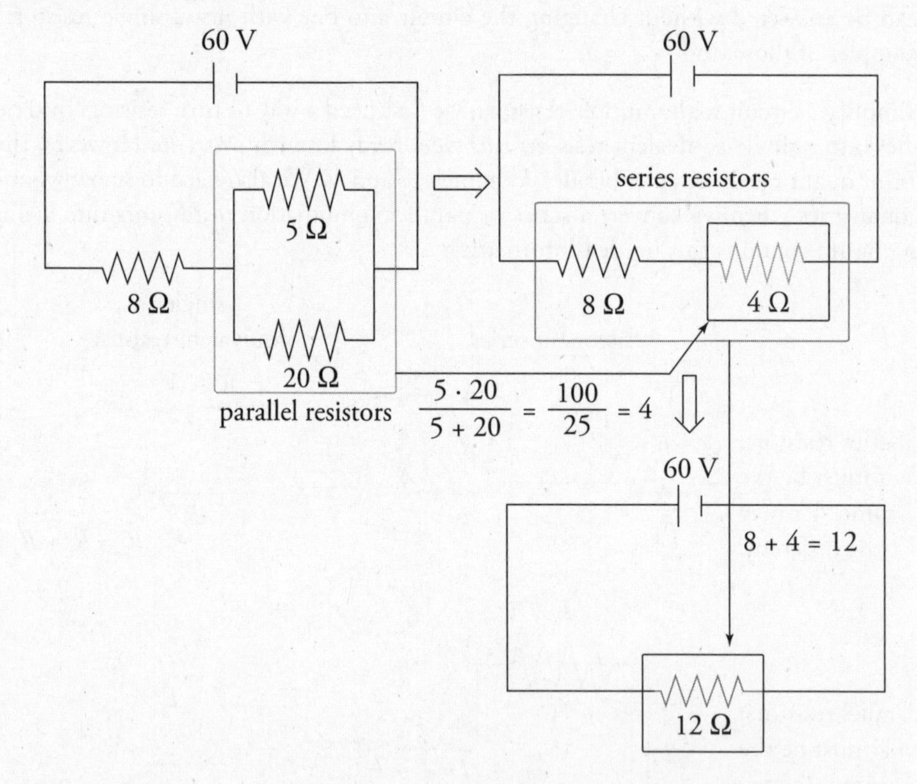

Now that we have an equivalent circuit with just one resistor, we can find the current:

$$I = \frac{V}{R} = \frac{60\,\text{V}}{12\,\Omega} = 5\,\text{A}$$

If we want to find the currents through (and the voltages across) the individual resistors in the original circuit, we have to work backward. The key to "working backward" is to ask at each stage: "What am I going back to?" If the answer is, "a *series* combination," then the value you bring back is the *current*, because series resistors share the same current. If the answer is, "a *parallel* combination," then the value you bring back is the *voltage*, because parallel resistors share the same voltage.

going back to series combination → bring *I*

going back to parallel combination → bring *V*

Let me illustrate this "working backward" technique with our circuit above. You should read this figure starting at the bottom, then up, then to the left... in other words, in the *reverse* order from what we did before because now we're working backward:

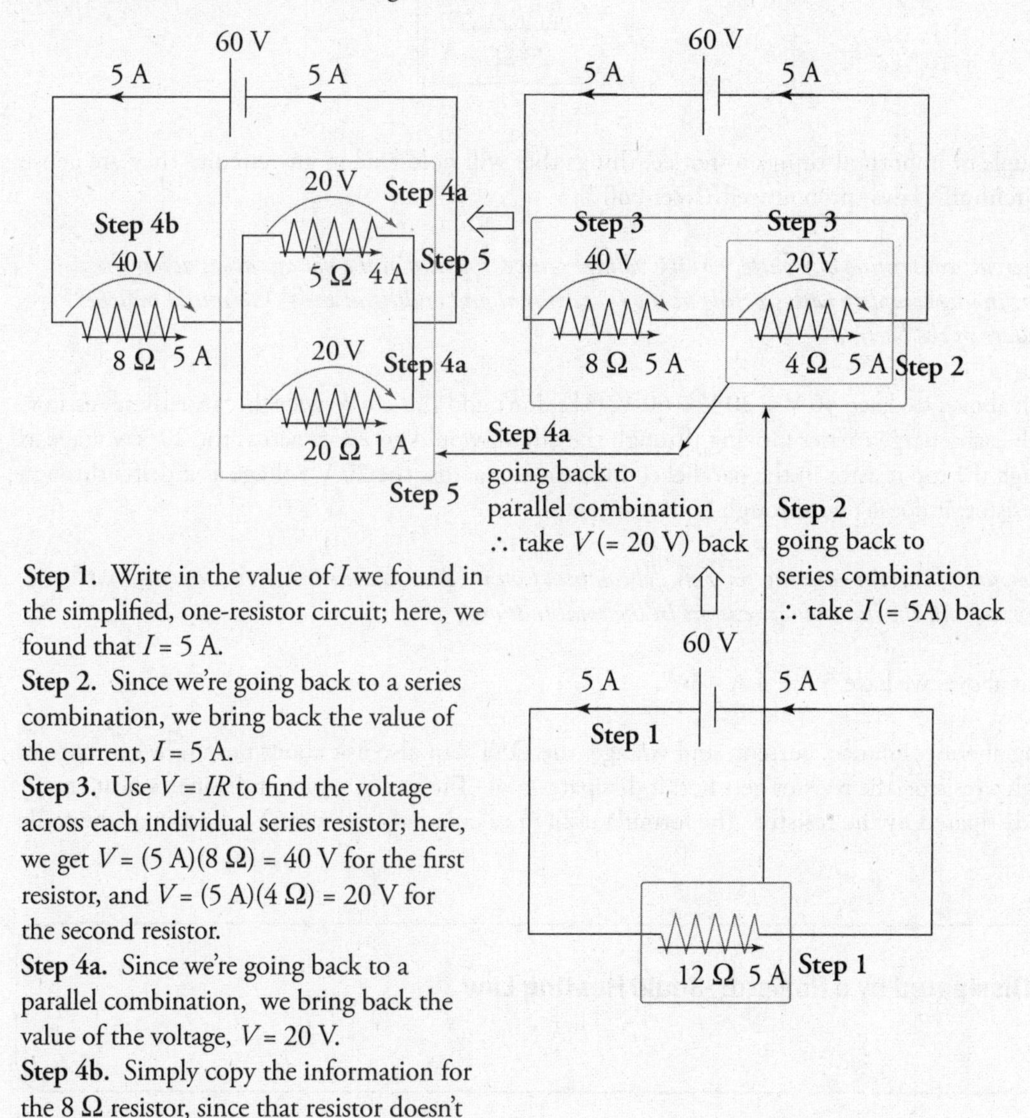

Step 1. Write in the value of I we found in the simplified, one-resistor circuit; here, we found that $I = 5$ A.
Step 2. Since we're going back to a series combination, we bring back the value of the current, $I = 5$ A.
Step 3. Use $V = IR$ to find the voltage across each individual series resistor; here, we get $V = (5\text{ A})(8\ \Omega) = 40$ V for the first resistor, and $V = (5\text{ A})(4\ \Omega) = 20$ V for the second resistor.
Step 4a. Since we're going back to a parallel combination, we bring back the value of the voltage, $V = 20$ V.
Step 4b. Simply copy the information for the 8 Ω resistor, since that resistor doesn't change when we go back.
Step 5. Use $I = V/R$ to find the current across each individual parallel resistor; here, we get $I = (20\text{ V})/(5\ \Omega) = 4$ A for the top resistor, and $I = (20\text{ V})/(20\ \Omega) = 1$ A for the bottom resistor.

Now that we have found all the information for the original circuit,

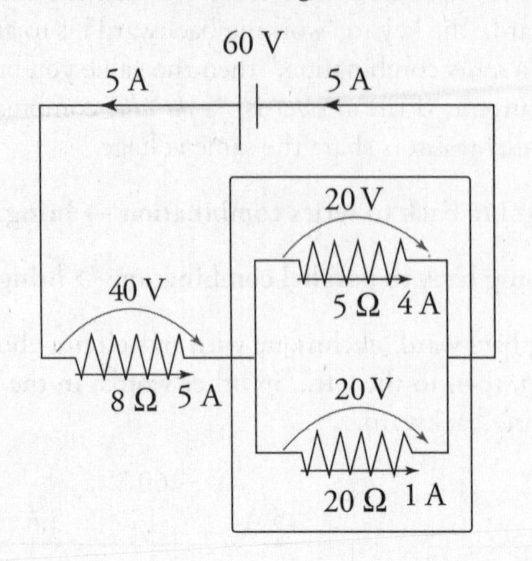

there are a couple of important things to notice, things that will hold true in any circuit. They are consequences of **Kirchhoff's laws** (pronounced "Keer-koff").

- *For a circuit containing one battery as the voltage source, the sum of the voltage drops across the resistors in any complete path starting at the (+) terminal and ending at the (–) terminal matches the voltage of the battery.*

For our circuit above, we have 40 V + 20 V = 60 V. (We don't add the 20 V twice, because these resistors are in parallel; each charge carrier moving through the circuit would go *either* across the 20 V voltage as it drifts through the top resistor in the parallel combination *or* across the 20 V voltage as it drifts through the bottom resistor; it doesn't go through both resistors.)

- *The amount of current entering the parallel combination is equal to the sum of the currents that pass through all the individual resistors in the combination.*

For our circuit above, we have 5 A = 4 A + 1 A.

Besides asking about resistance, current, and voltage, the OAT can also ask about power. When current passes through a resistor, the resistor gets hot: it dissipates heat. The rate at which it dissipates heat energy is the **power dissipated by the resistor**. The formula used to calculate this power, P, is known as the **Joule heating law.**

Power Dissipated by a Resistor: Joule Heating Law

$$P = I^2 R$$

So, for our circuit above, we find that:

the power dissipated by the 8 Ω resistor is $I^2R = (5\text{ A})^2(8\ \Omega) = 200$ W
the power dissipated by the 5 Ω resistor is $I^2R = (4\text{ A})^2(5\ \Omega) = 80$ W
the power dissipated by the 20 Ω resistor is $I^2R = (1\text{ A})^2(20\ \Omega) = 20$ W
the total power dissipated by all resistors is the sum: 300 W

The power *supplied* to the circuit by the voltage source (like a battery) is given by this formula: $P = IV$. So, for our circuit above, we find that

power supplied by the 60 V battery is $P = IV = (5\text{ A})(60\text{ V}) = 300$ W

Notice that these answers match:

power dissipated by all resistors = 300 W = power supplied by the battery

This is simply a consequence of Conservation of Energy, so it will be true in general:

- *The total power dissipated by the resistors is equal to the power supplied by the battery.*

Sometimes, a circuit may contain more than one battery, and in some of these cases, the battery with the lower voltage will be *absorbing* power from the battery with the higher voltage (that is, from the "boss battery" that supplies the power to the circuit). The power *absorbed* by a battery is also given by the formula $P = IV$, and the italicized statement above should then read:

- *The total power dissipated by the resistors and absorbed by other voltage sources (i.e., the total power used by the circuit) is equal to the power supplied to the circuit by the highest-voltage power source.*

One more note: The Joule heating law, $P = I^2R$, can be written as $P = I(IR) = IV$, so, in fact, we need just one formula for the power dissipated or supplied by *any* component in a circuit:

Power

$$P = IV$$

However, if you use the formula $P = IV$ to find the power dissipated by a resistor, *be careful* that you only use the V *for that resistor*, and not the V for the entire circuit. So, for our circuit above, we'd find that:

the power dissipated by the 8 Ω resistor is $IV = (5\text{ A})(40\text{ V}) = 200$ W
the power dissipated by the 5 Ω resistor is $IV = (4\text{ A})(20\text{ V}) = 80$ W
the power dissipated by the 20 Ω resistor is $IV = (1\text{ A})(20\text{ V}) = 20$ W

giving us the same answers we found before when we used the formula $P = I^2R$.

Along with questions about power, there could also be questions about energy. Simply remember the definition: power = energy/time, so

$$\text{energy} = \text{power} \times \text{time}$$

For example, how much energy is dissipated in 5 seconds by the 5-ohm resistor in the circuit above? We calculated that the power dissipated by this resistor is $P = 80$ W = 80 J/s; so the energy dissipated in $t = 5$ seconds is $Pt = (80 \text{ J/s})(5 \text{ s}) = 400$ J.

In some circuits (in practice, most of them), one or more of the resistors are actually doing something useful besides just heating up. However, the circuit diagrams and the calculations we do will be the same. For example, a motor will be shown as a resistor in an OAT circuit; so will a light bulb (which is really just a resistor that happens to get so hot that some of the energy dissipated is emitted as light rather than heat). In either case, the calculations for these components are the same as treating each as a regular resistor. Notice that if you want to calculate the work that can be done by a motor, you'll wind up multiplying power by time.

Finally, a common and useful model/analogy for an electric circuit is a stream of water traveling down a series of waterfalls, with a pump in the collecting pool at the bottom to take the water back up to the top again. The battery (voltage source) is like the pump, and the voltage of the battery is the height it lifts the water. The current is the water, and each resistor is a waterfall. Resistors in series share the same current, because however much water drops down one waterfall must drop down the next one in the line (it has nowhere else to go); the heights of these waterfalls can of course be different, which is why the voltage drops for series resistors may be different. Parallel resistors are parallel waterfalls: They provide different paths for the water to drop from one point in the stream to a lower point. Because such waterfalls connect the same higher point to the same lower point, their heights must be the same; this is why parallel resistors always share the same voltage drop. One waterfall in parallel might be very narrow and only allow a small amount of water to flow down, while another waterfall in the same parallel (side-by-side) combination might be wide and thus allow more water to flow down; this is why resistors in parallel may have different currents. However, the total amount of water entering the top of the parallel waterfall combination must go down all the waterfalls in that combination (again, the water has nowhere else to go); this illustrates why the amount of current entering the parallel combination is equal to the total amount of current that passes through all the resistors in the combination. Finally, the total height of the waterfalls must be the same as the height through which the pump lifts the water from the collecting pool at the bottom; this illustrates why the total voltage drop across the resistors matches the voltage of the battery.

circuit	stream of water flowing down waterfalls with pump at the bottom
current	the flow rate of the water
resistor	waterfall
series	one waterfall after another
parallel	side-by-side waterfalls
voltage	for resistor: height of waterfall (distance water falls) for battery: total height the pump lifts the water to start a new cycle
resistance	relative width of channel in the water circuit (narrower width = higher resistance; wider = lower resistance)

Here's a diagram of the water stream and waterfalls that would be analogous to the circuit we analyzed above.

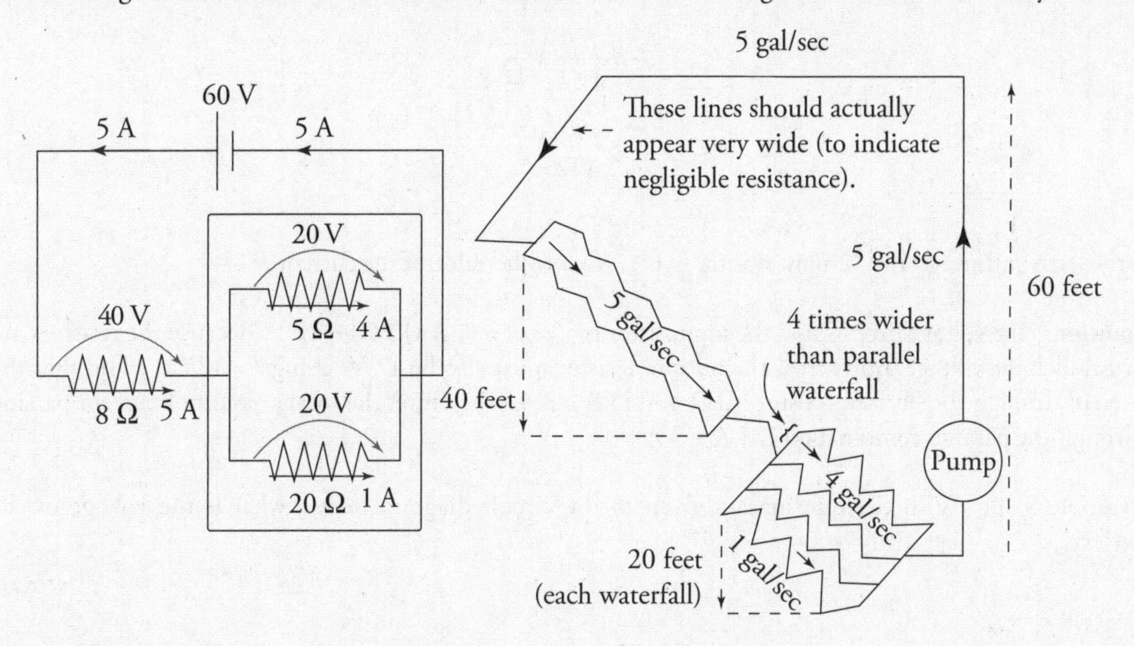

Example 9-7: Verify that the formulas $P = IV$ and $P = I^2R$ are dimensionally correct by showing that the product of current and voltage (IV) and the product of current squared and resistance (I^2R), both have the units of power.

Solution: First, because $[I]$ = C/s and $[V]$ = J/C, we have

$$[IV]=[I][V]=\frac{\text{C}}{\text{s}}\cdot\frac{\text{J}}{\text{C}}=\frac{\text{J}}{\text{s}}=\text{W}=\text{watt}=[P]$$

Next, because $[I]$ = C/s and $[R]$ = Ω = V/A, we have

$$[I^2R]=[I]^2[R]=\left(\frac{\text{C}}{\text{s}}\right)^2\cdot\frac{\text{V}}{\text{A}}=\frac{\text{C}^2}{\text{s}^2}\cdot\frac{\frac{\text{J}}{\text{C}}}{\frac{\text{C}}{\text{s}}}=\frac{\text{C}^2}{\text{s}^2}\cdot\frac{\text{J}\cdot\text{s}}{\text{C}^2}=\frac{\text{J}}{\text{s}}=\text{W}=\text{watt}=[P]$$

Example 9-8: A portion of a circuit is shown below:

If the current through the 10-ohm resistor is 1 A, what is the current through the 20-ohm resistor?

A. 0.25 A
B. 0.5 A
C. 1 A
D. 2 A

Solution: Because these resistors are in series, they all share the same current. If the current in the first resistor is 1 A, then the current through each of the other resistors is also 1 A. The answer is C.

Example 9-9: A portion of a circuit is shown below:

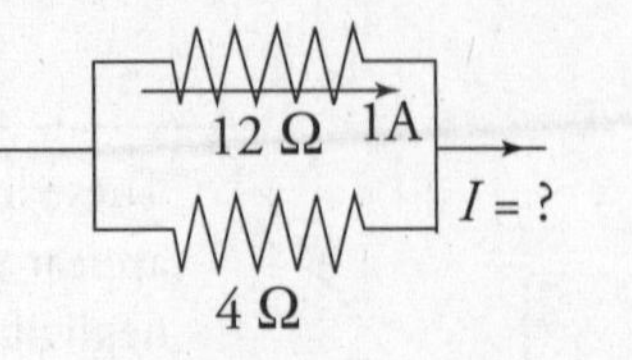

If the current through the 12-ohm resistor is 1 A, what is the value of the current I?

Solution: The voltage drop across the top resistor is $V = IR$ = (1 A)(12 Ω) = 12 V. Because the resistors are in parallel, the voltage drop across the bottom resistor must also be 12 V. Using $I = V/R$, we find that the current through the bottom resistor is (12 V)/(4 Ω) = 3 A. Therefore, the total amount of current passing through the parallel combination is 1 A + 3 A = 4 A.

Example 9-10: With the information given in the circuit diagram below, what is the voltage of the battery?

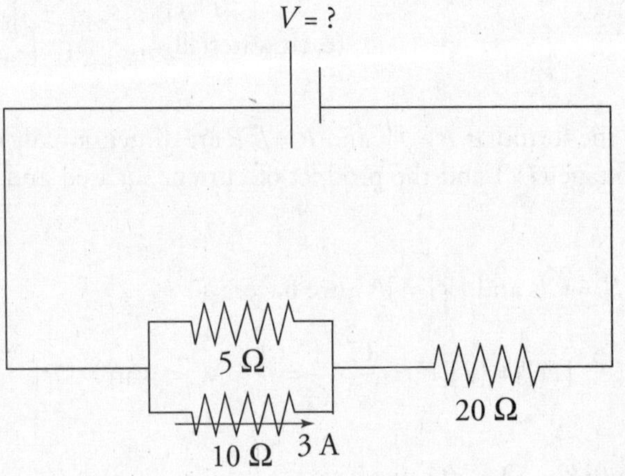

A. 150 V
B. 210 V
C. 240 V
D. 300 V

Solution: The voltage drop across the bottom resistor in the parallel combination is $V = IR$ = (3 A)(10 Ω) = 30 V. Because the top and bottom resistors in this combination are in parallel, the voltage drop across the top resistor must also be 30 V. Using $I = V/R$, we find that the current through the top resistor is (30 V)/(5 Ω) = 6 A. Therefore, the total amount of current passing through the parallel combination is 6 A + 3 A = 9 A. Since this much current flows through the 20-ohm resistor, the voltage drop across the 20-ohm resistor is $V = IR$ = (9 A)(20 Ω) = 180 V. Because the total voltage drop across the resistors must match the voltage of the battery, we have V = 30 V + 180 V = 210 V, so the answer is B. (Remember: We don't add the 30 V voltage drop twice here; choice C is a trap.)

Example 9-11: A portion of a circuit is shown below:

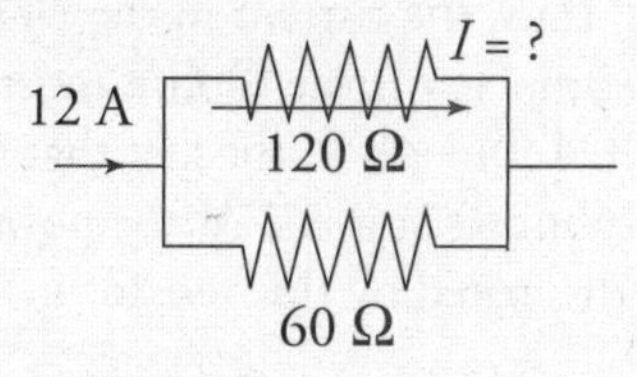

If the current entering the parallel combination is 12 A, how much current flows through the 120-ohm resistor?

Solution: Because the 60-ohm bottom resistor has half the resistance of the 120-ohm top resistor, twice as much current will flow through the bottom resistor as through the top one. So, if we let X stand for the current in the top resistor, then the current in the bottom resistor is $2X$. Because 12 A enters the parallel combination, we must have $X + 2X = 12$ A, so $X = 4$ A. Therefore, the current in the top resistor is 4 A (and the current in the bottom resistor is 8 A). Notice that the voltage drop across the top resistor is $V = IR = (4\text{ A})(120\ \Omega) = 480$ V, and the voltage drop across the bottom resistor is $V = IR = (8\text{ A})(60\ \Omega) = 480$ V. The fact that these voltages match (as they must for parallel resistors) verifies that our answer is correct.

Example 9-12: How much energy is dissipated in 10 seconds by the 24-ohm resistor in the following circuit?

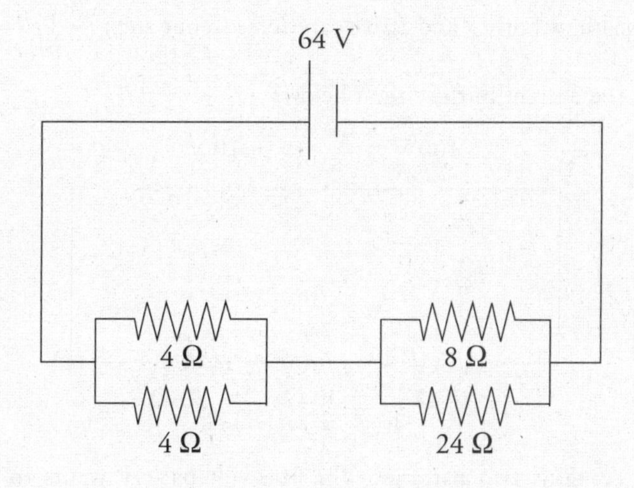

A. 480 J
B. 640 J
C. 720 J
D. 960 J

Solution: The pair of parallel 4-ohm resistors is equivalent to a single 2-ohm resistor [because $(4 \times 4)/(4 + 4) = 2$], and the parallel 8-ohm and 24-ohm resistors are equivalent to a single 6-ohm resistor [because $(8 \times 24)/(8 + 24) = 192/32 = 6$]. These equivalent resistors are in series, so the overall equivalent resistance for the circuit is $2\ \Omega + 6\ \Omega = 8\ \Omega$. This means the current in the circuit is $I = V/R_{eq} = 64/8 = 8$ A. When these 8 amps enter the second parallel combination (the one with the 8-ohm and 24-ohm resistors), it must split up in such a way that the current through the 8-ohm resistor is 3 times the current through the 24-ohm resistor. (Because the 8-ohm resistor has 1/3 the resistance of the 24-ohm resistor, it will get 3 times the current.)

So, if we let X stand for the current in the 24-ohm resistor, then the current through the 8-ohm resistor is $3X$; this gives $X + 3X = 8$ A, so $X = 2$ A. Thus, the current in the 24-ohm resistor is 2 A. [The current in the 8-ohm resistor is $3X = 6$ A. The voltage drop across the 8-ohm resistor is (6 A)(8 Ω) = 48 V, and the voltage drop across the 24-ohm resistor is (2 A)(24 Ω) = 48 V; the fact that these match verifies that our calculation is correct.] Since the current in the 24-ohm resistor is 2 A, the power dissipated by this resistor is $P = I^2R = (2^2)(24) = 96$ W. Therefore, the energy dissipated by this resistor in 10 seconds is (96 W)(10 s) = 960 J, and the answer is D.

Example 9-13: What is the current in the 100-ohm resistor shown below?

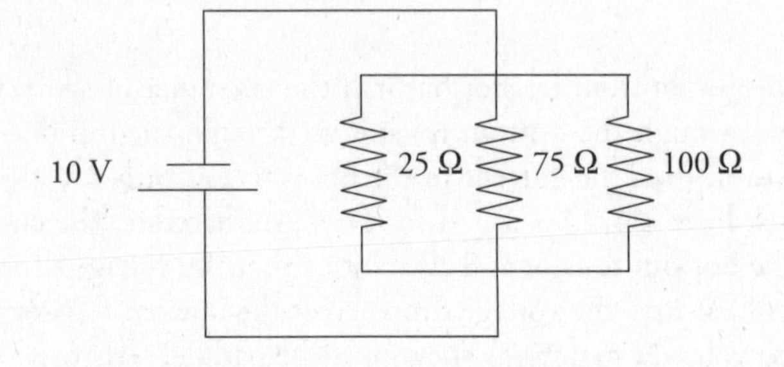

Solution: For this question, we don't need to begin by finding the single equivalent resistance of the given parallel combination, because we already know the voltage across the 100-ohm resistor. The parallel combination is attached directly to the terminals of the battery, so the voltage across each of the resistors must be 10 V. Because we know both V and R, we can find I in one step: $I = V/R$ = (10 V)/(100 Ω) = 0.1 A.

Example 9-14: What is the current in the circuit below?

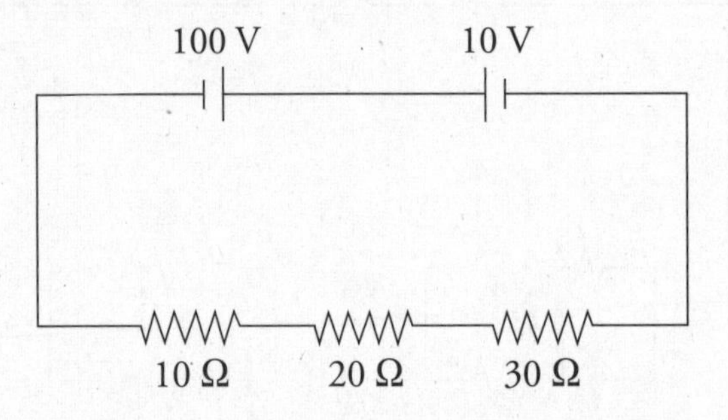

Solution: This circuit contains two batteries. The 100-volt battery wants to send current clockwise. (Remember: We consider current as the directed motion of positive charge, and positive charge carriers would move away from the positive terminal, around the circuit to the negative terminal.) However, the 10-volt battery would want to send current the opposite way: counterclockwise. Since the 100-volt battery has the higher voltage (or, equivalently, the greater emf), it's the "boss" battery. Therefore, current will flow clockwise, but the effective emf will be reduced to 100 – 10 = 90 V, because the 10-volt battery is opposing the 100-volt boss battery. The equivalent resistance is 10 + 20 + 30 = 60 Ω (the resistors are in series), so the current in the circuit will be $I = V/R_{eq}$ = (90 V)/(60 Ω) = 1.5 A. (Note: The 10-volt battery is being charged by the 100-volt boss battery.)

Example 9-15: A toaster oven is rated at 720 W. If it draws 6 A of current, what is its resistance?

Solution: Here, we're given P and I, and asked for R. Since $P = I^2R$, we find that

$$R = \frac{P}{I^2} = \frac{720\text{ W}}{(6\text{ A})^2} = 20\ \Omega$$

Example 9-16: Current passes through an insulated resistor of resistance R, mass m, and specific heat c. The voltage across this resistor is V. If the resistor absorbs all the heat it generates, find an expression for the increase in temperature of the resistor after a time t. (All values are expressed in SI units.)

Solution: The amount of heat energy generated (and absorbed) by the resistor is $q = Pt$, where $P = IV = (V/R)V = V^2/R$. (Here, q stands for "heat energy," not "charge.") Now, using the fundamental equation $q = mc\Delta T$ (from general chemistry), we have

$$\Delta T = \frac{q}{mc} = \frac{Pt}{mc} = \frac{\frac{V^2}{R}t}{mc} = \frac{V^2 t}{Rmc}$$

All real batteries have **internal resistance**, which we denote by r. Let ε denote the emf of the battery; this is its "ideal" voltage (i.e., the voltage between its terminals when there's no current). Once a current is established, the internal resistance causes the voltage between the terminals to be different from ε. If the battery is supplying current I to the circuit, then the **terminal voltage**, V, is less than ε and given by $V = \varepsilon - Ir$. (On the other hand, if the circuit is *supplying* current to the battery [charging it up] then the terminal voltage is greater than ε and given by the equation $V = \varepsilon + Ir$.) The internal resistance is actually *between* the terminals in a real battery, but in circuit diagrams, the internal resistance is drawn next to the battery, like this:

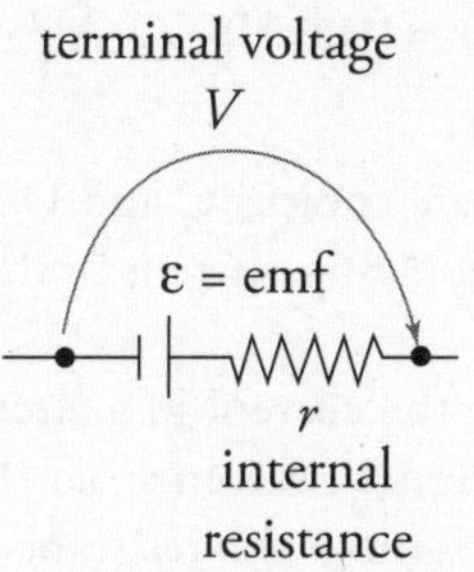

However, unless you are told otherwise, you may assume that all batteries are ideal and have no internal resistance.

Example 9-17: The battery shown in the circuit below has an emf of 100 V and an internal resistance of 5 Ω. What is its terminal voltage in this circuit? (*Note*: It's not uncommon to see a dashed box drawn around the battery and its internal resistance; this emphasizes that *r* is actually inside the battery.)

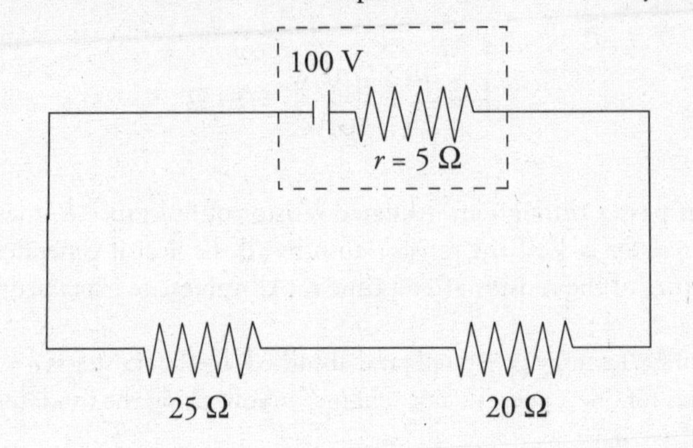

A. 80 V
B. 90 V
C. 100 V
D. 110 V

Solution: The three resistors in this circuit are in series, so the equivalent resistance for the circuit is 5 + 25 + 20 = 50 Ω. Because the emf is 100 V, the current in the circuit is

$$I = \varepsilon / R = (100\text{ V})/(50\ \Omega) = 2\text{ A}$$

The terminal voltage is therefore

$$V = \varepsilon - Ir = (100\text{ V}) - (2\text{ A})(5\ \Omega) = 90\text{ V}$$

The answer is B. (*Note*: You could eliminate choices C and D immediately; the terminal voltage must be *less* than the emf because the battery is supplying current to the circuit.)

Example 9-18: A device used to measure the current in a circuit is called an **ammeter** (denoted by A in a circuit diagram). It has a very small internal resistance, so that it only negligibly affects the current it's trying to measure; for most purposes, we ignore the resistance of an ammeter. What would an ammeter read if it were placed as shown in the following circuit?

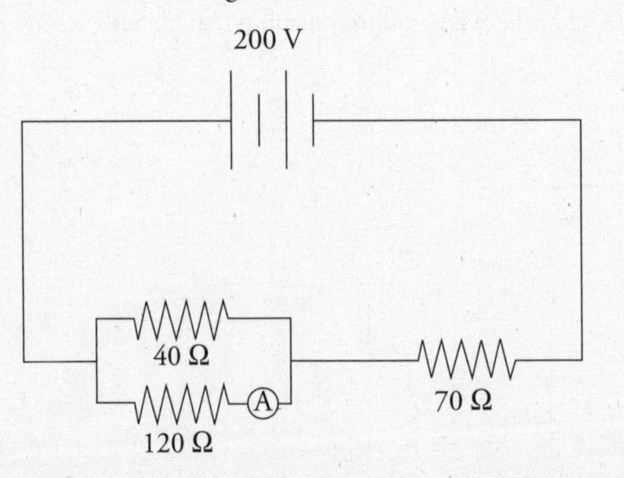

Solution: (The symbol for the battery in this circuit consists of two pairs of parallel lines, rather than the usual one pair. Batteries can be denoted by one *or more* pairs of parallel lines, as long as one "end" is a long line (representing the positive terminal) and the opposite "end" of the battery is a short line (representing the negative terminal). The two parallel resistors are equivalent to a single 30 Ω resistor (because (40 × 120)/(40+120) = 4800/160 = 30). This, in series with the 70 Ω resistor, means the overall resistance of the circuit is 30 + 70 = 100 Ω, so the current is $I = V/R_{eq}$ = (200 V)/(100 Ω) = 2 A. The voltage drop across the 30 Ω equivalent resistance is therefore (2 A)(30 Ω) = 60 V, so this is the voltage across each of the individual parallel resistors. The ammeter is placed in the branch with the 120 Ω resistor, so it will measure a current of V/R = (60 V)/(120 Ω) = 0.5 A.

Example 9-19: A device used to measure the voltage between two points in a circuit is called a **voltmeter** (denoted by V in a circuit diagram). It has a very large internal resistance so that it won't draw much current and thus affect the voltage it's trying to measure. What would a voltmeter read if it were placed as shown in the following circuit?

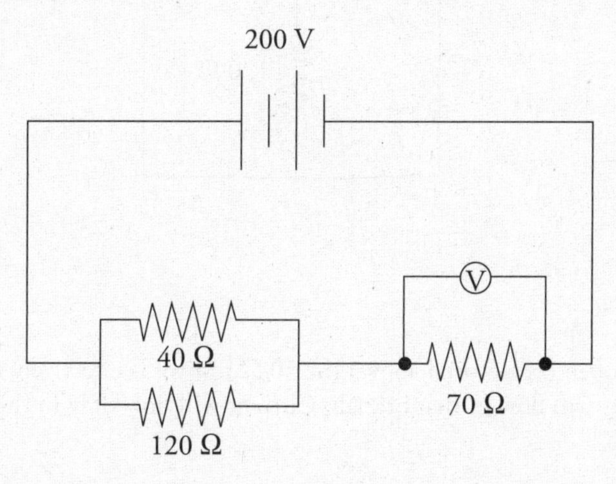

Solution: This is the same circuit we analyzed in the preceding example. Because the current in the circuit is 2 A, the voltage across the 70 Ω resistor will be $V = IR$ = (2 A)(70 Ω) = 140 V.

Example 9-20: The diagram below shows a point X held at a potential of $\phi = 60$ V connected by a combination of resistors to a point (denoted by G) that is **grounded.** ***The ground** is considered to be at potential zero.* What is the current through the 100-ohm resistor?

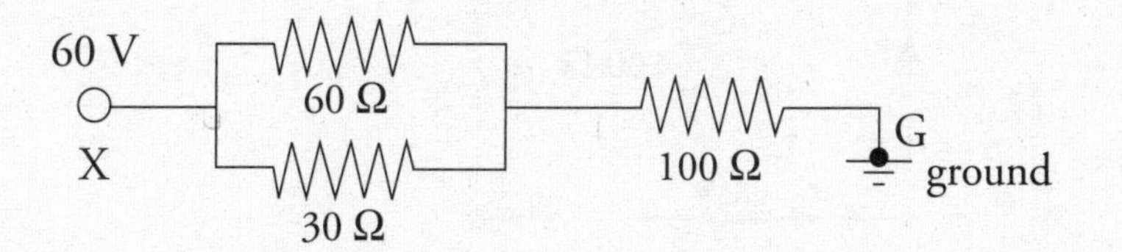

Solution: The parallel resistors are equivalent to a single 20 Ω resistor, which is then in series with the 100 Ω resistor, giving an overall equivalent resistance of 20 + 100 = 120 Ω. Since the potential difference between points X and G is $V = \phi_X - \phi_G = 60 - 0 = 60$ V, the current in the circuit (and through the 100-ohm resistor) is

$$I = V / R_{eq} = (60\text{ V})/(120\ \Omega) = 0.5\text{ A}$$

Example 9-21: The diagram below shows a battery with an emf of 100 V connected to a circuit equipped with a switch, S.

a) What is the current in the circuit when the switch is open?
b) What is the current in the circuit when the switch is closed?

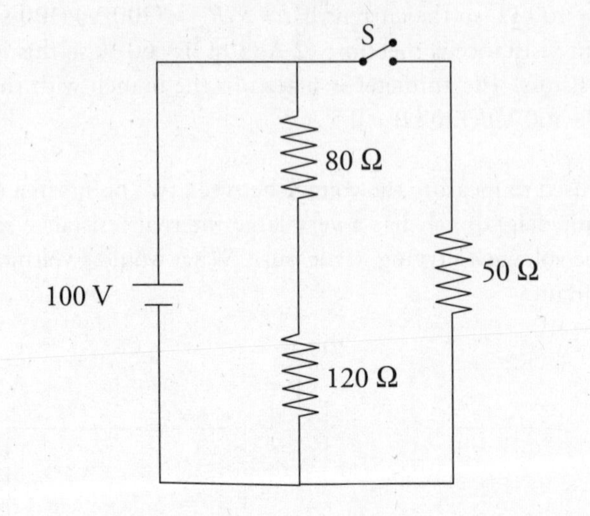

Solution:

a) With the switch open (as pictured above) the 50 Ω resistor is effectively taken out of the circuit; no current will flow in that branch. Current will flow only in the part of the circuit shown below:

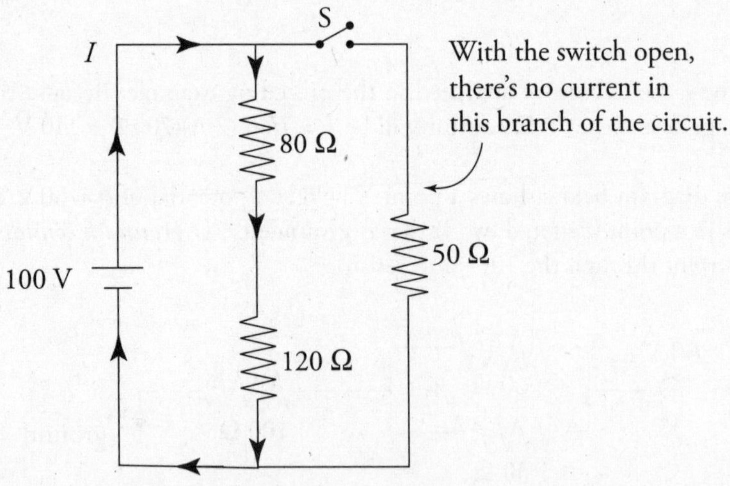

The two resistors that *are* in the circuit when the switch is open are in series, so the total equivalent resistance is 80 + 120 = 200 Ω; thus, the current is

$$I = V / R_{eq} = (100 \text{ V})/(200\ \Omega) = 0.5 \text{ A}$$

b) With the switch closed, all the resistors are part of the circuit, and there will be current in all the branches. Let's find the equivalent resistance. The 80 Ω and 120 Ω resistors are in series, so they're equivalent to a single 80 + 120 = 200 Ω resistor, which is then in parallel with the 50 Ω resistor. This gives an overall equivalent resistance of 40 Ω because (200 × 50)/(200 + 50) is equal to 40. Therefore, the current supplied to the circuit in this case is $I = V/R_{eq}$ = (100 V)/(40 Ω) = 2.5 A.

Example 9-22: Three identical light bulbs are connected to a battery, as shown:

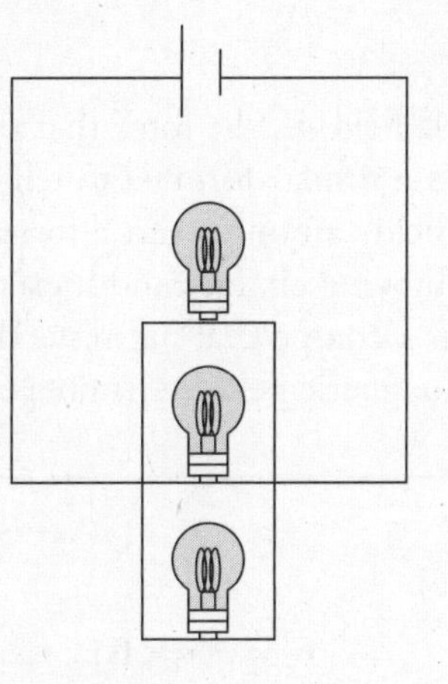

What will happen if the middle bulb burns out?

A. The other two bulbs will go out.
B. The light intensity of the other two bulbs will decrease, but they won't go out.
C. The light intensity of the other two bulbs will increase.
D. The light intensity of the other two bulbs will remain the same.

Solution: Let V be the voltage of the battery, and let R be the resistance of each light bulb. The current through each light bulb (that is, through each resistor) is $I = V/R$. If the middle bulb burns out, then the middle branch of the parallel combination is severed; but current can still flow through the top and bottom bulbs, and the current through each will still be $I = V/R$. Because the intensity of the light is directly related to the power each one dissipates, the fact that the current doesn't change means that $P = I^2R$ won't change, so the light intensity of the other two bulbs will remain the same. The answer is D. [What *will* change if the middle bulb burns out? Before the middle bulb burns out, the current through each of the three bulbs is $I = V/R$, so the battery must be providing a total current of $3I = 3V/R$. After the middle bulb burns out, the current through each of the other two bulbs is still $I = V/R$, so the battery need only provide a total current of $2I = 2V/R$. That is, the total current through the circuit will decrease (since, after all, there are only two bulbs to light, not three). In addition, the power supplied by the battery will also decrease, from $P = (3I)(V) = 3V^2/R$ to $P = (2I)(V) = 2V^2/R$, and the battery will last longer. Finally, notice that if the three bulbs were wired in *series* rather than in parallel, then if any one of the bulbs burned out, they'd all go out because the circuit would be broken.]

9.2 MAGNETIC FIELDS AND FORCES

Electric fields are created by electric charges; **magnetic fields** are created by *moving* electric charges. If a charge is at rest, it produces an electric field in the surrounding space. If this charge were to move, it would create an additional force field, a magnetic field, in the surrounding space. Since charge in motion constitutes a current, we can also say that magnetic fields are produced by electric currents. A permanent bar magnet is a source of a magnetic field because of the multitude of microscopic currents due to motions of the orbiting electrons within the metal; therefore, even a bar magnet's magnetic field is ultimately due to charges in motion.

If we place a charge q in a given electric field, **E**, the force that the field will exert on this charge is given by the equation $\mathbf{F}_E = q\mathbf{E}$. We now need a similar formula to tell us the force that a magnetic field would exert on a charge q. First, a magnetic field can only exert a force on a charge that is *moving* through the field. A magnetic field is produced by moving charges and it exerts a force only on other moving charges. A magnetic field will exert no force on a charge that's at rest. The letter **B** is used to denote a magnetic field. The formula for the force that a magnetic field exerts on a charge q is as follows:

Magnetic Force

$$\mathbf{F}_B = q(\mathbf{v} \times \mathbf{B})$$

where **v** is the velocity of the charge q. Notice that if $\mathbf{v} = 0$ (that is, if the charge is at rest), then $\mathbf{F}_B$ will also be 0.

The formula $\mathbf{F}_B = q(\mathbf{v} \times \mathbf{B})$ involves the *cross product* of **v** and **B**. You don't need to worry about calculating the vector components of the cross product; there is a much simpler way of finding $\mathbf{F}_B$ that is more than adequate for the OAT. First, the magnitude of $\mathbf{F}_B$ is given by this equation:

Magnitude of Magnetic Force

$$F_B = |q|vB\sin\theta$$

where θ is the angle between **v** and **B**. Notice that if **v** is parallel to **B**, then $\theta = 0$, and, since $\sin 0 = 0$, we get $\mathbf{F}_B = 0$. So, a charge could be moving through a magnetic field and yet feel no force if its direction of motion is parallel to the magnetic field lines. The same will be true if **v** is anti-parallel to **B** (that is, if the direction of **v** is exactly opposite to the direction of **B**), since in this case, we have $\theta = 180°$ and $\sin 180° = 0$, so again we get $\mathbf{F}_B = 0$. If $\mathbf{v} \perp \mathbf{B}$, then $\theta = 90°$, and since $\sin 90° = 1$, the magnitude of $\mathbf{F}_B$ becomes simply $F_B = |q|vB$. From this equation, we can find the SI unit for magnetic field strength:

$$[B] = \frac{[F_B]}{[q][v]} = \frac{\text{N}}{\text{C}\cdot\frac{\text{m}}{\text{s}}} = \frac{\text{N}}{\frac{\text{C}}{\text{s}}\cdot\text{m}} = \frac{\text{N}}{\text{A}\cdot\text{m}}$$

One newton per amp-meter (1 N/A·m) is renamed one **tesla**, abbreviated T. That is, B is measured in teslas.

Now that we know how to find the magnitude of $\mathbf{F}_B$, all we need is a way to find the direction. The direction of $\mathbf{F}_B$ will depend on whether the charge q that moves through the field is positive or negative. Just like the force due to an electric field, the force due to a magnetic field also depends on the sign of the charge: If **B** exerts a force in a particular direction on a charge $+q$ moving with velocity **v**, then it would exert a force in the opposite direction on $-q$ moving with velocity **v**. In addition, magnetic forces have the following strange property: *The direction of* $\mathbf{F}_B$ *is always perpendicular to both* **v** *and* **B**. For example, if we had a magnetic field whose field lines pointed across this page (say, from left to right), and a positive charge q travels down the page, then the direction of the force $\mathbf{F}_B$ that q feels would be out of the plane of the page. The direction of $\mathbf{F}_B$ will always be perpendicular to the plane containing the vectors **v** and **B**, since we're now dealing with a situation in which we'll have vectors in *three* dimensions, we need a notation to indicate when a vector points into, or out of, the plane of the page. Here are the symbols:

● *or* ⊙	× *or* ⊗
means **out of** the plane of the page	means **into** the plane of the page

Now let's learn how to find the direction of the magnetic force, $\mathbf{F}_B$, acting on a particle of charge q moving with velocity **v** through a magnetic field **B**. It involves the **right-hand rule** and the **left-hand rule**. You use the right-hand rule if the charge q moving through the field is positive, and the left-hand rule if q is negative.[3] Here's how the rules work.

First, determine whether the charge moving through the magnetic field is positive or negative.

If q is *positive*, use your *right* hand and the *right*-hand rule.

If q is *negative*, use your *left* hand and the *left*-hand rule.

Whether you use the right-hand rule or the left-hand rule, you will always follow these steps:

1. Orient your hand so that your thumb points in the direction of the velocity **v**.
2. Point your fingers in the direction of **B**.
3. The direction of $\mathbf{F}_B$ will then be perpendicular to your palm.

[3] Another method which many people prefer is always to use the right-hand rule, and then reverse the result (in other words, solve for the direction of the force on a positive charge, and then realize that the force on a negative charge is in exactly the opposite direction).

Think of your palm pushing with the force F_B; the direction it pushes is the direction of F_B.

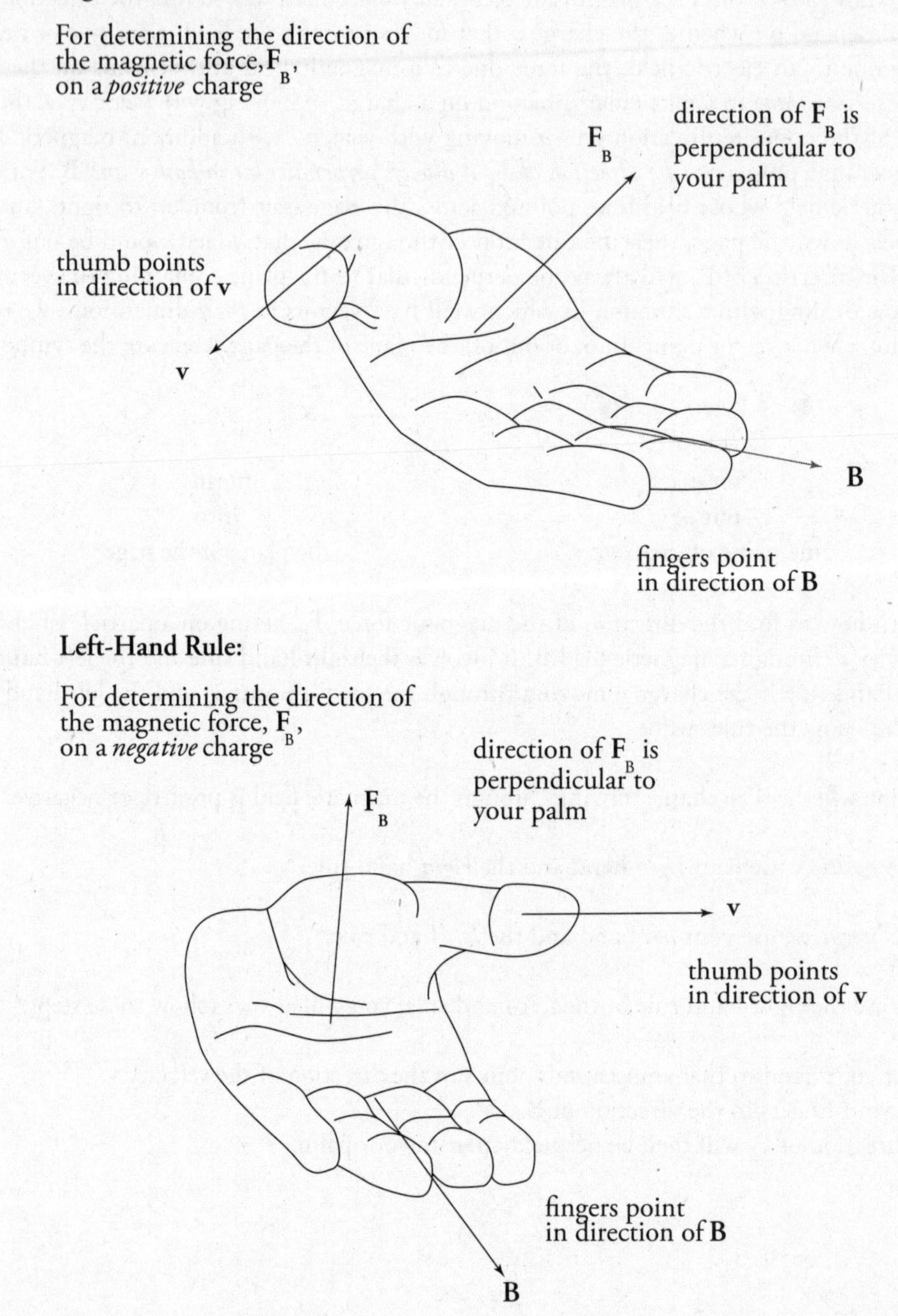

For example, let's say we have a positive charge q moving with velocity **v** to the right across the plane of this page through a magnetic field **B** directed toward the top of the page. How would you find the direction of the resulting magnetic force on this moving charge? Since q is positive, use your right hand, and lay it flat on this page with your palm facing up; notice that in this orientation, your thumb points to the right (as it should since your thumb always points in the direction of the particle's velocity, **v**) and your fingers point up toward the top of the page (as they should since your fingers always point in the direction of the magnetic field, **B**). The direction of $\mathbf{F}_B$ is perpendicular to your palm, pointing out of the plane of the page, and so we symbolize the direction of $\mathbf{F}_B$ by ◉. In this case, the charged particle would start curling out of the plane of the page as a result of the magnetic force it feels.

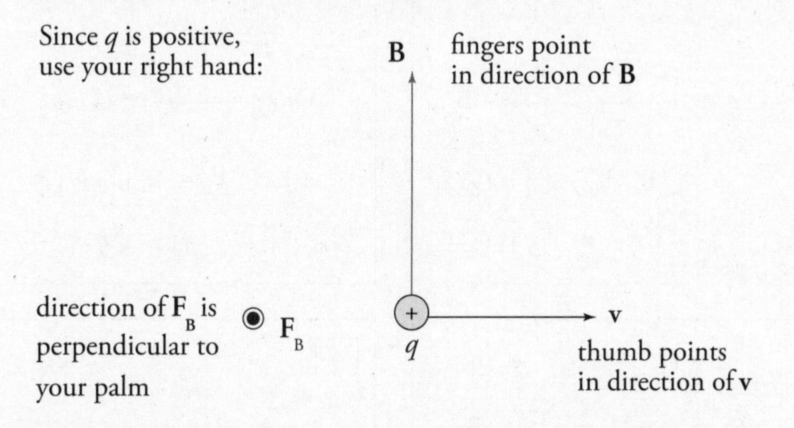

Now let's examine what would happen in the previous example if the charged particle had been *negative*. That is, we have a *negative* charge q moving with velocity **v** to the right across the plane of this page through a magnetic field **B** directed toward the top of the page. How would you find the direction of the resulting magnetic force on this moving charge? Since q is negative, use your *left* hand, and lay it flat on this page with your palm facing *down*; notice that in this orientation, your thumb points to the right (as it should since your thumb always points in the direction of the particle's velocity, **v**) and your fingers point up toward the top of the page (as they should since your fingers always point in the direction of the magnetic field, **B**). The direction of $\mathbf{F}_B$ is perpendicular to your palm, pointing *into* the plane of the page, and so we symbolize the direction of $\mathbf{F}_B$ by ⊗. In this case, the charged particle would start curling into the plane of the page as a result of the magnetic force it feels.

Since q is negative, use your left hand:

B fingers point in direction of **B**

direction of $\mathbf{F}_B$ is perpendicular to your palm, into the plane of the page ⊗ $\mathbf{F}_B$

− q **v**

thumb points in direction of **v**

Practice the right- and left-hand rules and verify each of the following:

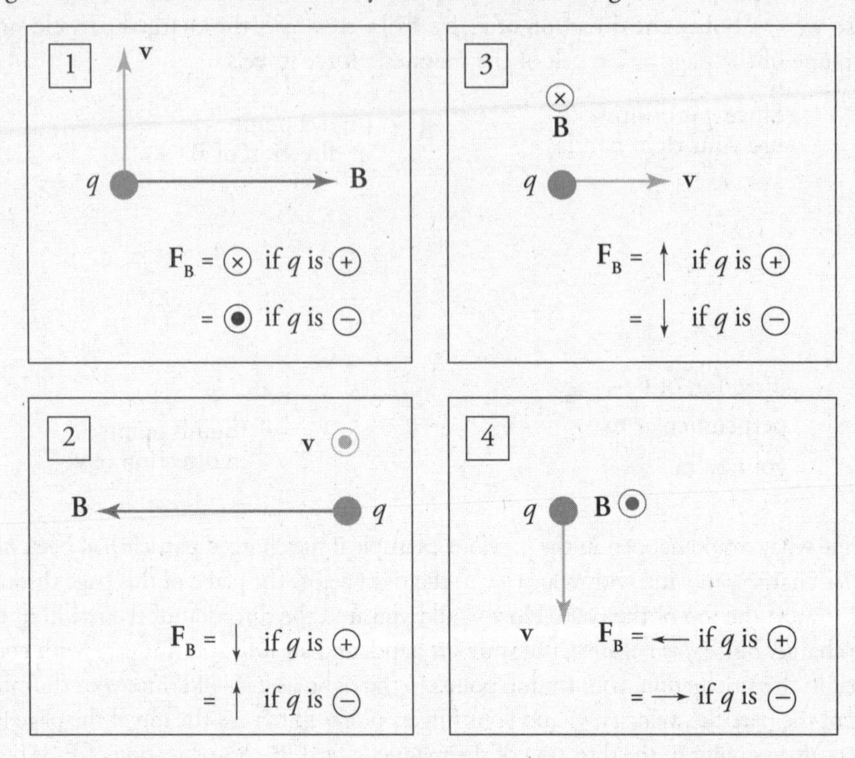

Because the magnetic force a charge feels is always perpendicular to the velocity of the charge, *magnetic forces do no work*. Recall that if a force **F** is perpendicular to the displacement **d** of an object, then this force **F** does zero work, because $W = Fd \cos \theta$ and $\theta = 90°$; since $\cos 90° = 0$, we get $W = 0$. Since magnetic forces never do work, they can never change the kinetic energy of a particle, meaning that KE is constant. (This follows from the work-energy theorem, $W = \Delta KE$.) Since magnetic forces cannot change the kinetic energy of a particle, they can't change the speed of a particle. All magnetic forces can do is make charged particles change their direction; they can't make them speed up or slow down.

The formula given earlier for the magnitude of the magnetic force is $|q| v B \sin\theta$, where θ is the angle between **v** and **B**. On the OAT, it's most common to have a constant magnetic field and **v** ⊥ **B**; in this case, $\theta = 90°$, and because $\sin 90° = 1$, the magnitude of $\mathbf{F}_B$ becomes $F_B = |q| vB$. Further, if **v** ⊥ **B**, the subsequent motion of the charged particle will be uniform circular motion, with the magnetic force providing the centripetal force. Recall that in uniform circular motion, the centripetal force is always perpendicular to the particle's velocity and the particle's speed is constant; all the particle does is continuously change direction as it moves in a circular path. This is consistent with what we said in the previous paragraph about magnetic forces: they don't change the speed of a particle, only its direction. The case of a charged particle executing uniform circular motion in a constant magnetic field is so important for the OAT, that we'll do the following example in detail.

Example 9-23: A proton is injected with velocity **v** into a region of constant magnetic field **B** that points out of the plane of the page. The direction of **v** is to the right, in the plane of the page, as shown in the diagram below:

proton

v

B

a) Describe the subsequent motion of the proton.
b) Find the radius of the circular trajectory it follows.

Solution:

a) Because the proton is a positive charge, we use the *right*-hand rule to find the direction of the magnetic force it feels. With **v** to the right and **B** out of the page, we find that $\mathbf{F}_B$ points downward in the plane of the page:

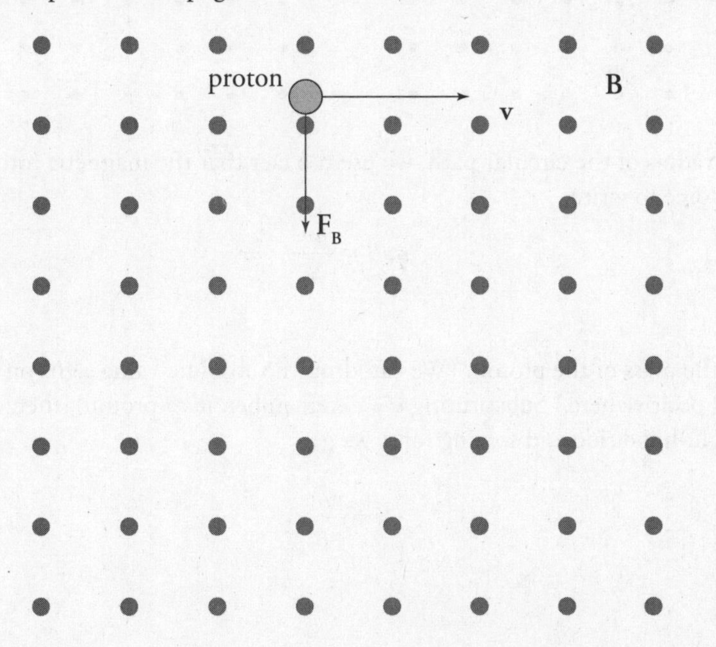

As a result, the proton will curve downward, and as it does, it is still continuously acted on by the magnetic force, but because the direction of **v** changes, so will the direction of $\mathbf{F}_B$. For example, when the proton is at the position shown in the following figure, the direction of $\mathbf{F}_B$ will be to the left:

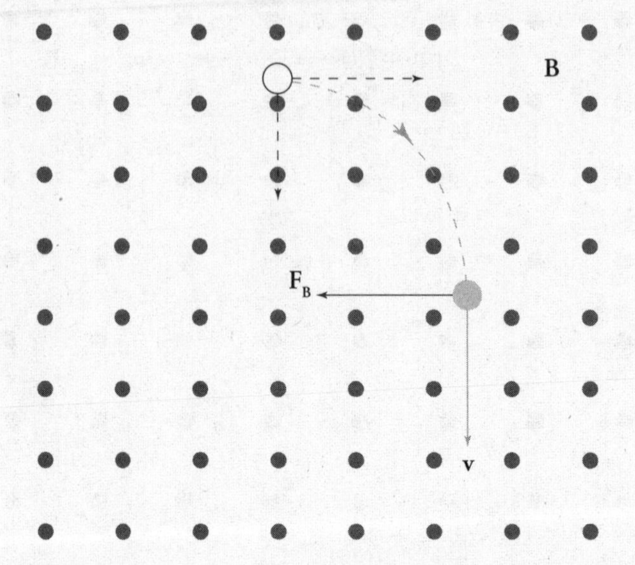

We can now see that the proton will continue to curve in a circular path, traveling clockwise:

b) To find the radius of the circular path, we use the fact that the magnetic force provides the centripetal force to write

$$qvB = \frac{mv^2}{r}$$

where m is the mass of the proton. (We can drop the absolute value signs on the charge q because q is positive here.) Substituting $q = e$ (remember, it's a proton), then canceling one v from the right-hand side and solving for r, we get

$$r = \frac{mv}{eB}$$

Example 9-24: A particle with positive charge q and mass m moving with speed v undergoes uniform circular motion in a constant magnetic field **B**. If the radius of the particle's path is r, which one of the following expressions gives the magnitude of the momentum of the particle?

A. qB/r
B. r/qB
C. rB/q
D. qBr

Solution: Since the magnetic force provides the centripetal force, we have

$$qvB = \frac{mv^2}{r}$$

Canceling one v from the right-hand side, we get $qB = mv/r$, so $mv = qBr$. The answer is D.

Example 9-25: A particle with positive charge q and mass m moving with speed v undergoes uniform circular motion in a constant magnetic field **B**. If the radius of the particle's path is r, which of the following expressions gives the particle's orbit period; in other words, the time required for the particle to complete one revolution?

A. $2\pi/qvB$
B. $2\pi m/qB$
C. $qvB/2\pi m$
D. $qB/2\pi m$

Solution: Since the magnetic force provides the centripetal force, we have

$$qvB = \frac{mv^2}{r}$$

Canceling one v from the right-hand side and solving for r, we get $r = mv/qB$. The time required for the particle to complete one revolution is equal to the total distance traveled by the particle in one revolution (the circumference, $2\pi r$) divided by the particle's speed, v. This gives

$$T = \frac{2\pi r}{v} = \frac{2\pi \cdot \frac{mv}{qB}}{v} = \frac{2\pi m}{qB}$$

Therefore, the answer is B. (*Note*: T is called the *cyclotron period*. Notice that it does *not* depend on r or v. Whether the particle moves rapidly in a large circle or more slowly in a smaller circle, it doesn't matter: the orbit period is determined solely by the mass and charge of the particle, and the magnitude of the magnetic field.)

Example 9-26: A sulfide ion, S^{2-}, moving with speed v_0, enters a region containing a uniform magnetic field **B**. If the vector $\mathbf{v}_0$ makes an angle of 30° with **B**, what is the magnitude of the initial magnetic force on this ion?

A. $ev_0B/4$
B. $ev_0B/2$
C. ev_0B
D. $2ev_0B$

Solution: The charge on this ion is $-2e$, so the initial magnetic force the ion feels has magnitude

$$F_B = |q|vB\sin\theta = |-2e|\cdot v_0B\sin 30° = 2e\cdot v_0B\cdot \tfrac{1}{2} = ev_0B$$

The answer is C.

Example 9-27: A particle with negative charge $-q$ moving with speed v_0 enters a region containing a uniform magnetic field **B**. If the vector $\mathbf{v}_0$ makes an angle of 30° with **B**, what is the particle's speed 8 seconds after entering the field?

A. $v_0/4$
B. v_0
C. $2v_0$
D. $4v_0$

Solution: Since magnetic forces do no work, the kinetic energy (and thus the speed) of the particle will be unchanged. The answer is B.

Example 9-28: A particle with charge q moves with velocity **v** through a region of space containing a uniform electric field, **E**, *and* a uniform magnetic field, **B**. Which of the following expressions gives the total electromagnetic force on the particle?

A. $q(\mathbf{E} + \mathbf{B})$
B. $q(\mathbf{v} \times \mathbf{E} + \mathbf{B})$
C. $q\mathbf{v} \times (\mathbf{E} + \mathbf{B})$
D. $q(\mathbf{E} + \mathbf{v} \times \mathbf{B})$

Solution: The electric force on the particle is $\mathbf{F}_E = q\mathbf{E}$, and the magnetic force is $\mathbf{F}_B = q(\mathbf{v} \times \mathbf{B})$. Therefore, the *total* electromagnetic force is

$$\mathbf{F}_E + \mathbf{F}_B = q\mathbf{E} + q(\mathbf{v} \times \mathbf{B}) = q(\mathbf{E} + \mathbf{v} \times \mathbf{B})$$

The answer is D.

Note: The total electromagnetic force is known as the **Lorentz force**.

Example 9-29: The figure below shows a charged parallel-plate capacitor with a uniform electric field, E, in the space between its plates. A uniform magnetic field, **B**, is also produced in the space between the capacitor plates by another device.

At what speed would an electron need to travel between the plates in order to pass through undeflected? (Ignore gravity.)

A. E/B
B. B/E
C. EB
D. EB^2

Solution: In between the plates, the direction of the electric force, $\mathbf{F}_E$, on the electron is upward. Using the left-hand rule (because the particle carries a negative charge), we find that the direction of the magnetic force, $\mathbf{F}_B$, is downward.

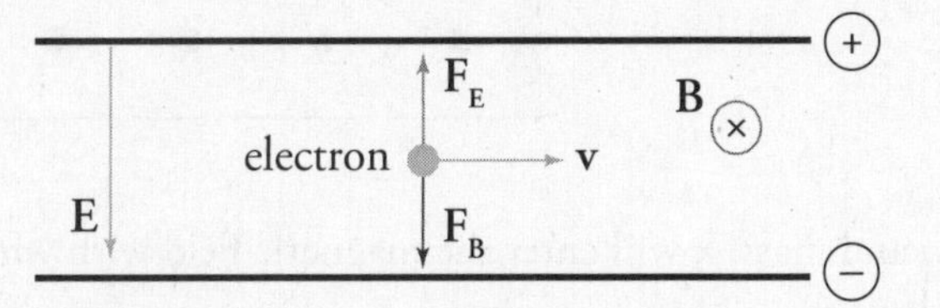

Therefore, these two forces point in opposite directions. They'll cancel (giving $\mathbf{F}_{net} = 0$) and allow the particle to pass through undeflected if these forces have the same magnitude. The magnitude of the electric force is $F_E = |q|E = |-e|E = eE$, and the magnitude of the magnetic force is $F_B = |q|vB = |-e|vB = evB$. Therefore, we'll have $F_B = F_E$ when $evB = eE$. Solving this equation for v, we find that $v = E/B$, choice A.

Example 9-30: A uniform magnetic field **B** exerts a force $\mathbf{F}_B$ on a particle with charge q moving with velocity **v** through the field. Which of the following gives the magnetic force that the same field would exert on a particle of charge $2q$ moving with velocity –2**v**?

A. $-8\mathbf{F}_B$
B. $-4\mathbf{F}_B$
C. $4\mathbf{F}_B$
D. $8\mathbf{F}_B$

Solution: If **B** exerts a force of $\mathbf{F}_B$ on a charge q moving with velocity **v**, then it would exert a force of $-\mathbf{F}_B$ on a charge q moving with velocity –**v**. Now, because F_B is proportional to q and to v, if q and v both double, then F_B will be multiplied by a factor of $2 \cdot 2 = 4$. Therefore, the force that **B** would exert on a particle of charge $2q$ moving with velocity –2**v** is $-4\mathbf{F}_B$, choice B.

Example 9-31: The figure below shows a simple mass spectrometer. It consists of a source of ions that are accelerated from rest through a potential difference V, and then enter a region containing a uniform magnetic field **B**, that points out of the plane of the page and is perpendicular to the initial velocity, **v**, of the ion as it enters. Once an ion enters the magnetic field, it travels in a semicircular path until it strikes the detector, which records its arrival and the distance, d, from the opening.

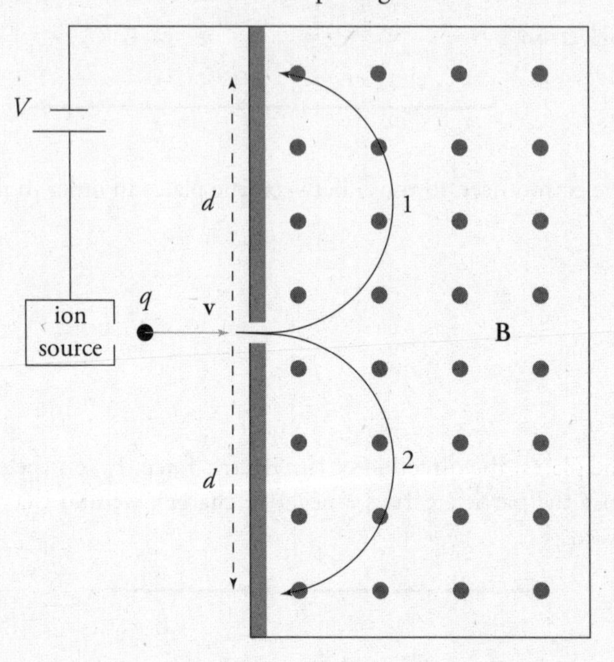

a) An ion of charge $+q$ and mass m will enter the magnetic field with what speed? Write v in terms of q, m, and V.
b) Which semicircular path would a cation follow: 1 or 2?
c) If you were using this device in a lab to analyze a sample containing various isotopes of an element, how would you find the mass of a cation striking the detector if all you knew were q, V, B, and d?

Solution:

a) The ion loses electrical potential energy in the amount qV, and as a result, gains kinetic energy, $\frac{1}{2}mv^2$. Therefore, $\frac{1}{2}mv^2 = qV$, so $v = \sqrt{2qV/m}$.

b) The right-hand rule (for a positive charge) tells us that if **v** points to the right and **B** points out of the plane of the page, then $\mathbf{F}_B$ points downward:

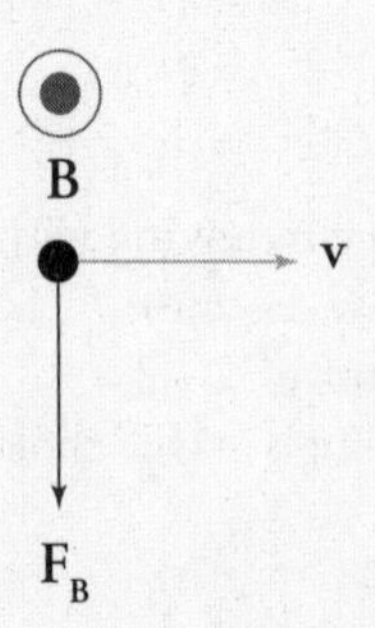

Since F_B points downward when the particle is at the opening, a cation would follow path 2, because F_B provides the centripetal force and thus points toward the center of the path. The following diagram illustrates this:

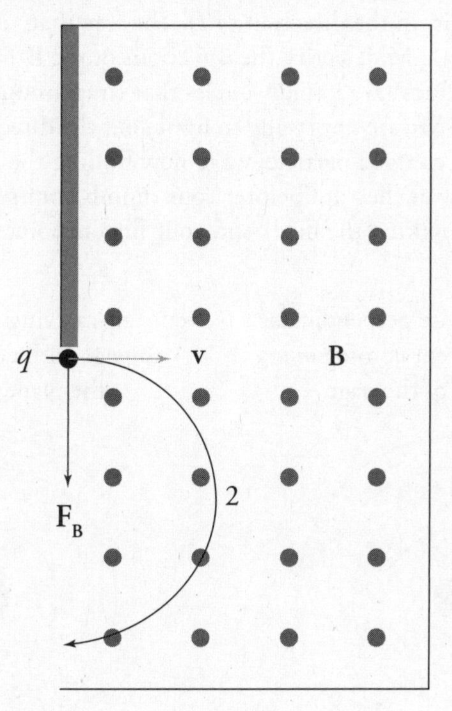

c) Since the magnetic force provides the centripetal force, we have

$$qvB = \frac{mv^2}{r}$$

Canceling one v from the right-hand side and solving for m (the mass of the cation) gives

$$m = \frac{qBr}{v}$$

From the diagram, we see that $r = \frac{1}{2}d$, and from part (a), $v = \sqrt{2qV / m}$, so we get

$$m = \frac{qB \cdot \frac{1}{2}d}{\sqrt{2qV / m}}$$

Squaring both sides and solving for m, we find that the mass of the cation is

$$m = \frac{qB^2 d^2}{8V}$$

Sources of Magnetic Fields

Now that we know how a given magnetic field affects a charged particle, we'll now look at how the magnetic field was created in the first place. Recall that charges *in motion* produce a magnetic field. A current is charge in motion, so electric currents produce magnetic fields. Let's take the simplest possible case: An electric current moving in a straight line. The magnetic field lines created by the current wrap around the current, forming closed loops. To find the direction of these magnetic field loops, we use the right-hand rule because by convention we consider a current I to be the direction that positive charges would move.[4] Imagine grabbing the wire in your right hand in such a way that your thumb points in the direction of the velocity of the charges (that is, in the direction of I). The way that your fingers wrap around the wire gives the direction of the magnetic field. Verify the directions of the **B**-field loops for the wires shown below; remember, magnetic field "lines" are actually circles that wrap around the wire. (That's the end of the right-hand rule in this situation. We are not trying to figure out the direction of the magnetic force that a given magnetic field exerts on a charged particle; we're now finding the magnetic field. Your thumb and fingers mean the same thing now as they did before: Your thumb points in the direction of the motion of the relevant charge (the charge making the field) and your fingers point in the direction of the magnetic field, **B**.)

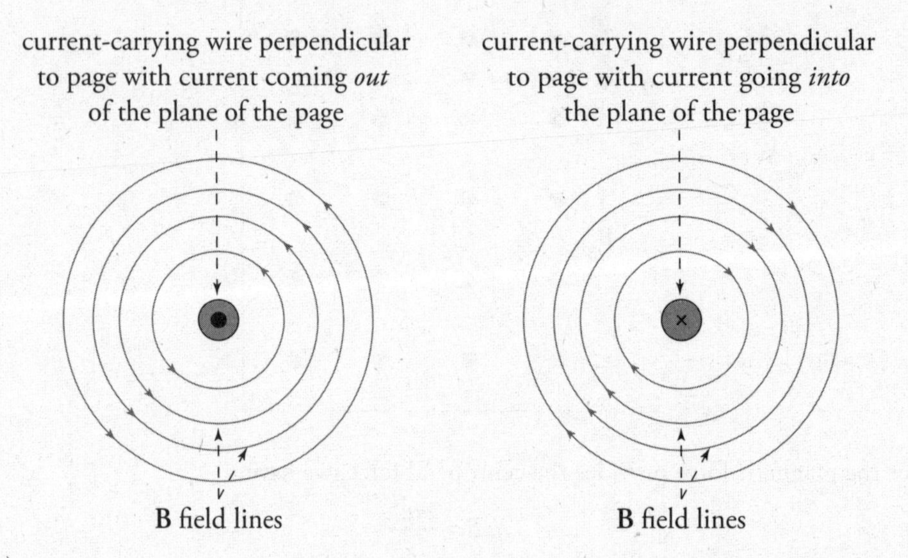

In these next two diagrams, the **B**-field circles look like ellipses because of perspective; here the current-carrying wires lie in the plane of the page, and the **B**-field circles are perpendicular to the page, going into (or out of) the page above the wire and out of (or into) the page below the wire.

With the current pointing to the left, the **B** field lines go into the page above the wire . . .

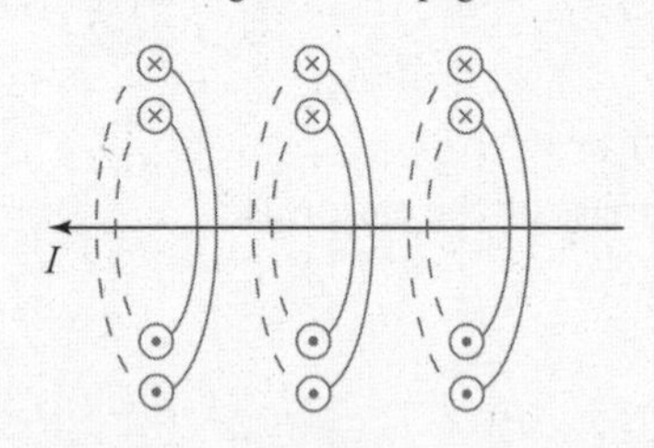

and come out of the page below the wire.

With the current pointing to the right, the **B** field lines come out of the page above the wire . . .

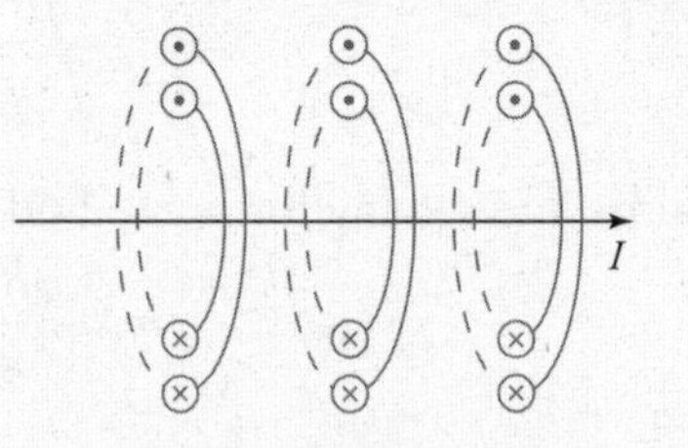

and go into the page below the wire.

---

[4] Though it's uncommon on the OAT, it's possible you'll be asked about the field produced by a single moving charge, not a current. If the charge is positive you simply use the method given here; if the charge is negative you could use the left-hand rule, or use the right-hand rule and then reverse the direction of the answer; in other words, the field lines created by a negative charge circle in the opposite direction from those created by a positive charge.

The magnitude of the magnetic field created by a straight wire carrying a current I is proportional to I and inversely proportional to the distance r from the wire:

$$B \propto \frac{I}{r}$$

Hence, the magnetic field will be stronger if the current is increased or if we are positioned closer to the wire.

Circular wire loops that carry current also create magnetic fields. In the figure below, notice that the field lines are nearly vertical near the center of the circular wire loop that lies along the central axis. At the center of the loop, the magnitude of **B** is proportional to the current, I, and inversely proportional to the radius of the wire loop ($B \propto I/r_{loop}$). If the current in the wire loop had been traveling in the opposite direction (that is, clockwise), then each of the arrows on the **B**-field lines would point in the opposite direction.

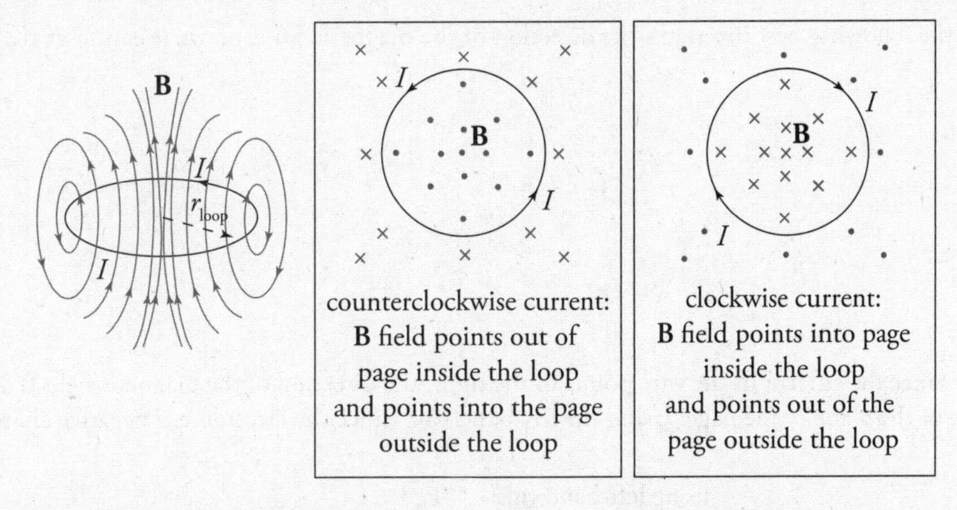

counterclockwise current: **B** field points out of page inside the loop and points into the page outside the loop

clockwise current: **B** field points into page inside the loop and points out of the page outside the loop

Imagine taking a long wire and wrapping it tightly around a cylinder, like a paper-towel tube. The result will look like a spring; we can also consider it to be like a lot of circular loops close together. Such a helical coil of wire is called a **solenoid**. The magnetic field it produces inside the cylinder is parallel to the central axis and achieves its maximum magnitude *on* the central axis, getting weaker as we move away from the center, closer to the coils:

portion of a current-carrying solenoid

Imagine this section above the plane of the page, with the current flowing down . . .

I

B

I

. . .and this section behind the plane of the page, with the current flowing up.

9.2

If the solenoid has many windings and if the length is much greater than its diameter, then the magnetic field down the center of a long solenoid is nearly uniform and is proportional to the current (I) and to the number of turns per unit length (N/L): $B \propto I(N/L)$. Hence, the magnetic field will be stronger if the current is increased or if the solenoid wire loops are tightly packed.

Example 9-32: The figure below shows a long, straight wire carrying a current, I. An electron is projected above the wire and initially parallel to it.

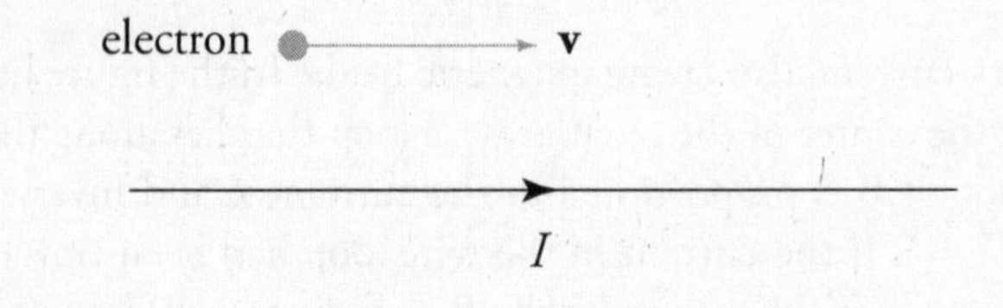

Which of the following best illustrates the direction of the magnetic force on the electron at the position shown?

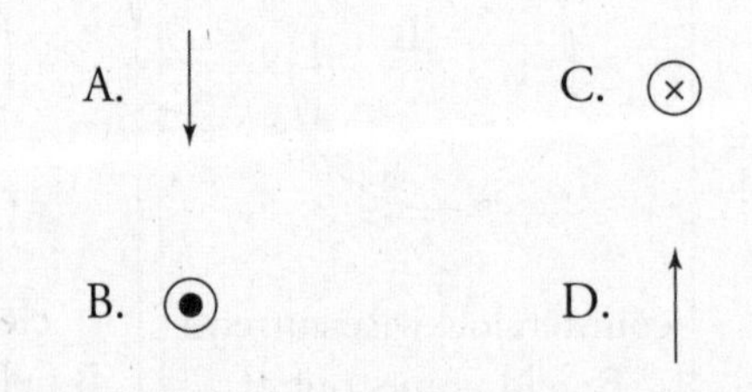

Solution: Since the current in the wire points to the right, the direction of the magnetic field **B** above the wire is out of the plane of the page. Using the left-hand rule (since the electron is a negative charge),

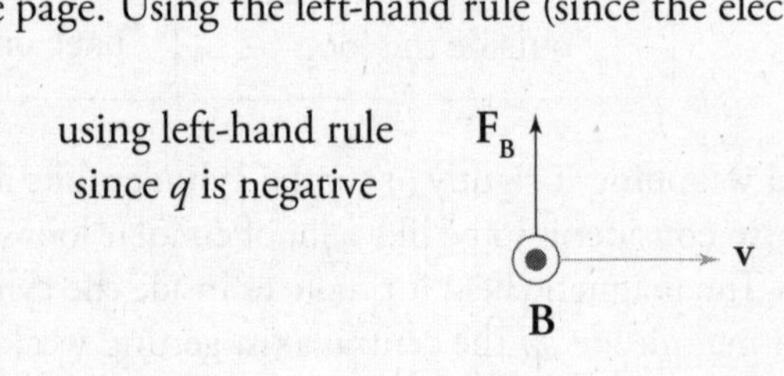

we find that the direction of the magnetic force $\mathbf{F}_B$ is upward, away from the wire, so choice D is correct.

Example 9-33: The figure below shows two long, straight wires carrying current. The top wire carries a current $I_1 = I$ to the left, while the bottom wire carries a current $I_2 = 2I$ to the right.

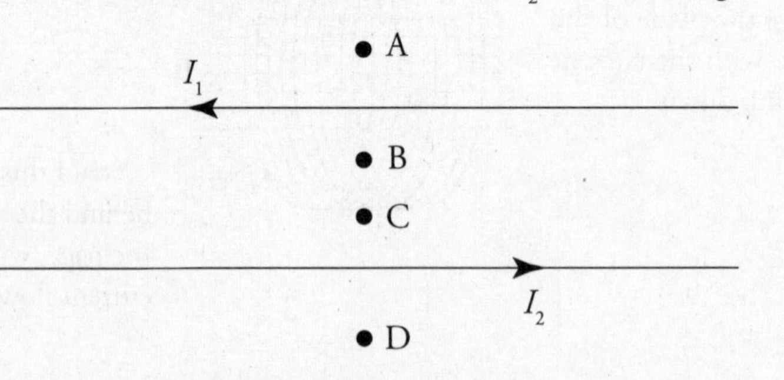

Points A and B are equidistant from the top wire, and Points C and D are equidistant from the bottom wire. Furthermore, the distance between Points B and C is the same as the distance between B and the top wire, which is also the same as the distance between C and the bottom wire. Of these four points, where is the total magnetic field the weakest?

Solution: First, we notice that the magnetic field created by the top wire, $\mathbf{B}_1$, encircles the wire, with the magnetic field circles centered on the top wire and pointing into the plane of the page above the wire and out of the page below it. Similarly, the magnetic field created by the bottom wire, $\mathbf{B}_2$, also encircles the wire, with the magnetic field circles centered on the bottom wire and pointing out of the plane of the page above the wire and into the page below it:

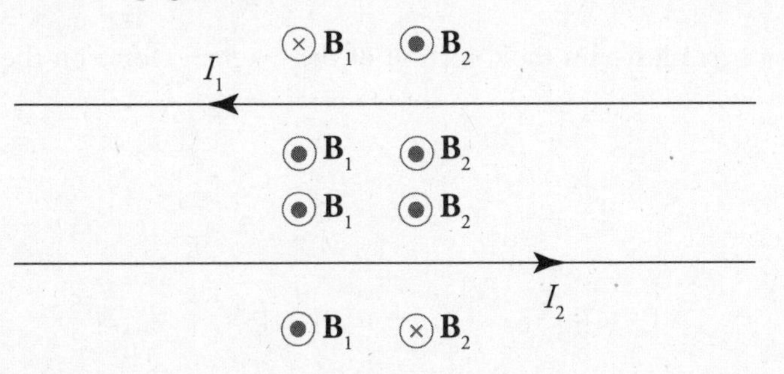

So, we can immediately rule out choices B and C; between the wires, the individual magnetic fields point in the same direction, so their magnitudes add, giving a strong field in this region. However, above the top wire and below the bottom wire, the individual magnetic fields point in opposite directions, so their magnitudes subtract; therefore, of the choices given, the field is weakest at either Point A or Point D. Because $I_2 = 2I$, Point D is closer to the higher-current wire, so to calculate the net **B** field at Point D, we'd subtract a small quantity (the contribution from the weaker-current, which is also farther away) from a large quantity (the contribution from the close higher-current). By contrast, to calculate the net **B** field at Point A, the quantity we'd subtract is larger than the one we subtracted to find the field at Point D and the positive term here is smaller than the positive term in the calculation of the field at Point D. Therefore, we expect the field at Point A to be weaker than at Point D. If this "intuitive" argument is unconvincing, let's do some math to back it up:

$$B_{\text{at A}} = B_{1\text{A}} - B_{2\text{A}} \propto \frac{I_1}{r_{1\text{A}}} - \frac{I_2}{r_{2\text{A}}} = \frac{I}{d} - \frac{2I}{4d} = \frac{2I}{4d}$$

A, B, C, D; I_1, I_2; d, d, d, d, d

$$B_{\text{at D}} = B_{2\text{D}} - B_{1\text{D}} \propto \frac{I_2}{r_{2\text{D}}} - \frac{I_1}{r_{1\text{D}}} = \frac{2I}{d} - \frac{I}{4d} = \frac{7I}{4d}$$

Example 9-34: The figure below shows a circular loop of wire in the plane of the page, carrying a current I. A proton is projected with velocity **v**, such that **v** lies in a plane slightly above and parallel to the plane of the loop, as shown:

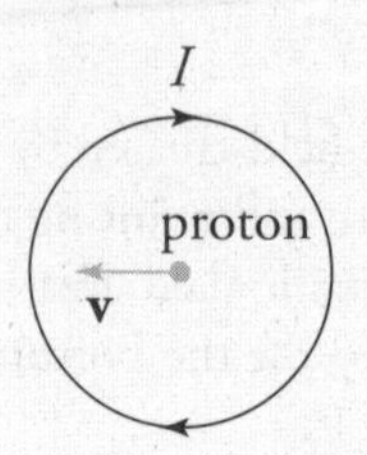

Which of the following best illustrates the direction of the magnetic force on the proton at the position shown?

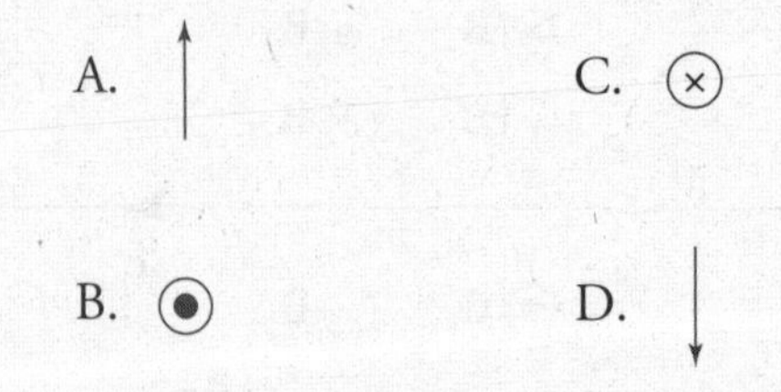

Solution: Since the current in the loop travels clockwise, the direction of the magnetic field **B** above the center of the loop points *into* the plane of the page. Using the right-hand rule (since the proton is a positive charge),

using right-hand rule
since q is positive

B

v

$\mathbf{F}_B$

we find that the magnetic force $\mathbf{F}_B$ is in the plane above and parallel to the plane of the loop, and with a direction as illustrated by choice D.

Example 9-35: The figure below shows a portion of a long, narrow solenoid carrying a current, I. An alpha particle (α) is projected with velocity **v** down the central axis of the solenoid, as shown:

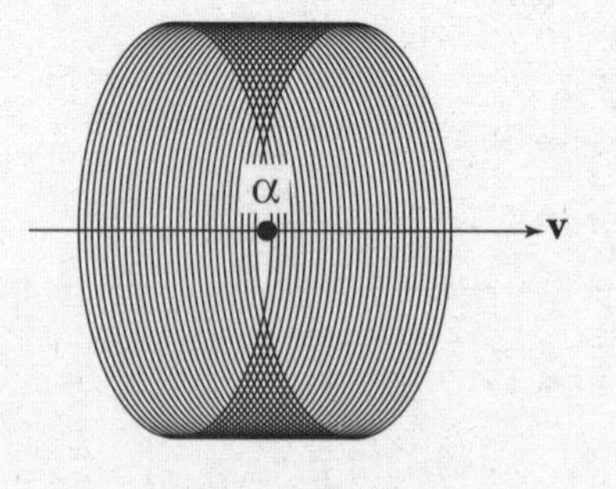

Which of the following best illustrates the direction of the magnetic force on the alpha particle?

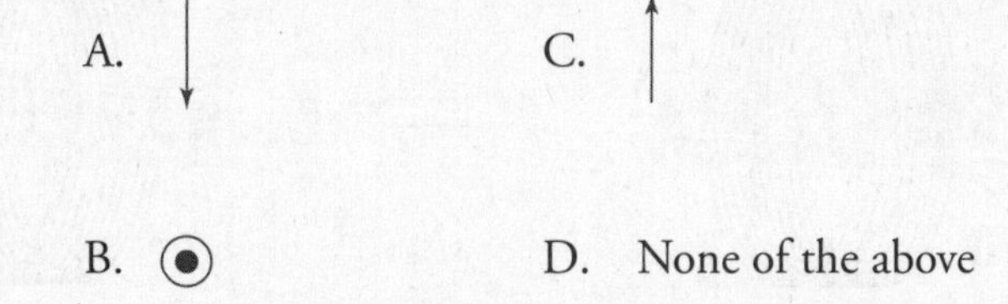

Solution: At the position of the alpha particle, the magnetic field **B** created by the current-carrying solenoid is directed along the central axis; that is, either in the same direction as **v** or in the opposite direction from **v**, depending on the direction of the current in the wire loops. In either case, though, the magnetic force will be zero. (Remember that if **v** is parallel [or anti-parallel] to **B**, then $\mathbf{F}_B = 0$.) The answer is D.

Magnets

A permanent bar magnet creates a magnetic field that closely resembles the magnetic field produced by a circular loop of current-carrying wire:

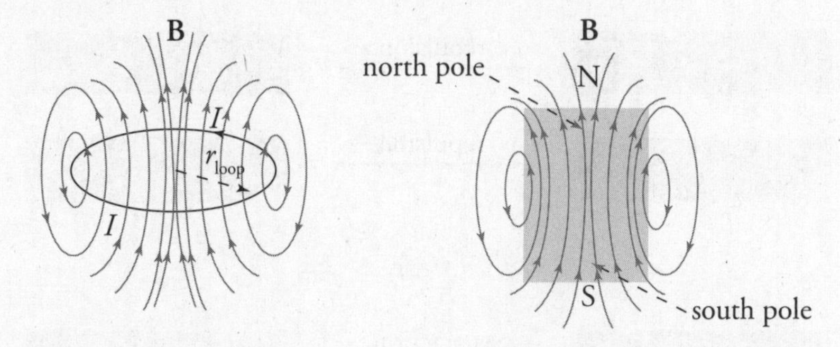

By convention, the magnetic field lines emanate from the end of the magnet designated the **north pole** (**N**) and then curl around and re-enter the magnet at the end designated the **south pole** (S). The magnetic field created by a permanent bar magnet is due to the electrons; they have an intrinsic spin (remember the spin quantum number, m_s, from general chemistry?) and they orbit their nuclei; therefore, they are charges in motion, the ultimate source of all magnetic fields. If a piece of iron is placed in an external magnetic field (for example, the one created by a current-carrying solenoid) the individual magnetic dipole moments of the electrons will be forced to more or less line up. Because iron is *ferromagnetic*, these now-aligned magnetic dipole moments tend to retain this configuration, thus permanently magnetizing the bar and causing it to produce its own magnetic field.

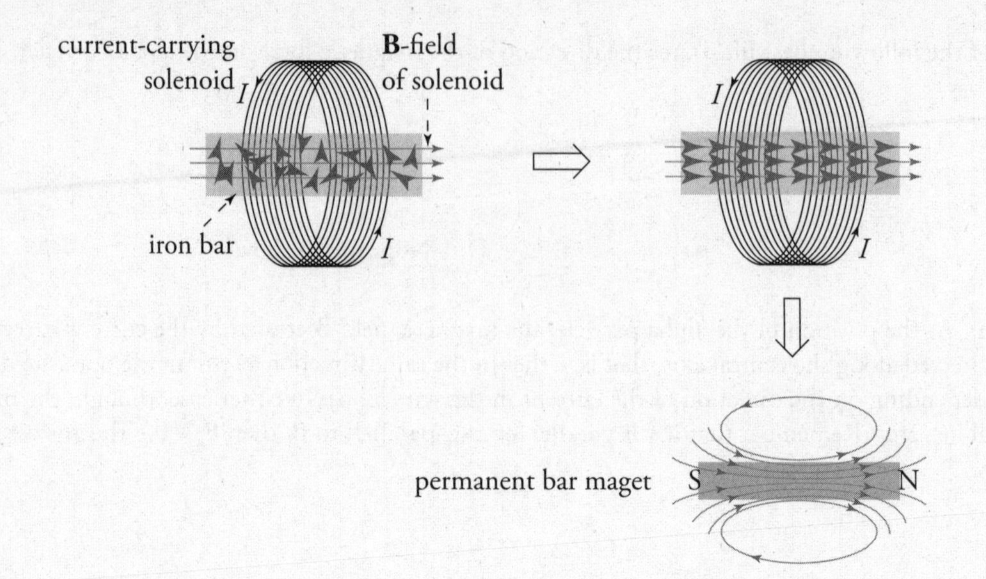

As with electric charges, like magnetic poles repel each other, while opposite magnetic poles attract each other:

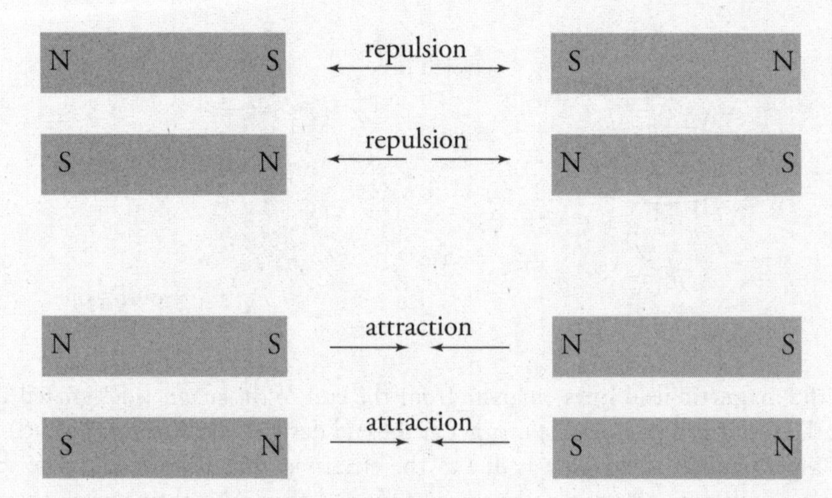

However, while you can have a positive electric charge all by itself, you can't have a single magnetic pole all by itself: the existence of a lone magnetic pole has never been confirmed. That is, there are no magnetic *monopoles*; magnetic poles always exist *in pairs*. If you cut a bar magnet into two pieces, you wouldn't get a piece with just an N and another piece with just an S; you'd get two separate and complete magnets, each with a N–S *pair*:

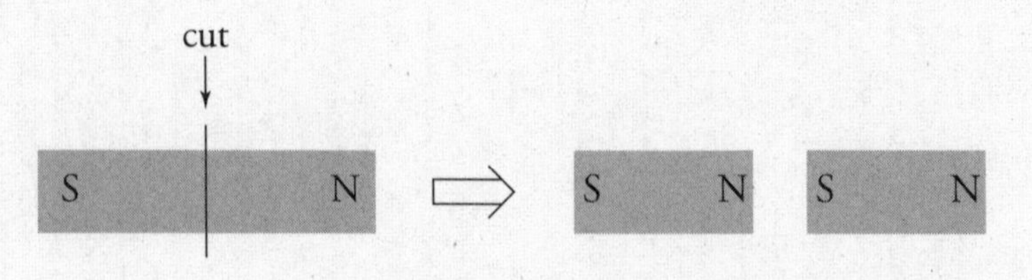

Example 9-36: When a magnet is placed in a magnetic field, it tends to align with the field, so that the vector from the S pole to the N pole of the magnet is parallel to the field lines.

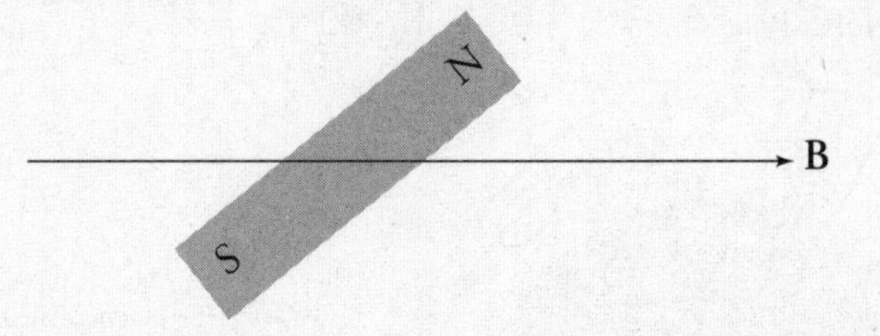

Given that the uniform magnetic field **B** in the figure above exerts the same magnitude of force on the N pole as it does on the S pole, and the magnetic force on a pole is along the field line, what can you say about the net force and net torque on the magnet?

Solution: Because the **B** field will exert a force $\mathbf{F}_B$ on the N pole and a force of $-\mathbf{F}_B$ on the S pole, the net force on the magnet will be zero ($\mathbf{F}_B + -\mathbf{F}_B = 0$). However, the net torque will not be zero, since the magnetic force produces a clockwise torque on each pole, tending to align the magnet parallel to the field line.

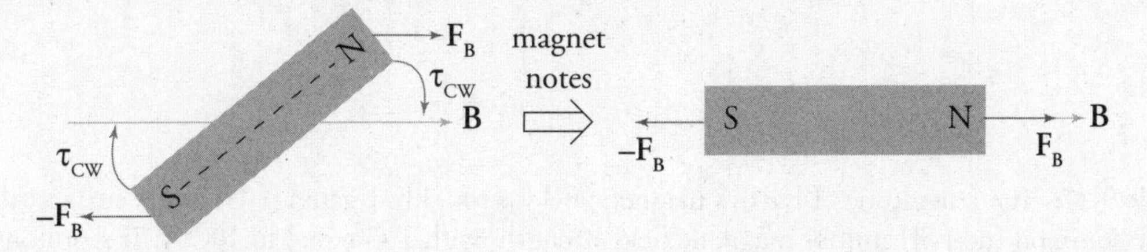

The rotating Earth itself is the source of a (nonuniform) magnetic field, which surrounds the planet and traps electrons and protons emitted by the Sun, making them spiral throughout curved regions called the Van Allen belts. (Protons tend to be confined in Van Allen belts close to Earth's surface, while electrons spiral around in belts farther from the surface. These energetic trapped protons can ionize nitrogen and oxygen in the upper atmosphere, creating cations and electrons. When these cations and electrons recombine, energy is emitted. This is the source of the light that produces the aurora borealis [and, in the southern hemisphere, the aurora australis].) The magnetic poles are *near*, but not *at*, the geographic poles; also notice that it's the magnetic *south* pole that's near the geographic North Pole, and the magnetic *north* pole that's near the geographic South Pole. After all, the magnetic north pole of a compass needle points (roughly) toward geographic north, but we know that it's *opposite* magnetic poles that attract, so the compass needle must be attracted to the magnetic south pole.

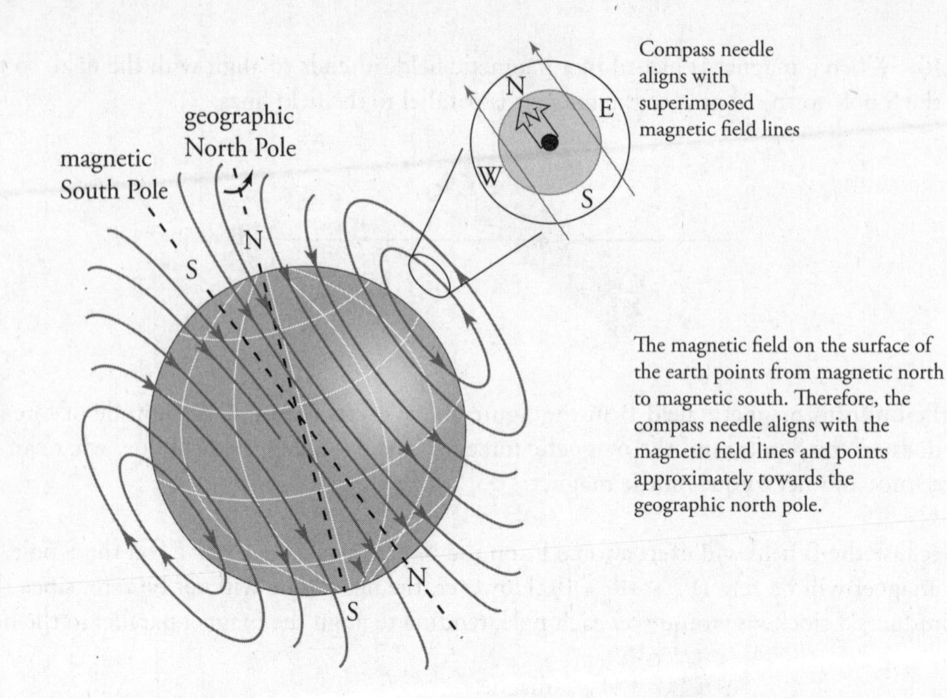

Example 9-37: The magnitude of Earth's magnetic field is roughly 1 gauss (1 G) at the surface; the **gauss** is a very common (non-SI) unit of magnetic field strength, with 1 G equal to 10^{-4} T. If a proton moving with speed $v = 5 \times 10^6$ m/s in the atmosphere experiences a magnetic field strength of 0.5 G, what force (magnetic or gravitational) has the greater effect? (*Note*: mass of proton ≈ 1.7×10^{-27} kg.)

Solution: The gravitational force on the proton is

$$F_{\text{grav}} = mg = (1.7 \times 10^{-27} \text{ kg})(10 \text{ N/kg}) = 1.7 \times 10^{-26} \text{ N}$$

The maximum magnetic force on the proton is

$$F_{\text{B}} = qvB = evB = (1.6 \times 10^{-19} \text{ C})(5 \times 10^{6} \text{ m/s})(0.5 \times 10^{-4} \text{ T}) = 4 \times 10^{-17} \text{ N}$$

Since $F_{\text{B}} >> F_{\text{grav}}$, we see that it's the magnetic force that is chiefly responsible for the proton's motion through Earth's atmosphere.

Example 9-38: Two bar magnets are fixed in position, and a proton is projected with velocity **v** into the region between adjacent opposite poles, as shown below:

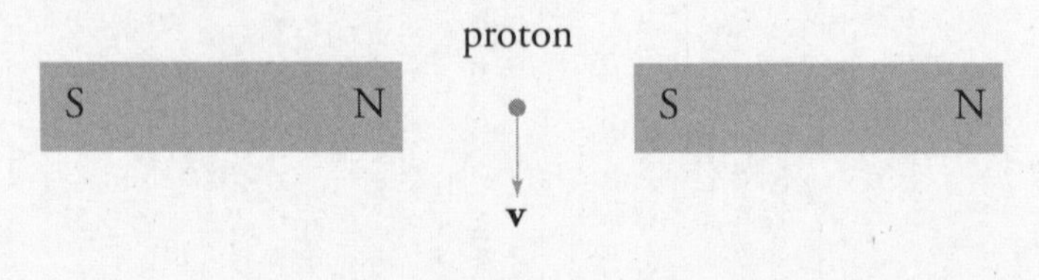

Which of the following best illustrates the direction of the magnetic force on the proton at the position shown?

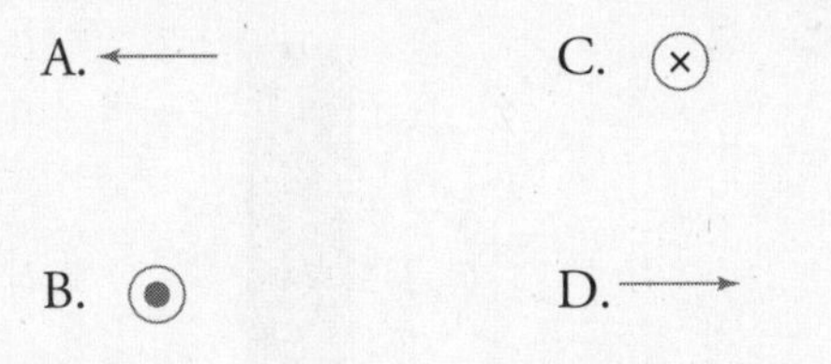

Solution: On the outside of the magnet(s), **B** points from the N pole to the S pole.

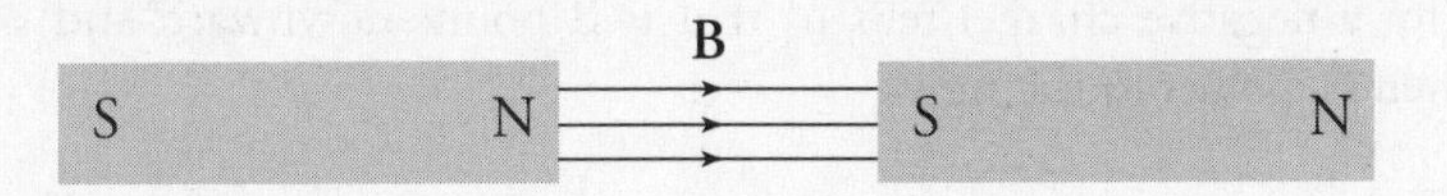

Using the right-hand rule (for a positive charge) where **B** points to the right and **v** is downward, then $\mathbf{F}_B$ points out of the plane of the page:

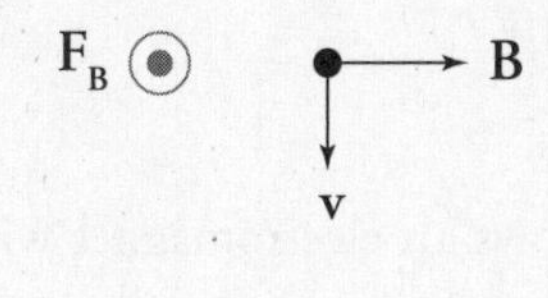

Therefore, the answer is B.

Example 9-39: An electron initially travels with velocity **v**, directed into the plane of the page, near a bar magnet, as illustrated below:

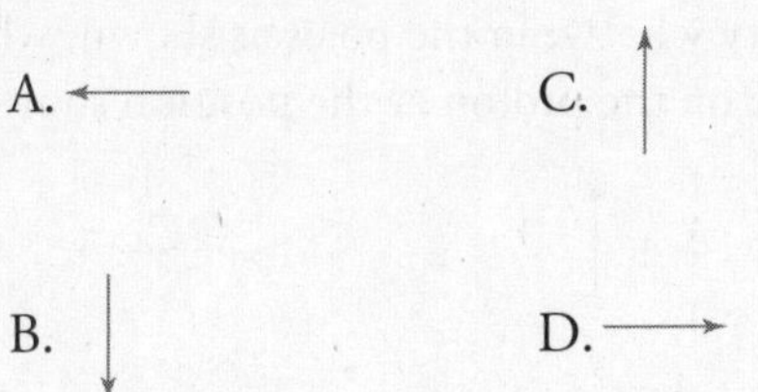

Which of the following arrows best illustrates the direction of the magnetic force on the electron at the position shown?

A. ←

C. ↑

B. ↓

D. →

Solution: Because the **B** field points from the N pole to the S pole (*outside* the magnet), the direction of the **B** field at the position of the electron is downward:

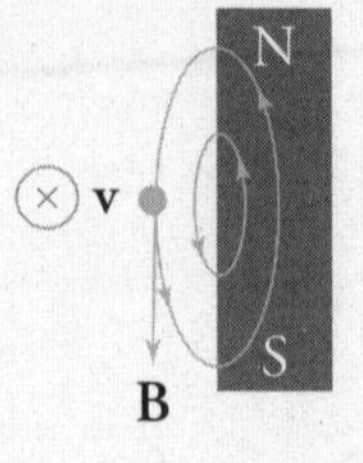

The left-hand rule (for a negative charge) tells us that if **B** points downward and **v** is directed into the plane of the page, then $\mathbf{F}_B$ points to the right:

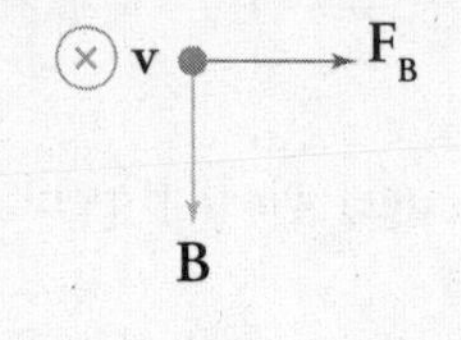

Therefore, the answer is D.

Example 9-40: The following figure shows an electromagnet with an iron core. Since iron is ferromagnetic, the magnetic field created by the current-carrying coil aligns the magnetic dipole moments of electrons in the iron, creating a magnetic field throughout the iron.

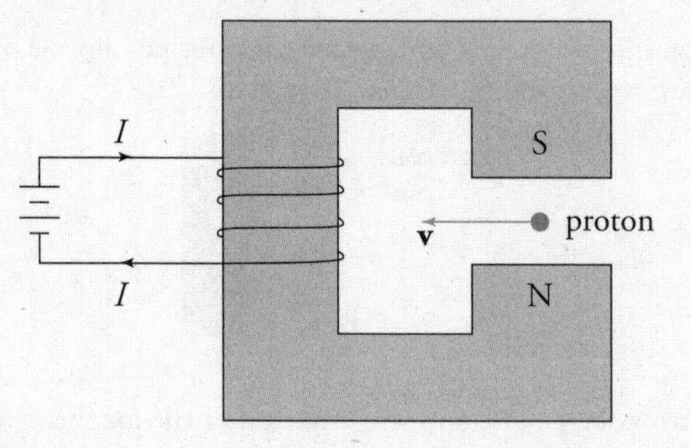

If a proton is projected with velocity **v** between the poles as shown, which of the following best illustrates the direction of the magnetic force on the proton at the position shown?

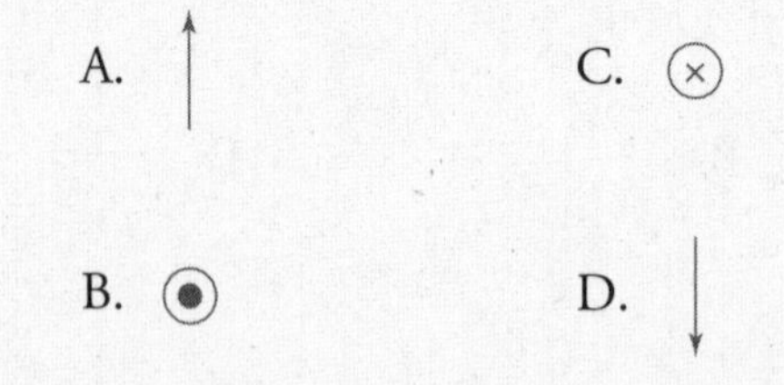

Solution: Because outside the magnet the B field always points from the N pole to the S pole, the direction of the **B** field at the position of the proton is upward:

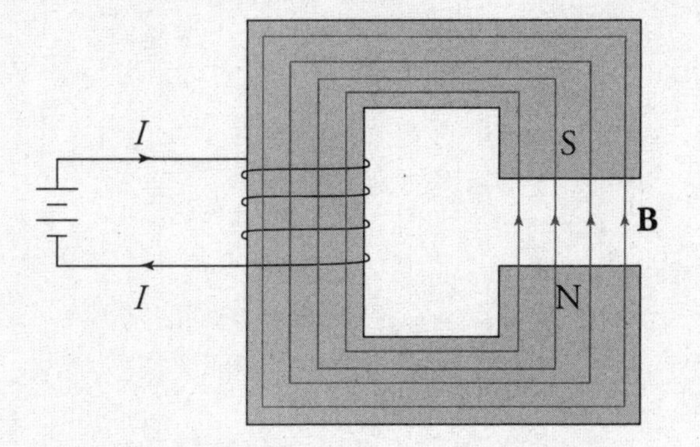

The right-hand rule (for a positive charge) tells us that if **B** points upward and **v** is directed to the left, then $\mathbf{F}_B$ points into the plane of the page:

B

v proton

$\otimes$

$\mathbf{F}_B$

Therefore, the answer is C.

Summary Of Formulas

CIRCUITS

Current: $I = \dfrac{Q}{t}$

– in the direction of "flow of positive charge"

– actual flow of electrons is in the opposite direction

Resistance: $R = \rho \dfrac{L}{A}$ (ρ = resistivity, not density)

Ohm's law: $V = IR$ (where R is constant as V varies)

Resistors in series: $R_{eq} = R_1 + R_2 + \ldots$

Resistors in parallel: $\dfrac{1}{R_{eq}} = \dfrac{1}{R_1} + \dfrac{1}{R_2} + \ldots$ or $R_{eq} = \dfrac{R_1 R_2}{R_1 + R_2}$ (two at a time)

Current is the same for resistors in series; voltage is the same for resistors in parallel.

Kirchhoff's Rules:

– The sum of the voltage-drops across the resistors in any complete path is equal to the voltage of the battery.

– The amount of current entering a parallel combination of resistors is equal to the sum of the currents that pass through the individual resistors.

Power of circuit element: $P = IV = I^2R = \dfrac{V^2}{R}$

Total power supplied by a battery equals the total power dissipated by the resistors.

The ground is at potential zero (potential = 0).

MAGNETIC FORCE AND FIELD

Magnetic force on moving charge q:

$$\mathrm{F_B} = q(\mathrm{v} \times \mathrm{B})$$

$F_B = |q| vB \sin\theta$ (θ = angle between **v** and **B**)

Direction of $\mathbf{F}_B$: use right-hand rule if q is positive; use left-hand rule if q is negative (or use right-hand rule and reverse the answer)

$\mathbf{F}_B$ is always perpendicular to both **v** and **B**

B created by long, straight current carrying wire: $B \propto I / r$

B created by a solenoid: $B \propto I \frac{N}{L}$ (L = length of solenoid, N = number of coils)

- The magnetic force never changes the speed of a particle, and does NO work on the particle.
- Magnetic field lines created by a magnet will point North to South.
- The North pole of a magnet wants to line up with the direction of an external magnetic field; the South pole wants to line up opposite the field.

Chapter 10
Oscillations and Waves

10.1 SIMPLE HARMONIC MOTION (SHM)

The spring in the series of diagrams below is fixed at its left-hand end and has a block attached to its right-hand end. When the spring is neither stretched nor compressed (i.e., when it's at its natural length, as shown in Diagram 1 below), we say the spring is at its **equilibrium position**. In general, the point at which the net force on the block is zero, which in this case is when the spring is at its natural length, is called the equilibrium position, and we label it the zero position.

Now, imagine that we stretch the spring (Diagram 1 to Diagram 2), and let go. Once released, the spring pulls back to the left, going through its equilibrium position and then to the point of maximum compression. From here, the spring pushes back to the right, passing again through its equilibrium position, and returning to the point of maximum extension. If friction is negligible, this back-and-forth motion (the **oscillations**) will continue indefinitely, and the time it takes for the block to go through one oscillation, for example, from Diagram 2 to Diagram 6, is a constant. The oscillations of the block at the end of this spring provide us with a physical example of **simple harmonic motion** (often abbreviated **SHM**).

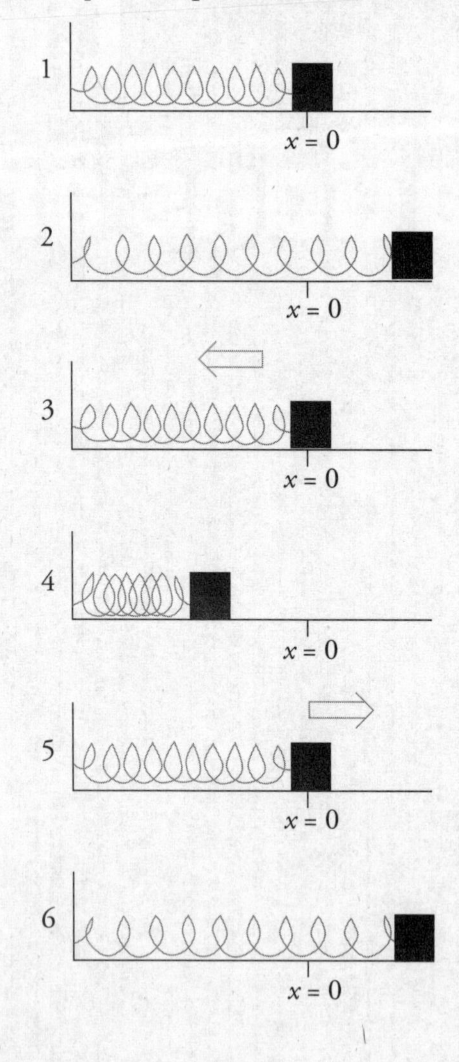

The Dynamics of SHM

Force

Let's first describe the motion of the block attached to the spring from the point of view of the force it feels. The spring exerts a force on the block that's proportional to its displacement. If we call the equilibrium position $x = 0$, then the force exerted by the spring is given by

Hooke's Law

$$\mathbf{F} = -kx$$

The proportionality constant, k, called the **spring constant**, tells us how strong the spring is; the greater the value of k, the stiffer (and stronger) the spring.

What is the role of the minus sign in Hooke's law? Look back at the diagrams on the previous page. Since we're calling the equilibrium position $x = 0$, when the block is to the right of equilibrium, its position, x, is positive. At this point, the stretched spring wants to pull back to the left; because the direction of the force of the spring is to the left, we indicate this direction by calling it negative. Similarly, when the block is to the left of equilibrium, its position, x, is negative. At this point, the compressed spring wants to push back to the right; because the direction of the force of the spring is to the right, we indicate this direction by calling it positive. We see that the direction of the spring force is always directed opposite to its displacement from equilibrium, and for this reason, the minus sign is needed in Hooke's law. Furthermore, because the spring is always trying to restore the block to equilibrium, we say that the spring provides the **restoring force**; it's this force that maintains the oscillations.

Energy

Unfortunately, knowing an equation for the force doesn't allow us to solve directly for other things, such as the speed of the block at some later time: The force changes as the block moves, so acceleration is not uniform. However, there is a way to figure out how fast the block moves using conservation of energy. When we pull on the spring to get the oscillations started, we're exerting a force over a distance; that is, we're doing work. Because we're doing work against the spring, the spring stores potential energy, called **elastic potential energy.** If we once again call the equilibrium position of the spring $x = 0$, then the potential energy of a stretched or compressed spring is given by this equation:

Elastic Potential Energy

$$PE_{\text{elastic}} = \tfrac{1}{2}kx^2$$

When we release the block from rest in Diagram 2 above, the spring is stretched and the block isn't moving, so all the energy is in the form of elastic potential energy. This potential energy turns into kinetic energy, until at $x = 0$ (equilibrium), all the energy has been converted to kinetic energy. As the block rushes past equilibrium, this kinetic energy gradually turns back into elastic potential energy until the point where the spring is at maximum compression and it's all transformed back to potential energy. The compressed spring then pushes outward, converting its potential energy back to kinetic; the block rushes through equilibrium again, and kinetic energy is transformed back to potential energy, until it reaches its starting point (Diagram 6 above) at maximum extension. At this instant, we're back to our full reserve of elastic potential energy (and no kinetic energy), and the process is ready to repeat.

As a result, we can look at the motion of the block from the point of view of the back-and-forth transfer between elastic potential energy and kinetic energy.

The maximum displacement of the block from equilibrium is called the **amplitude**, denoted by A. This positive number tells us how far to the left and right of equilibrium the block will travel. So, in the series of diagrams above, the block's position at maximum extension is $x = +A$, and its position at maximum compression is $x = -A$.

We can summarize the dynamics of the oscillations in this table:

	at $x = -A$	at $x = 0$	at $x = +A$
magnitude of restoring force	max	0	max
magnitude of acceleration	max	0	max
$PE_{elastic}$ of spring	max	0	max
KE of block	0	max	0
speed (v) of block	0	max	0

$x = -A$ $x = 0$ $x = +A$

$x = -A$ $x = 0$ $x = +A$

$x = -A$ $x = 0$ $x = +A$

Because we're ignoring any frictional forces during the oscillations of the block, total mechanical energy will be conserved. That is, the sum of the block's kinetic energy, $\frac{1}{2}mv^2$, and the spring's potential energy, $\frac{1}{2}kx^2$, will be a constant. We can use this fact to figure out the maximum speed of the block. At the instant the block is passing through equilibrium, all the potential energy of the spring has been transformed into kinetic energy of the block. If the amplitude of the oscillations is A, then the maximum elastic potential energy, $\frac{1}{2}kA^2$ (the value of $\frac{1}{2}kx^2$ when $x = \pm A$), is completely converted to maximum kinetic energy at $x = 0$. This gives us:

$$PE_{\text{elastic, max}} \rightarrow KE_{\text{max}}$$

$$\frac{1}{2}kA^2 = \frac{1}{2}mv_{\text{max}}^2$$

$$\therefore v_{\text{max}} = A\sqrt{\frac{k}{m}}$$

Example 10-1: A block of mass 200 g is oscillating on the end of a horizontal spring of spring constant 100 N/m and natural length 12 cm. When the spring is stretched to a length of 14 cm, what is the acceleration of the block?

Solution: When the spring is stretched by 2 cm, Hooke's law tells us that the force exerted by the spring has a magnitude of $F = kx = (100 \text{ N/m})(0.02 \text{ m}) = 2 \text{ N}$. Therefore, by Newton's second law, the acceleration of the block will have a magnitude of $a = F/m = (2 \text{ N})/(0.2 \text{ kg}) = 10 \text{ m/s}^2$.

Example 10-2: If the block in Example 10-1 above were replaced with a block of mass 800 g, how would its maximum speed change?

Solution: The equation derived above, $v_{max} = A\sqrt{k/m}$, tells us that v_{max} is inversely proportional to the square root of the mass of the oscillator. Therefore, if m increases by a factor of 4, v_{max} will decrease by a factor of 2.

So far, we have examined the simple harmonic motion of a horizontal spring. However, SHM can be demonstrated with a vertical spring that is fixed at one end. Consider a horizontal spring with a natural length of l_0 and a block of mass m attached to one end. When turned 90° to make the spring oscillate in the vertical dimension, the spring will stretch/compress to establish a new "natural length." To find this new equilibrium point, we apply Newton's first law to balance the restoring force (caused by the spring) with the force of gravity being exerted on the block. Once this equilibrium is established, a new applied force can initiate simple harmonic motion with $x = 0$ at the newly established natural length point.

The Kinematics of SHM

Period

An oscillation of the block is known as a **cycle**. One cycle is one *round trip*. For example, in the series of diagrams shown earlier, as the block moves from Diagram 2 through to Diagram 6, it completes one round trip; this is one cycle. The amount of time required for the block to complete one cycle is called the **period** of the motion, denoted by T. The period T is measured in seconds, and the longer the period, the slower the oscillations.

Frequency

Rather than timing one cycle (to give the period), we can instead count the number of cycles that take place in one second. This is known as the **frequency**, denoted by f. The units of f are cycles per second, and 1 cycle/second is renamed 1 **hertz** (Hz). The lower the frequency, the slower the oscillations.

Now the first thing we notice is that period and frequency are reciprocals. After all, the period is "the number of seconds per cycle," and the frequency is "the number of cycles per second." So, we have these fundamental relationships:

Period and Frequency

$$f = \frac{1}{T} \text{ and } T = \frac{1}{f}$$

What isn't so obvious is that both the frequency and the period can be figured out (using calculus) just from the spring constant, k, and the mass of the block, m. Here are the formulas:

$$f = \frac{1}{2\pi}\sqrt{\frac{k}{m}} \text{ and } T = 2\pi\sqrt{\frac{m}{k}}$$

Notice that neither f nor T depends on A, the amplitude. This is why we call the motion of the block on the spring *simple* harmonic motion. It turns out that this follows from the fact that the restoring force is directly proportional to the displacement (from Hooke's law).

It's possible for a system to oscillate because of a restoring force that is not directly proportional to the displacement. If this were the case, the frequency and period would depend on the amplitude; we'd still call the motion *harmonic*, which just means back-and-forth, but we wouldn't call it *simple* harmonic.

Example 10-3: Suppose that the block shown in the series of diagrams on the first page of this chapter requires 0.25 sec to move from Diagram 4 to Diagram 6. What is the frequency of the oscillations?

Solution: The interval from Diagram 4 to Diagram 6 represents *half* a cycle, which requires *half* a period to complete. If half a period is 0.25 sec, then the period is 0.5 sec. Therefore, the frequency, f, is $1/T = 1/(0.5 \text{ s}) = 2$ Hz.

Pendulums

Besides the spring-block simple harmonic oscillator, there's another oscillator that the OAT will expect you to know about: the simple pendulum. If the connecting rod or string between the suspension point and the object at the end of a pendulum has negligible mass (so that all the mass is in the object at the end of the rod or string), and if there is no friction at the suspension point during oscillation, we say the pendulum is a **simple pendulum**.

The displacement of the mass is not taken as a distance from equilibrium (as in the spring-block case), but rather as the angle it makes with the vertical. The vertical (shown as a dashed line in the figure below) is the equilibrium position, $\theta = 0$. The restoring force here is gravity; specifically, it's equal to $mg \sin\theta$, which is the component of the object's weight in the direction toward equilibrium.

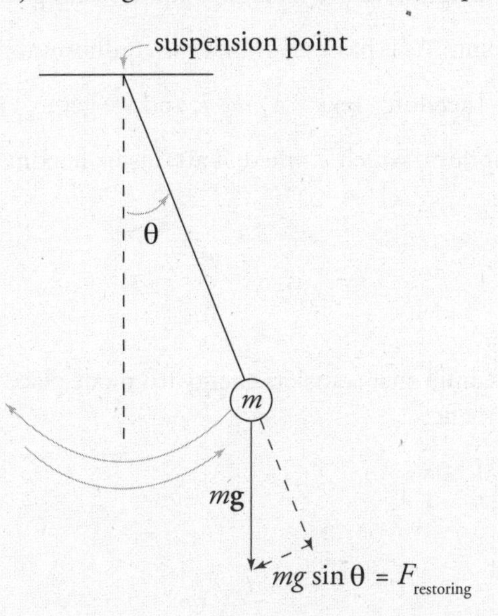

Strictly speaking, a pendulum does not undergo simple harmonic motion because the restoring force is not proportional to the displacement ($mg \sin\theta$ is not exactly proportional to θ). However, if the angle is small, then $\sin\theta \approx \theta$ (in radians), so the restoring force can be approximated as $mg\theta$, which is proportional to θ.[1] In this case, we can treat the motion as simple harmonic, and the frequency and period are given by the following equations:

$$f = \frac{1}{2\pi}\sqrt{\frac{g}{l}} \quad \text{and} \quad T = 2\pi\sqrt{\frac{l}{g}}$$

where l is the length of the pendulum and g is the acceleration due to gravity. Observe that in the case of simple harmonic motion of a simple pendulum, the mass of the swinging object does not affect the frequency or period of oscillation.

[1] The conversion between degrees and radians is as follows: 180 degrees = π radians. If the angle is given in degrees, the restoring force is approximately $mg\theta(\pi/180°)$, which is still proportional to θ.

Example 10-4: The bob (mass = *m*) of a simple pendulum is raised to a height *h* above its lowest point and released. Find an expression for the maximum speed of the pendulum.

Solution: When the bob is at height *h* above its lowest point, it has gravitational potential energy equal to *mgh* (relative to its lowest point). As it passes through the equilibrium position, all this potential energy is converted to kinetic energy. Therefore, $mgh = \frac{1}{2}mv_{max}^2$, and we get $v_{max} = \sqrt{2gh}$. This is the speed of the bob as it passes through equilibrium, which is where it attains its maximum speed.

10.2 WAVES

A **wave** is a disturbance in a medium that transfers energy from one place to another. The medium itself is not transported, just the disturbance.

Transverse Waves

Perhaps the simplest example of a wave is one we can create by wiggling one end of a long rope:

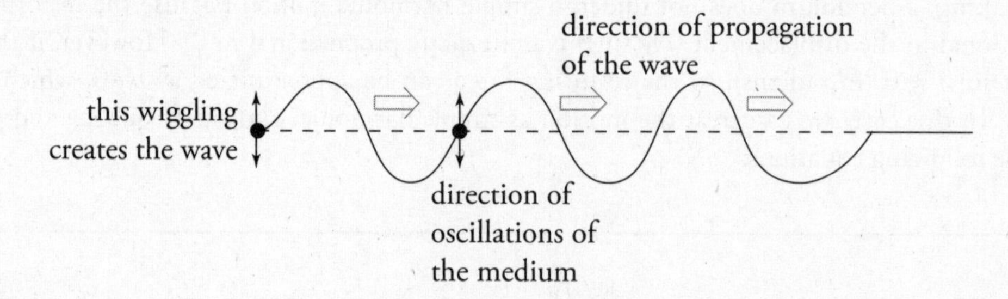

This wave uses the rope as the medium, traveling from one end to the other. Notice that the wave is moving horizontally, but the rope itself is moving up and down. That's why this is called a **transverse** wave: The wave travels (propagates) in a direction that's *perpendicular* to the direction in which the medium is vibrating.

Frequency and Period

The most fundamental characteristic of a wave is its frequency. If we pick a spot on the rope and count how many times it moves up and down (the number of round trips it makes) in one second, we've just measured the **frequency**, *f*, which we express in hertz (cycles per second).

The **period** of a wave, *T*, is the reciprocal of the frequency, and is the amount of time it takes any spot on the rope to complete one cycle (in this case, one up-and-down round trip).

Wavelength and Amplitude

The figure below identifies the **crests (peaks)** and **troughs** of the wave. The distance from one crest to the next (i.e., the length of one cycle of the wave) is called the **wavelength**, denoted by λ, the Greek letter lambda. We can also measure the wavelength by measuring the distance from one trough to the next, or, in fact, between any two consecutive corresponding points along the wave.

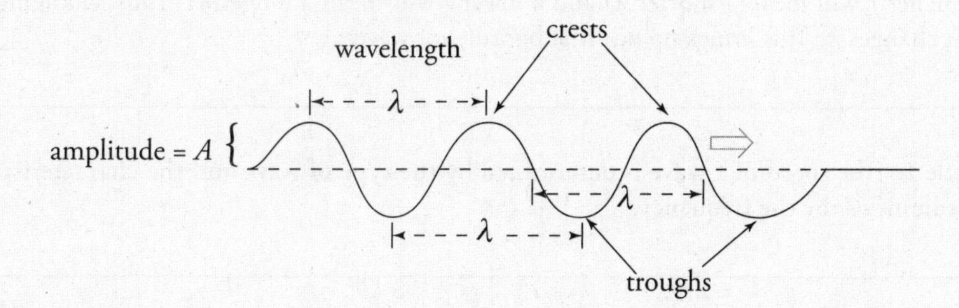

The **amplitude** of a wave, A, is the maximum displacement from equilibrium that any point in the medium makes as the wave goes by. In the case of a wave on a rope, the amplitude is the distance from the original horizontal position of the rope up to a crest; it's also the distance from the horizontal position down to a trough.

Wave Speed

To figure out how fast the wave travels, we just notice that the wave travels a distance of λ in time T; that is, λ is the length of one wave cycle, and T, the period, is the time required for one wave cycle to go by. Since distance = rate × time, we get $\lambda = vT$. Solving this for v gives us $\lambda(1/T) = v$, and since $f = 1/T$, the equation becomes $v = \lambda f$. *This is the most important equation for waves and one of the most important equations for the OAT.*

Wave Equation

$$v = \lambda f$$

For a transverse wave on a rope, there's another equation we can use to figure out the wave speed:

$$v = \sqrt{\frac{\text{tension}}{\text{linear density}}}$$

The linear density of a rope is its mass per unit length.

Two Big Rules for Waves

Notice that the second equation for the wave speed shows that v does not depend on f (or λ). While this may seem to contradict the first equation, $v = \lambda f$, it really doesn't. The speed of the wave depends on the characteristics of the rope; how tense it is, and what it's made of. We can wiggle the end at any frequency we want, and the speed of the wave we create will be a constant. However, because $\lambda f = v$ must always be true, a higher f will mean a shorter λ (and a lower f will mean a longer λ). Thus, changing f doesn't change v: It changes λ. This brings up our first big rule for waves:

Big Rule 1: The speed of a wave is determined by the type of wave and the characteristics of the medium, *not* by the frequency.

Notice that two different types of wave can move with different speeds through the same medium; for example, sound and light move through air with very different speeds. There are exceptions to Big Rule 1, but the only one the OAT will expect you to know about is *dispersion*, which is discussed in the last physics chapter, on Optics. Any other exception would be discussed in the passage; otherwise, you can assume the rule applies.

Our second big rule for waves concerns what happens when a wave passes from one medium into another. Because wave speed is determined by the characteristics of the medium, a change in the medium implies a change in wave speed, but the frequency won't change.

Big Rule 2: When a wave passes into another medium, its speed changes, but its frequency does *not*.

Because f is constant, Rule 2 tells us that the wavelength is proportional to wave speed.

Notice that Rule 1 applies to different waves in one medium, while Rule 2 applies to a single wave in different media. Memorize these rules. The OAT loves waves.

Example 10-5: A transverse wave of frequency 4 Hz travels at a speed of 6 m/s along a rope. What would be the speed of a 12 Hz wave along this same rope?

Solution: Big Rule 1 for waves says that the speed of a wave is determined by the type of wave and the characteristics of the medium, not by the frequency. If all we do is change the frequency, the wave speed will not change: The wave speed will still be 6 m/s. (What *will* change? The wavelength. Because $\lambda = v/f$, a change in f with no change in v will change λ.)

Example 10-6: Which one of the following statements is true concerning the amplitude of a wave?

A. Amplitude increases with increasing frequency.
B. Amplitude increases with increasing wavelength.
C. Amplitude increases with increasing wave speed.
D. None of the above.

Solution: The amplitude is determined by how much energy we put into the wave to get it started. If we wiggle the rope up and down through a large distance (a large amplitude), this takes more energy on our part, and as a result, the wave carries more energy. However, the amplitude doesn't depend on f, λ, or v. The answer is D.

Example 10-7: A wave of frequency 12 Hz has a wavelength of 3 m. What is the speed of this wave?

Solution: Using the equation $v = \lambda f$, we find that v = (3 m)(12 Hz) = 36 m/s.

Example 10-8: The horizontal distance between each crest and the closest trough of a transverse traveling wave along a long horizontal rope is 2 m. If the wave speed is 8 m/s, what is the period of this wave?

Solution: If the horizontal distance between each crest and the closest trough for a transverse traveling wave is 2 m, then the wavelength is 4 m. Now, using $v = \lambda f$, we find that $f = v/\lambda$ = (8 m/s)/(4 m) = 2 Hz, so $T = 1/f$ = 1/(2 Hz) = 0.5 sec.

Example 10-9: What happens when the wave shown below passes from the thick, heavy rope into the thinner, lighter rope?

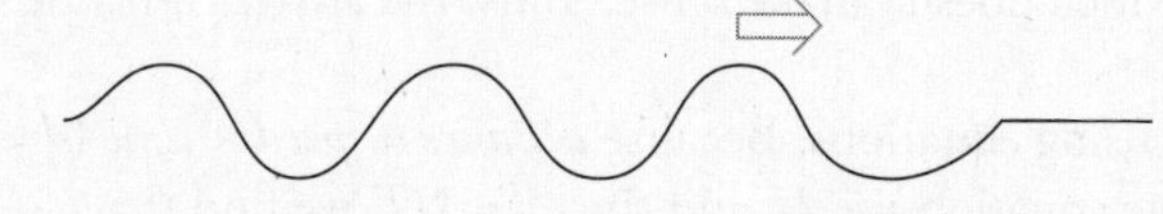

Solution: According to Big Rule 2 for waves, when a wave passes into another medium, its speed changes, but its frequency does not. How does the speed change? Because the rope is lighter (i.e., it has a lower linear density), the equation for wave speed on a string (given above) tells us that v will *increase*. So, if v increases but f doesn't change, then λ will also increase because $\lambda = v/f$.

Example 10-10: A certain rope transmits a 2 Hz transverse wave of amplitude 10 cm with a speed of 1 m/s. What would be the wavelength of a 5 Hz transverse wave of amplitude 8 cm on this same rope?

Solution: First, ignore the amplitudes; they're included in the question only to make things seem more complicated than they are. The amplitude of a wave indicates how much energy the wave transports, but it has nothing to do with wavelength, period, frequency, or wave speed (recall Example 10-6 above). Now, if a 2 Hz transverse wave has a speed of 1 m/s on this rope, then a transverse wave of *any* frequency will have a speed of 1 m/s on this rope; that's what Big Rule 1 for waves tells us. Thus, if f = 5 Hz and v = 1 m/s, then

$$\lambda = \frac{v}{f} = \frac{1\text{ m/s}}{5\text{ Hz}} = 0.2\,\text{m}$$

Example 10-11: How long will it take a wave of wavelength λ and period T to travel a distance d?

A. λTd

B. $\dfrac{\lambda d}{T}$

C. $\dfrac{Td}{\lambda}$

D. $\dfrac{\lambda T}{d}$

Solution: First, let's see if we can eliminate any choices because the units don't work out correctly. We're being asked for an amount of time, so the answer must have the dimension (and units) of time. Choice A can't be correct, since it has units of $[\lambda][T][d]$ = m·sec·m = m^2·sec. Notice that both λ and d have units of meters, which we don't want in the answer, so these units must cancel. Therefore, B can't be correct either since λ and d are multiplied by each other, rather than being divided as they should to make their units cancel.

One difference between the two remaining choices is that in C, the distance d is in the numerator, while in D, the distance d is in the denominator. Now, let's think about this: More time will be required for the wave to travel a greater distance. In other words, the bigger d is, the greater the travel time should be. Therefore, we can eliminate D; after all, since d is in the denominator in choice D, a larger d will result in a smaller amount of time, which doesn't make sense. Thus, the answer must be C.

Here's an alternate solution using equations. Because *distance* = *speed* × *time* ($d = vt$), we know that $t = d/v$. We can find v using the wave equation $v = \lambda f$, and since $f = 1/T$, we find that

$$t = \frac{d}{v} = \frac{d}{\lambda f} = \frac{d}{\lambda} \times \frac{1}{f} = \frac{d}{\lambda} \times T = \frac{Td}{\lambda}$$

The answer is indeed C, just as we figured out by checking units and using logic.

10.3 INTERFERENCE OF WAVES

When two or more waves are superimposed on each other, they will combine to form a single resultant wave. This is called **interference.** The amplitude of the resultant wave will depend on the amplitudes of the combining waves *and* on how these waves travel relative to each other.

If crest meets crest, and trough meets trough, we say that the waves are **in phase** with each other. Their amplitudes will *add*, and we say the waves interfere **constructively.** However, if the crest of one wave coincides with the *trough* of the other (and vice versa), we say that the waves are exactly **out of phase** with each other. In this case, their amplitudes *subtract*, and we say that the waves interfere **destructively.**

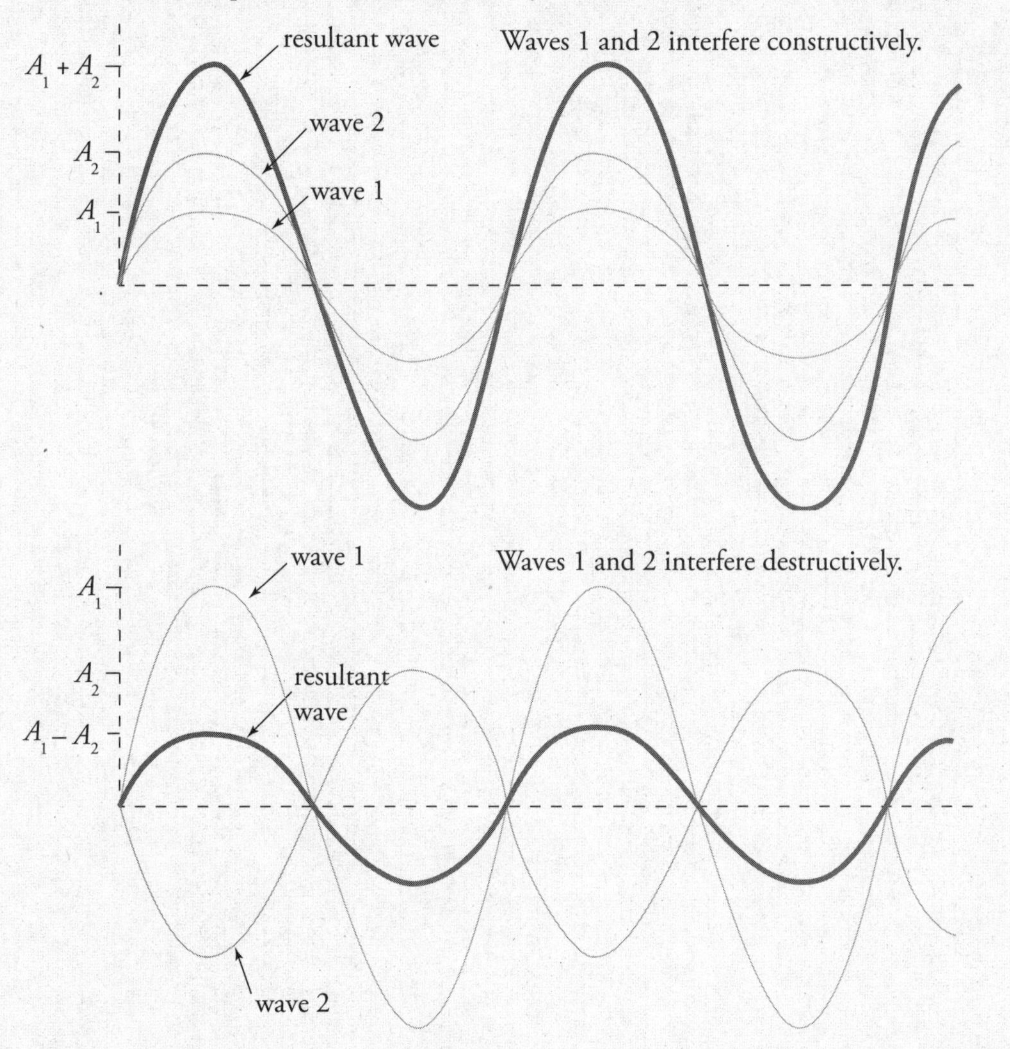

A passage might also say that waves that are directly opposite each other in amplitude are *180 degrees out of phase*, or *π radians out of phase*; it is common to refer to a whole cycle or wave as being 360 degrees or 2π radians, as if it were a circle. If the waves aren't exactly in phase (0°, 360°, or 2π radians) or exactly out of phase (180° or π radians), the amplitude of the resultant wave will be somewhere between the difference and the sum of the amplitudes of the interfering waves.

The interfering waves may also have different wavelengths. These waves will produce a more complicated-looking resultant wave, but we'd still say the waves interfere constructively where they reinforce each other, and destructively where they tend to cancel each other out.

Summary of Formulas

Simple Harmonic Motion (SHM) requires:

- dynamics condition: restoring force is directly proportional to displacement from equilibrium ($x = 0$) and points towards that equilibrium point
- kinematics condition: frequency and period are independent of the amplitude of oscillations

Hooke's law (spring): $\mathbf{F} = -kx$

Elastic potential energy (spring): $PE_{\text{elastic}} = \frac{1}{2}kx^2$

Spring-block oscillator frequency: $f = \dfrac{1}{2\pi}\sqrt{\dfrac{k}{m}}$

Simple pendulum frequency (small oscillations): $f = \dfrac{1}{2\pi}\sqrt{\dfrac{g}{l}}$

Period/frequency
(all harmonic motion and waves): $T = 1/f$

Wave equation: $v = \lambda f$

Two Big Rules for Waves to be used with wave equation:

1) Wave speed v depends on wave type and the medium, not on frequency

2) A single wave passing between media maintains a constant frequency

Standing wave on a rope (both ends fixed nodes)

Standing-wave wavelengths: $\lambda_n = \dfrac{2L}{n}$ $(n = 1, 2, 3, \ldots)$

$$\lambda_n = \frac{\lambda_1}{n}$$

Standing-wave frequencies: $f_n = \dfrac{n}{2L}v$ $(n = 1, 2, 3, \ldots)$

$$f_n = nf_1$$

Chapter 11
Light and Geometrical Optics

11.1 ELECTROMAGNETIC WAVES

We've seen that if we oscillate one end of a long rope, we generate a wave that travels down the rope and whose frequency is the frequency with which we oscillate.

You can think of an electromagnetic wave in a similar way: An oscillating electric charge generates an **electromagnetic** (EM) wave, which is composed of oscillating electric and magnetic fields. These fields oscillate with the same frequency at which the electric charge that created the wave oscillated. The fields oscillate in phase with each other, perpendicular to each other and to the direction of propagation. For this reason, electromagnetic waves are transverse waves. The direction in which the wave's electric field oscillates is called the direction of **polarization** of the wave.

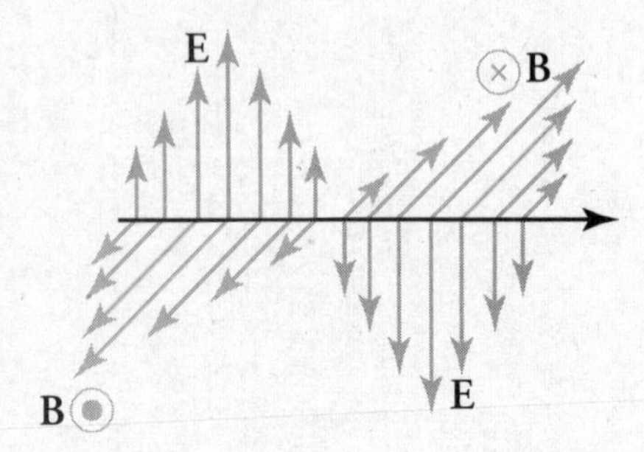

Most EM waves have electric fields oscillating in all perpendicular directions to propagation equally and are thus *unpolarized.*

Unlike waves on a rope or sound waves, electromagnetic waves do not require a material medium to propagate; they can travel through empty space (vacuum). When an EM wave travels through a vacuum, its speed is a constant. It is one of the fundamental constants of nature and a value you should memorize for the OAT:

Speed of Light in Vacuum

$$c = 3 \times 10^8 \text{ m/s}$$

All electromagnetic waves, regardless of frequency, travel through a vacuum at this speed.
The most important equation for waves, $v = \lambda f$, is also true for electromagnetic waves. For EM waves traveling through a vacuum, $v = c$, so the equation becomes $\lambda f = c$.

The frequencies for electromagnetic waves span a huge range, and different ranges have been given specific names. This assignment of names to specific regions based on frequency (or wavelength) is known as the **electromagnetic spectrum** and is shown here.

Notice that visible light occupies only a small part of the electromagnetic spectrum. When waves from all over the visible spectrum are mixed together, the resulting light is perceived as white. You should memorize the order of the colors of the visible spectrum from lowest frequency (longest wavelength) to highest frequency (shortest wavelength): ROYGBV ("Roy-Gee-Biv"), which stands for red, orange, yellow, green, blue, and violet. In terms of wavelengths, violet light has a wavelength (in vacuum) of about 400 nm and red light has a wavelength of about 700 nm; the other colors are in between.

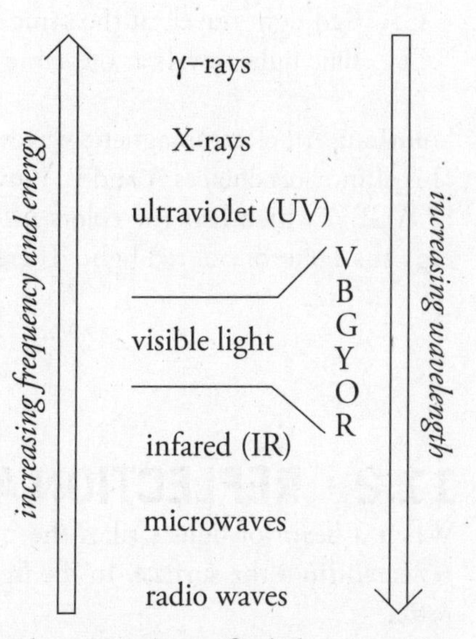

Photons

When electromagnetic radiation interacts with matter (absorption and emission), we find that it carries energy, and that the energy is quantized. That is, the energy associated with EM radiation is absorbed or emitted by matter in "packets"; individual bundles. Each such bundle of energy is called a **photon**, and the energy of a photon is directly proportional to the frequency:

Photon Energy

$$E = hf = h\frac{c}{\lambda}$$

The constant of proportionality, h, is called **Planck's constant**. (In SI units, its value is about 6.6×10^{-34} J·s. Don't worry about memorizing this constant; it would be given to you on the OAT if it were needed.)

The fact that electromagnetic radiation carries energy in packets (photons), which we can think of as "particles of light," gives rise to the idea of **wave-particle duality** for electromagnetic radiation: EM radiation travels like a wave but interacts with matter like a particle. One peculiarity of this duality is that, for waves, energy is proportional to the square of amplitude (recall the intensity relation from the previous chapter), whereas for particles (photons), energy is proportional to frequency. In Chapter 9, we noted that these two properties were independent of one another. Thus, the wave and particle models for light differ significantly in their predictions, and yet each is sometimes true.

Example 11-1: Which one of the following statements is true regarding red photons and blue photons traveling through a vacuum?

A. Red light travels faster than blue light and carries more energy.
B. Blue light travels faster than red light and carries more energy.
C. Red light travels at the same speed as blue light and carries more energy.
D. Blue light travels at the same speed as red light and carries more energy.

Solution: All electromagnetic waves, regardless of frequency, travel through vacuum at the same speed, *c*. This eliminates choices A and B. Now, because blue light has a higher frequency than red light (remember ROYGBV, which lists the colors in order of increasing frequency), photons of blue light have higher energy than photons of red light. Therefore, the answer is D.

11.2 REFLECTION AND REFRACTION

When a beam of light strikes the boundary between two transparent media, some of the light will be reflected from the surface. In the figure below, some of the sunlight will be reflected off the water in the tank.

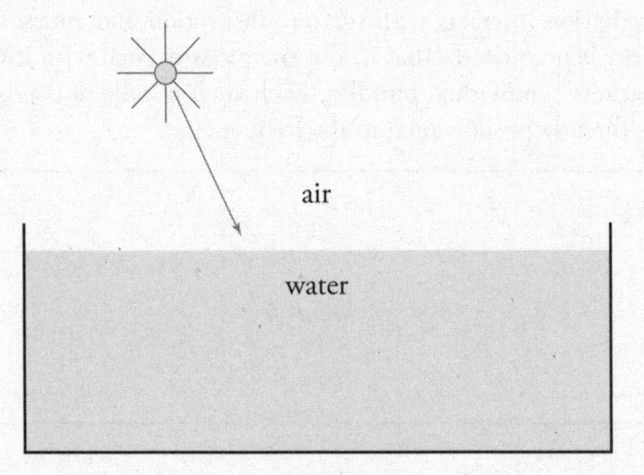

When a ray of light passing through one medium is reflected from the surface of another, the angle at which it bounces off the new medium is equal to the angle at which it strikes. In other words, *the angle of reflection is equal to the angle of incidence*. This fact is known as the **law of reflection**. Notice that, by definition, the angles of incidence and reflection are measured with reference to a line that's perpendicular to the plane of interface between the two media; that is, the angle of incidence and the angle of reflection are the angles that the incident and reflected rays make with *the normal*, not with the surface.

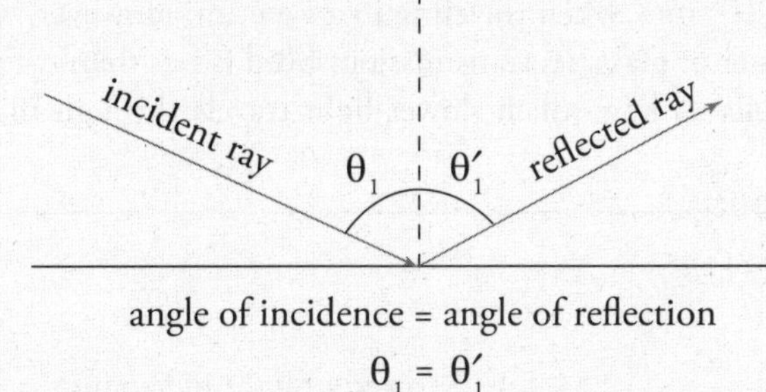

angle of incidence = angle of reflection

$$\theta_1 = \theta_1'$$

Example 11-2: In the figure above, assume that a ray of sunlight strikes the water, making an angle of 60° with the surface. What is the angle of reflection?

A. 15°
B. 30°
C. 60°
D. 90°

Solution: Be careful. If the incident ray makes an angle of 60° with the surface, then it makes an angle of 30° with the normal. Therefore, the angle of incidence is 30°. By the law of reflection, the angle of reflection is 30° also. Choice B is the answer.

In the figure below, not all of the sunlight that encounters the surface of the water is reflected; some is transmitted into the water. Unless the angle of incidence is 0°, the light will be *bent* as it enters the water. The bending is called **refraction.** The **angle of refraction** is the angle that the **transmitted** (or **refracted**) ray makes with the line that's perpendicular to the plane of interface between the two media.

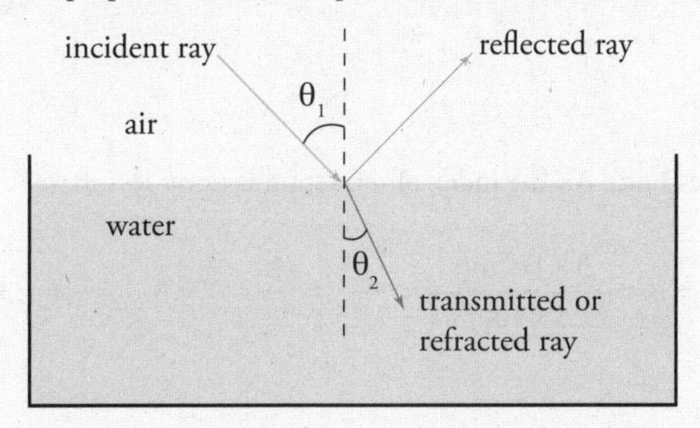

If $\theta_1 = 0°$ (that is, if the incident ray is perpendicular to the boundary), then $\theta_2 = 0°$. However, if θ_1 is any other angle, then θ_2 will be different from θ_1; that is, the ray bends as it's transmitted. In order to figure out the angle of refraction, we first need to discuss a medium's index of refraction.

11.2

Index of Refraction

Light travels at speed $c = 3 \times 10^8$ m/s when traveling in a vacuum. However, when light travels through a material medium such as water or glass, its transmission speed is less than c. Every medium, in fact, has an **index of refraction** that tells us how much slower light travels through that medium than through empty space.

Index of Refraction

$$\text{index of refraction} = \frac{\text{speed of light in vacuum}}{\text{speed of light in medium}}$$

$$n = \frac{c}{v}$$

The index of refraction of vacuum is, by definition, exactly equal to 1. Because the index for air is very close to 1, we simply use $n = 1$ for air as well. (The OAT will use this approximation unless otherwise specified.) Notice that n has no units, it's never less than 1, and the greater the value of n for a medium, the slower light travels through that medium. For most materials, the value of n is between 1 and 2.5. Glass has an index of refraction of about 1.5 (but varies depending on the type of glass) while a diamond has a particularly high value of n, about 2.4. Values of n above 2.5 are rare.

Example 11-3: Light travels through water at an approximate speed of 2.25×10^8 m/s. What is the refractive index of water?

A. 0.75
B. 1.33
C. 1.50
D. 2.25

Solution: First, eliminate choice A: The index of refraction is never less than 1. Now, by definition,

$$n = \frac{c}{v} = \frac{3 \times 10^8 \text{ m/s}}{2.25 \times 10^8 \text{ m/s}} = \frac{3}{2.25} = \frac{3}{2\frac{1}{4}} = \frac{3}{\frac{9}{4}} = 3 \cdot \tfrac{4}{9} = \tfrac{4}{3} \approx 1.33$$

Therefore, the answer is B.

Now that we know about the index of refraction, we can state the rule that's used to figure out the angle of refraction. It's called the law of refraction, or Snell's law:

Law of Refraction (Snell's Law)

$$n_1 \sin \theta_1 = n_2 \sin \theta_2$$

In this equation, n_1 is the refractive index of the medium through which the incident ray is traveling, and n_2 is the refractive index of the medium through which the transmitted (or refracted) ray is traveling.

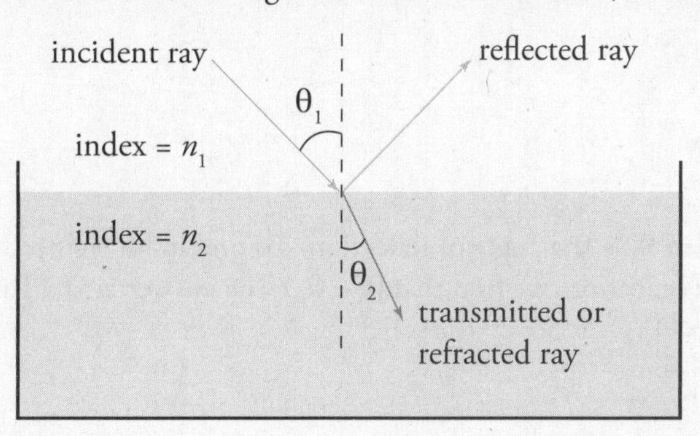

It follows from Snell's law that if $n_2 > n_1$, then $\theta_2 < \theta_1$. That is, if the transmitting medium has a higher index of refraction than the incident medium, then the ray will bend *toward* the normal. Similarly, if $n_2 < n_1$, then $\theta_2 > \theta_1$. That is, if the transmitting medium has a lower index of refraction than the incident medium, then the ray will bend *away from* the normal. You should memorize both of these facts.

Example 11-4: A ray of light traveling through air is incident on a piece of glass whose refractive index is 1.5. If the sine of the angle of incidence is 0.6, what's the sine of the angle of refraction?

Solution: Using the law of refraction, we find that

$$n_1 \sin\theta_1 = n_2 \sin\theta_2 \rightarrow (1)(0.6) = (1.5)(\sin\theta_2) \rightarrow \sin\theta_2 = \frac{0.6}{1.5} = \frac{\frac{3}{5}}{\frac{3}{2}} = \frac{2}{5} = 0.4$$

Notice that $\sin\theta_2$ is less than $\sin\theta_1$; this immediately tells us that $\theta_2 < \theta_1$. The light is traveling from air ($n_1 = 1$) into glass, whose refractive index is higher. If the transmitting medium (i.e., the second one) has a higher index of refraction than the incident medium (i.e., the first one), then θ_2 *will* be less than θ_1; that is, the ray will bend toward the normal.

Example 11-5: Consider the diagram below, showing an incident ray, reflected ray, and transmitted ray:

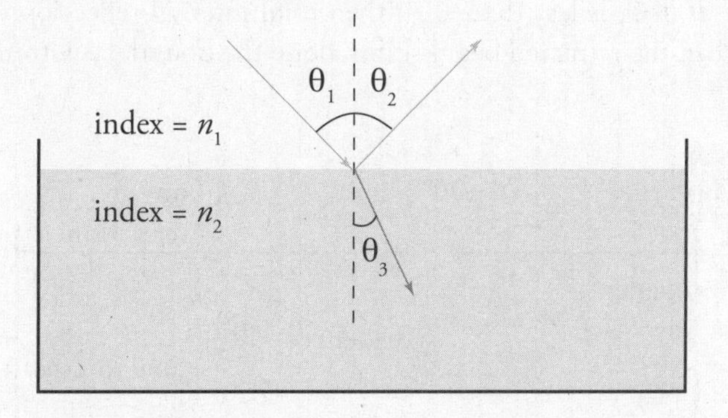

What information is needed to find θ_2?

A. n_1, n_2, and θ_1
B. n_1, n_2, and θ_3
C. n_1 only
D. θ_1 only

Solution: The angle labeled θ_2 is the angle of reflection. To find it, all we need to know is the angle of incidence, θ_1. (By the law of reflection, we find that $\theta_2 = \theta_1$.) The answer is D. (This unconventional labeling of the angles is a common OAT tactic, by the way.)

Total Internal Reflection

When a light ray traveling in a medium of high refractive index approaches a medium of lower refractive index (for example, a light ray traveling in water towards the interface with the air), it may or may not escape into the second medium. If the ray's angle of incidence exceeds a certain **critical angle**, the light ray will undergo **total internal reflection**: All of the incident ray's energy will be reflected back into its original medium; there will be no refracted ray.

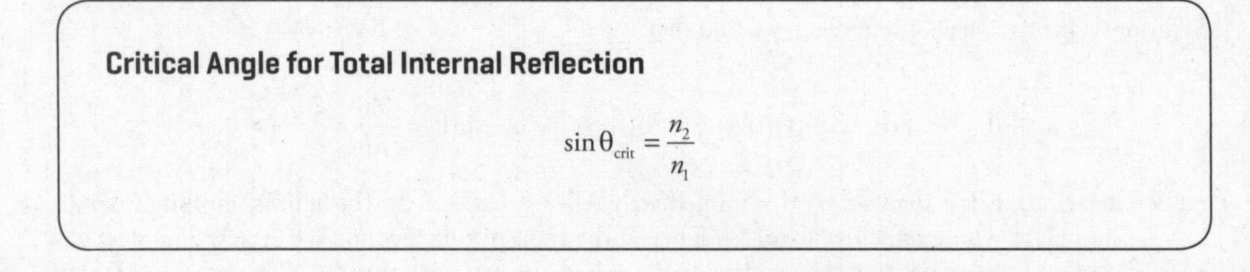

Critical Angle for Total Internal Reflection

$$\sin\theta_{crit} = \frac{n_2}{n_1}$$

In this equation, n_1 is the refractive index of the medium through which the incident ray is traveling, and n_2 is the refractive index of the medium on the other side of the boundary. The angle θ_{crit} is the critical angle. What this means is that if the angle of incidence, θ_1, is greater than θ_{crit}, then total internal reflection will occur.[1] However, if θ_1 is less than θ_{crit}, then total internal reflection will not occur. (If θ_1 just happens to equal θ_{crit}, then the refracted beam skims along the boundary with $\theta_2 = 90°$.)

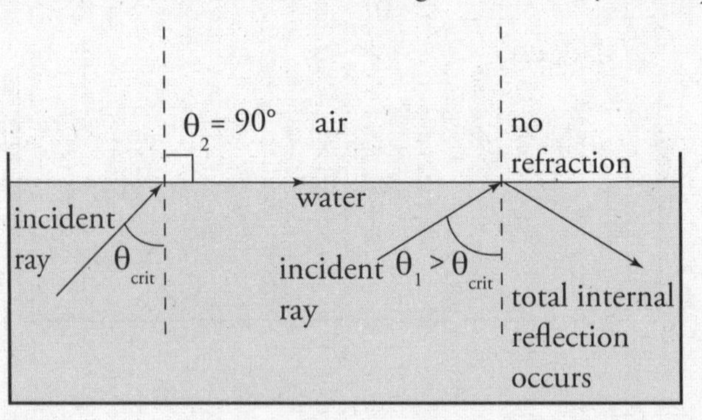

[1] If you forget the formula for the critical angle, there's another way to know that total internal reflection occurs: If you plug numbers into the law of refraction and find that sin θ > 1 (which is impossible), that tells you there is no angle of refraction, so there must be total internal reflection.

Notice that there can be a critical angle for total internal reflection *only if n_1 is greater than n_2*. For example, a beam of light incident in the air and striking the surface of the water can never experience total internal reflection because $n_1 < n_2$. In other words, there'll be some reflection and some refraction, as usual. In this case, some of the light's intensity will always be transmitted into the water.

Example 11-6: A beam of light is incident on the boundary between air and a piece of glass whose index of refraction is $\sqrt{2}$. When would total internal reflection (TIR, for short) of this beam occur?

Solution: First, in order to have TIR, the beam would have to start in the glass, trying to exit into the air. (If the beam were traveling in the air and incident on the glass, then TIR could not occur.) Furthermore, the angle of incidence would have to be greater than the critical angle, which we calculate as follows:

$$\sin\theta_{\text{crit}} = \frac{n_2}{n_1} = \frac{1}{\sqrt{2}} = \frac{\sqrt{2}}{2} \rightarrow \theta_{\text{crit}} = 45°$$

11.3 MIRRORS

A **mirror** is a surface, usually made of glass or metal, that forms an image of an object by *reflecting* light.

Plane Mirrors

A **plane** mirror is an ordinary flat mirror. If you put an object in front of a plane mirror, the image will appear to be behind the mirror. The image will be the same size as the object and will appear to be as far behind the mirror's surface as the object is in front of it. The image will also appear upright; it won't be inverted.

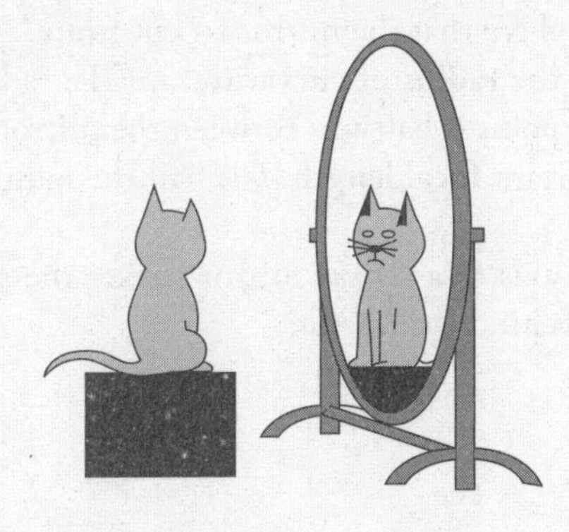

11.3

Curved Mirrors

We all have experience with plane mirrors, but a **curved** mirror presents us with images that are less familiar. The purpose of this section is to find a systematic way to describe the images formed by curved mirrors.

There are essentially two types of curved mirrors: concave and convex. The shiny (reflecting) surface of a **concave** mirror appears like the entrance to a "cave" from the point of view of the object. The reflecting surface of a **convex** mirror bends away from the object. As a simple demonstration of the difference, imagine holding a polished spoon. If you look into the spoon, you're looking at a concave surface; if you turn it around and look at the back of the spoon, you're looking at a convex surface.

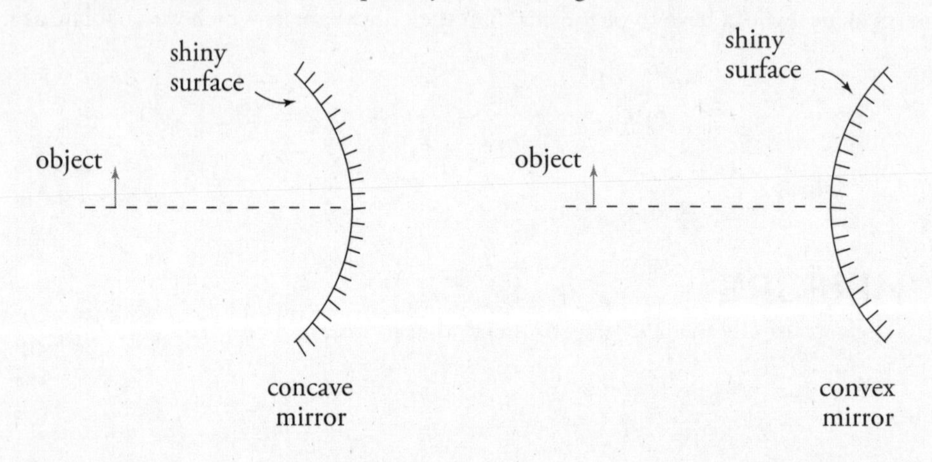

The curved mirrors we'll consider could be termed **spherical** mirrors, because near the center of the mirror, the surface is spherical (that is, part of a sphere).

When light parallel to the central **axis** of a concave mirror strikes the surface, it's reflected through a point called the **focus** (or **focal point**), denoted by F. This point is halfway to the **center of curvature**, C, of the mirror, which is the center of the sphere that the mirror is "cut from." The distance between the center of curvature and the mirror is called the **radius of curvature**, *r*. (The radius of curvature is also sometimes denoted by *RC*.) Because the focal point is halfway between the mirror and C, the distance from the mirror to the focal point, the all-important **focal length**, *f*, is half the radius of curvature: $f = \frac{1}{2}r$.

When light parallel to the central axis of a *convex* mirror strikes the surface, it's reflected directly *away from* the "imaginary" **focal point** behind the mirror.

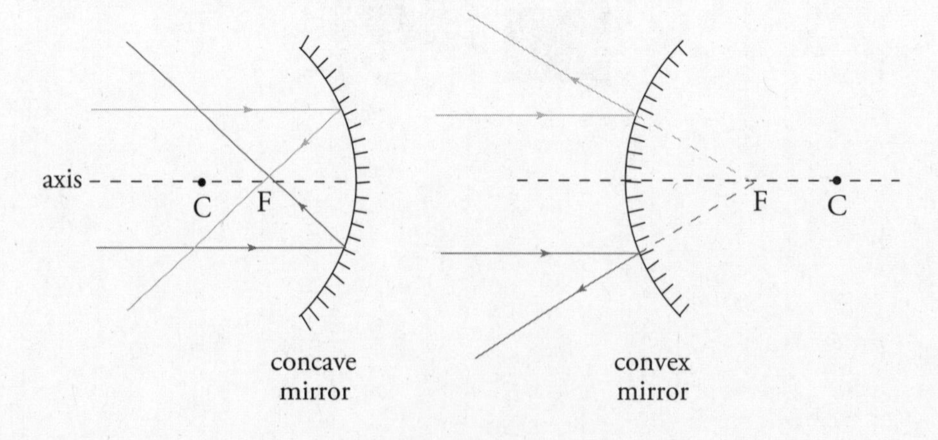

We see an image in a mirror at the point where the rays reflected off the mirror intersect *or* at the point from where the reflected rays seem to intersect (and therefore emanate from) behind the mirror. The following figures illustrate the process of image formation by curved mirrors:

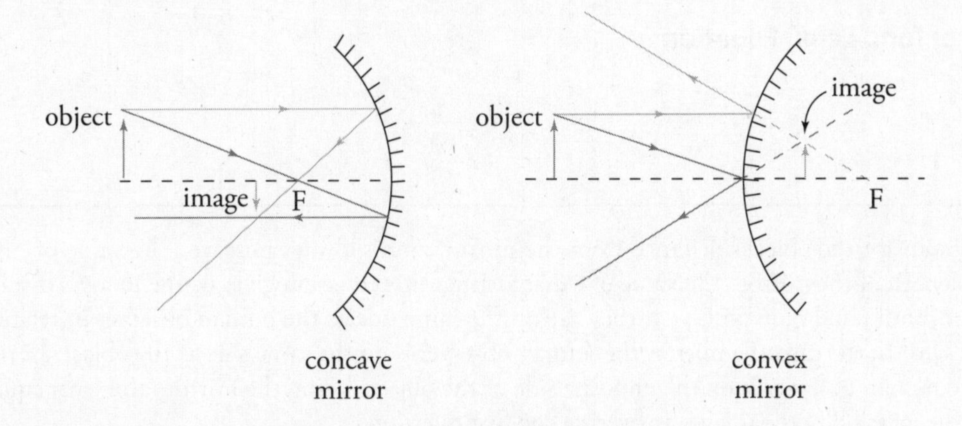

The ray diagram for the concave mirror shows two incident rays reflecting off the mirror. One ray, parallel to the axis, is reflected through the focal point. Another ray, which goes through the focal point, is reflected parallel to the axis. The intersection point of these reflected rays determines the location of the image.

The ray diagram for the convex mirror also shows two incident rays reflecting off the mirror. One ray, parallel to the axis, is reflected directly away from the focal point. Another ray, which hits the center of the mirror (the point where its axis of symmetry intersects the mirror surface), is reflected at the same angle below the axis. Following these reflected rays back behind the mirror, their intersection point determines the location of the image.

Ray diagrams (like the ones drawn in the figure above) can be used to determine the approximate location of the image, but they usually can't give precise answers to all the questions we may be asked about the image formed by a mirror. What we want is a systematic way to get precise answers to these four questions:

1. Where is the image?
2. Is the image real or is it virtual?
3. Is the image upright or is it inverted?
4. How tall is the image (compared to the object)?

Before we discuss how to answer these questions, let's first define the terms *real* and *virtual.* An image is said to be **real** if light rays actually focus at the position of the image. A real image can be projected onto a surface. An image is said to be **virtual** if light rays don't actually focus at the apparent location of the image. For example, look back at the figure above, showing the formation of images by a concave mirror and by a convex mirror. The image formed by the concave mirror in that diagram is real: light rays actually intersect at the image location. However, the image formed by the convex mirror is virtual: no light rays intersect at its location, they just seem to come from that location.

11.3

The Mirror Equation

To answer the first two questions given above, we use the mirror (and lens) equation:

Mirror (and Lens) Equation

$$\frac{1}{o} + \frac{1}{i} = \frac{1}{f}$$

Here, o stands for the object's distance from the mirror, and is always positive. The value of f represents the focal length of the mirror. The value of i that satisfies this equation gives us the image's distance from the mirror. Both f and i are positive if they are on the same side as the human observer in relation to the mirror or lens. In the case of a mirror, the human observer is on the same side as the object. In the case of a lens, the human observer is on the opposite side of the object. Using the mirror (and lens) equation, we can find the location of the image, answering the first question.

The second question is also answered using the mirror equation. If we get a *positive* value for i, that tells us that the image is in front of the mirror and it's *real*; a *negative* value for i means the image is behind the mirror and is *virtual*. For example, let's say that o = 2 cm and f = 6 cm. Substituting these values into the mirror equation, we find that i = –3 cm. Therefore, the image is 3 cm behind the mirror and it's virtual. Note that you can use any unit for the measurement of distance, as long as it is the same unit for o, i, and f.

The Magnification Equation

To answer the last two questions, we then use the magnification equation:

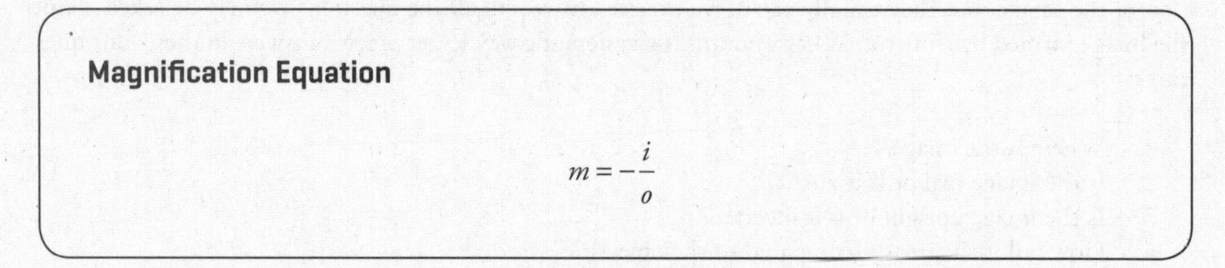

Magnification Equation

$$m = -\frac{i}{o}$$

The value of m is the **magnification factor**; multiplying the height of the object by m gives us the height of the image. The sign of m tells us whether the image is upright or inverted. If m is *positive*, the image is *upright*; if m is *negative*, the image is *inverted*. To illustrate this, let's continue our example above, with o = 2 cm and f = 6 cm. We found that i = –3 cm. Therefore, the magnification factor is m = –(–3 cm)/(2 cm) = +1.5. This tells us that the height of the image is 1.5 times the height of the object, and (because m is positive) the image is upright.

The object distance, o, is always positive. If i is positive, then m is negative; if i is negative, then m is positive. In other words,

Real images are inverted, and virtual images are upright.

Now, the only thing that's left to do is to find the way to "tell" the mirror equation whether we have a concave mirror or a convex mirror. The rule is simple: When using the mirror equation, we write the focal length of a *concave* mirror as a *positive* number, and we write the focal length of a *convex* mirror as a *negative* number. Here's a summary of mirrors:

Mirrors

Concave mirror	Convex mirror
f is positive	f is negative

$$\frac{1}{o} + \frac{1}{i} = \frac{1}{f}$$

i positive ⟶ real image (in front of mirror)

i negative ⟶ virtual image (behind mirror)

$$m = -\frac{i}{o}$$

m positive ⟶ image upright

m negative ⟶ image inverted

- Concave mirrors can create real and virtual images
- Convex mirrors can only create virtual images

Example 11-7: Describe the image formed in a plane mirror.

A. Real and upright
B. Real and inverted
C. Virtual and upright
D. Virtual and inverted

Solution: First, eliminate choices A and D; *real* always goes with *inverted*, and *virtual* always goes with *upright.* We know from common experience that the image formed in a flat mirror is upright, so the answer must be C.

Example 11-8: If an object is placed very far from a concave mirror, where will the image be formed?

A. Halfway between the focal point and the mirror
B. At the focal point
C. At the center of curvature
D. At infinity

Solution: Use the mirror equation. "The object is placed very far from a mirror" means that we take $o = \infty$, so $1/o = 0$. The mirror equation then says $1/i = 1/f$, so $i = f$. That is, the image is formed at the focal point of the mirror, choice B.

Example 11-9: An object is placed 40 cm in front of a concave mirror with a radius of curvature of 60 cm. Locate and describe the image.

Solution: Because $f = \frac{1}{2}r$, we know that f = 30 cm. The mirror equation now gives

$$\frac{1}{40\text{ cm}} + \frac{1}{i} = \frac{1}{30\text{ cm}} \rightarrow \frac{1}{i} = \frac{1}{30} - \frac{1}{40} = \frac{4-3}{120} = \frac{1}{120} \rightarrow \therefore i = 120\text{ cm}$$

(Be careful: The OAT often gives the radius of curvature, *r*. What you want is *f*, the focal length, which is half of *r*.) Since *i* is positive, we know the image is real; also, it's located 120 cm from the mirror on the same side of the mirror as the object. (*Virtual* images are located *behind* the mirror.) Since $m = -i/o = -(120\text{ cm})/(40\text{ cm}) = -3$, we know that the image is 3 times the height of the object and inverted.

Example 11-10: An object is placed 40 cm in front of a convex mirror with a radius of curvature of –60 cm. Locate and describe the image.

Solution: Because $f = \frac{1}{2}r$, we know that f = –30 cm. The mirror equation now gives

$$\frac{1}{40\text{ cm}} + \frac{1}{i} = \frac{1}{-30\text{ cm}} \rightarrow \frac{1}{i} = -\frac{1}{30} - \frac{1}{40} = \frac{-4-3}{120} = \frac{-7}{120} \rightarrow \therefore i = -\frac{120}{7}\text{ cm}$$

Since *i* is negative, we know the image is virtual; also, it's located $120/7 \approx 17$ cm from the mirror on the opposite side of the mirror from the object. Since $m = -i/o = -(-\frac{120}{7}\text{ cm})/(40\text{ cm}) = +3/7$, we know that the image is 3/7 times the height of the object and upright. Comparing this example to the preceding one, notice how critical the sign of *f* was. It changed everything about the image.

Example 11-11: A convex mirror forms an upright image 12 cm behind the mirror when an object of height 15 cm is placed 20 cm in front of it. What is the height of the image?

Solution: To find the height of the image, we need the magnification. We're given that o = 20 cm and i = –12 cm. (We know that *i* is negative because not only do convex mirrors only form virtual images [a good fact to remember, by the way] but the question also says that the image is formed "behind the mirror." Images formed behind the mirror are virtual.) Therefore, $m = -i/o = -(-12\text{ cm})/(20\text{ cm}) = 3/5$. Multiplying the height of the object by the magnification gives the height of the image. Therefore, the height of the image is (3/5)(15 cm) = 9 cm.

11.4 LENSES

A **lens** is a thin piece of clear glass or plastic that forms an image of an object by *refracting* light. The purpose of this section is to find a systematic way to describe the images formed by lenses.

There are essentially two types of lenses: converging and diverging. **Converging** lenses are thicker in the middle than they are at the ends, and they refract light rays that are parallel to the axis *toward* the focal point on the other side of the lens. **Diverging** lenses are thinner in the middle than they are at the ends, and they refract light rays that are parallel to the axis *away from* the "imaginary" focal point that's in front of the lens.

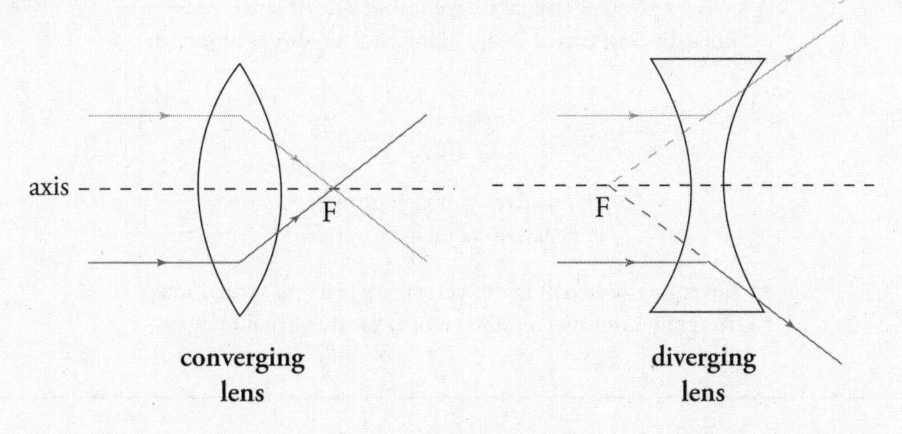

We want to be able to answer the same four questions for lenses as we did for mirrors. Fortunately, *virtually everything we did for mirrors carries over unchanged to lenses.* For example, the mirror equation is also the lens equation, and the magnification equation is also the same. The conventions for positive and negative i and m are also the same for lenses as they are for mirrors.

We distinguish between the two types of lenses in the same way we distinguished between the two types of mirrors. When using the lens equation, we write the focal length of a *converging* lens as a *positive* number, and we write the focal length of a *diverging* lens as a *negative* number.

Here's an important note. The OAT uses the terms *concave* and *convex* to refer to different mirrors and lenses. The diagrams above show us that the surfaces of a converging lens are convex, and the surfaces of a diverging lens are concave. Thus, a concave lens is the same as a diverging lens, and a convex lens is the same as a converging lens. Now for a warning: For a concave *mirror*, f is positive; and for a convex *mirror*, f is negative. When these terms are applied to lenses, things necessarily switch: For a concave *lens*, f is negative; and for a convex *lens*, f is positive. *Be careful* when you see the words *concave* or *convex*. Whether these terms describe a mirror or a lens will make a critically important difference in whether you write the focal length as a positive or as a negative number.

Besides the fact the lenses form images by refracting light (rather than by reflecting light, as is the case for mirrors), there's really only one difference: For lenses, *real* images are formed on the *opposite* side of the lens from the object while *virtual* images are formed on the *same* side of the lens as the object.

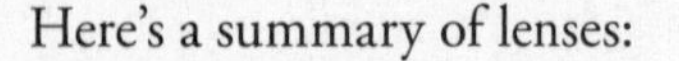

Here's a summary of lenses:

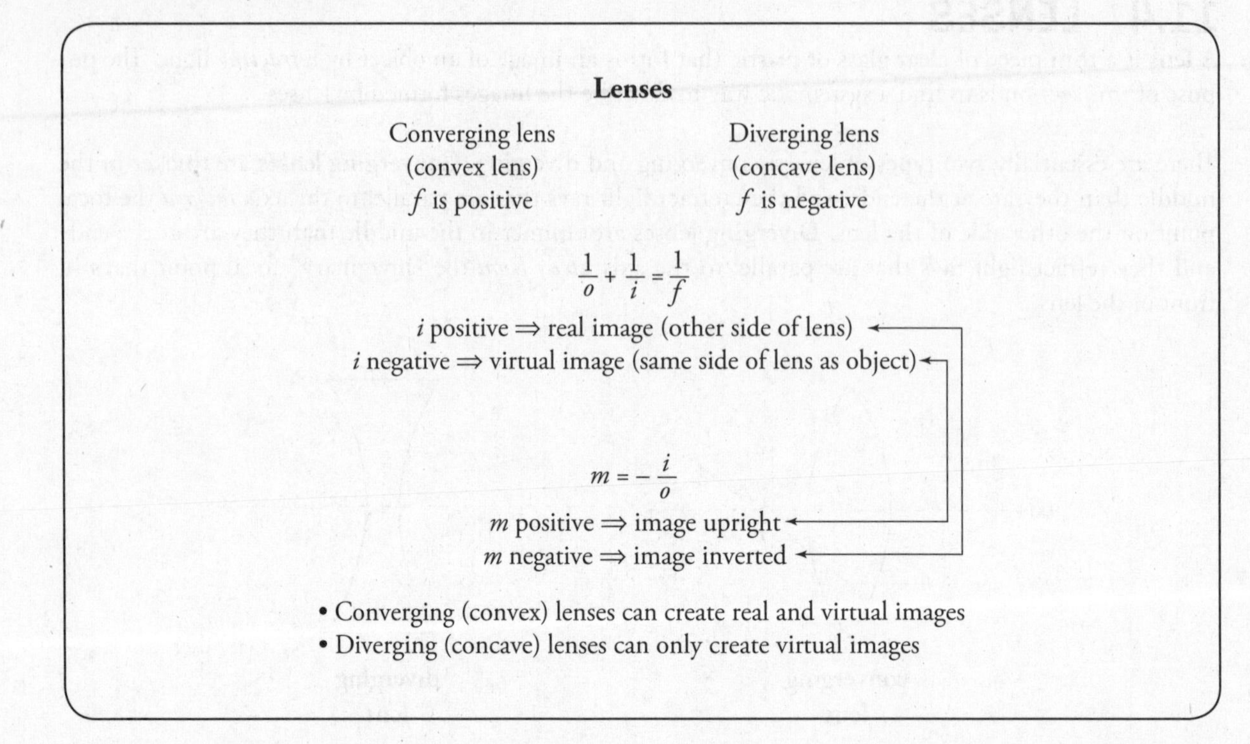

Example 11-12: An object is placed 10 cm in front of a diverging lens with a focal length of –40 cm, then the image will be located:

A. 5 cm in front of the lens.
B. 5 cm behind the lens.
C. 8 cm in front of the lens.
D. 8 cm behind the lens.

Solution: We use the lens equation to find i:

$$\frac{1}{10\text{ cm}}+\frac{1}{i}=\frac{1}{-40\text{ cm}} \rightarrow \frac{1}{i}=-\frac{1}{40}-\frac{1}{10}=\frac{-1-4}{40}=\frac{-5}{40}=-\frac{1}{8} \rightarrow \therefore i=-8\text{ cm}$$

This eliminates choices A and B. Because i is negative, the image is virtual, and for lenses, virtual images are formed on the same side of the lens as the object. Therefore, the answer is C.

Example 11-13: An object of height 10 cm is held 50 cm in front of a convex lens with a focal length of magnitude 40 cm. Describe the image.

Solution: The fact that the lens is convex means that it's a converging lens with a *positive* focal length; therefore, $f = +40$ cm. The lens equation now gives us i:

$$\frac{1}{50\text{ cm}}+\frac{1}{i}=\frac{1}{40\text{ cm}} \rightarrow \frac{1}{i}=\frac{1}{40}-\frac{1}{50}=\frac{5-4}{200}=\frac{1}{200} \rightarrow \therefore i=200\text{ cm}$$

Because i is positive, we know the image is real; also, it's located 200 cm from the lens on the *opposite* side of the lens from the object. Because $m = -i/o = -(200 \text{ cm})/(50 \text{ cm}) = -4$, we know that the image is 4 times the height of the object and inverted.

Lens Power

A lens with a short focal length refracts light more (i.e., through larger angles) than a lens with a longer focal length. We say that the lens of short focal length has a greater *power* than a lens with a longer focal length.

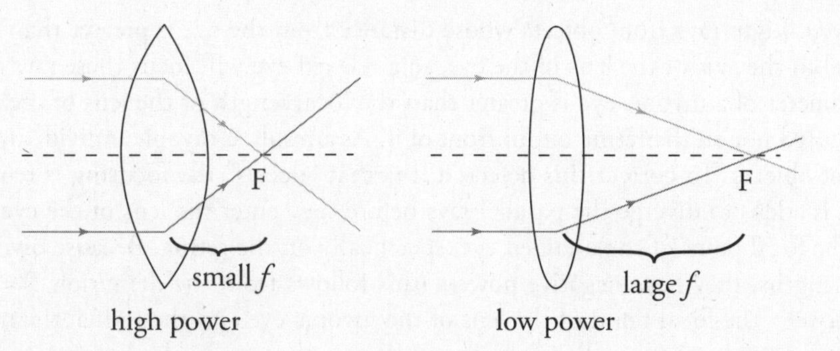

The **power** of a lens is defined to be the reciprocal of f, the focal length. When f is expressed in *meters*, the unit of lens power is called the **diopter** (abbreviated **D**).

Lens Power

$$P = \frac{1}{f} \quad \text{where } f \text{ is in meters}$$

For example, to find the power of a lens whose focal length is 40 cm, we first write f in meters: $f = 0.4$ m. Since $0.4 = 2/5$, the reciprocal of 0.4 is $5/2 = 2.5$. Therefore, the power of this lens is 2.5 diopters. Since the focal length of a converging lens is positive, the power of a converging lens is positive. Similarly, since the focal length of a diverging lens is negative, the power of a diverging lens is negative.

If two (or more) lenses are placed side by side, the power of the lens combination is equal to the sum of the powers of the individual lenses. In the case of two lenses, $P = P_1 + P_2$. For example, if we place a converging lens with a power of 3 D right next to a converging lens with a power of 1 D, then the power of the lens combination will be 4 D.

Example 11-14: A lens has a focal length of –20 cm. Is the lens converging or diverging? What is the power of this lens?

Solution: The fact that the lens has a negative focal length means that it's a diverging (or concave) lens. Rewriting f in meters, we have $f = -\frac{1}{5}$ m. Therefore, the power of this lens is

$$P = \frac{1}{f} = \frac{1}{-\frac{1}{5}\text{ m}} = -5\text{D}$$

The Basics of Eyesight Correction

Let's now look at the fundamental use of auxiliary lenses to correct the two most common types of eye defects: myopia and hyperopia. **Myopia** is the technical name for *nearsightedness*; myopic individuals cannot focus clearly on distant objects. **Hyperopia** (or **hypermetropia**) is the technical name for *far-sightedness*; in contrast to myopes, hyperopic individuals cannot focus clearly on objects that are near the eye. (As we age, most of us will be afflicted with *presbyopia*, in which the eyes' ability to *accommodate* is compromised by the loss of elasticity in the lens of the eye. **Accommodation** refers to the ability to focus on nearby objects through the action of the ciliary muscles, which essentially squeeze the lens of the eye, increasing its curvature and decreasing its focal length. However, the correction for presbyopia is the same as that for hyperopia.)

Correcting Myopia. Light rays from objects whose distance from the eye is greater than about 6 m are essentially parallel to the axis of the lens of the eye, so a relaxed eye will focus these rays at the focal point. Because the diameter of a myopic eye is greater than the focal length of the lens of the eye, the image of the object is focused not on the retina but in front of it. As a result, a myopic individual receives a blurred image of distant objects. To correct this defect, a lens that "delays" the focusing is required. In essence, what is needed is a lens to diverge the parallel rays before they enter the lens of the eye so that they will focus beyond the focal point of the unaided eye, specifically on the retina. Because diverging lenses have negative focal lengths, they have negative powers (this follows from the definition $P = 1/f$). The greater the distance between the focal point of the lens of the myopic eye and the retina, the more the auxiliary lens must diverge the incoming parallel rays; that is, the more powerful the corrective lens (and the more negative the lens power).

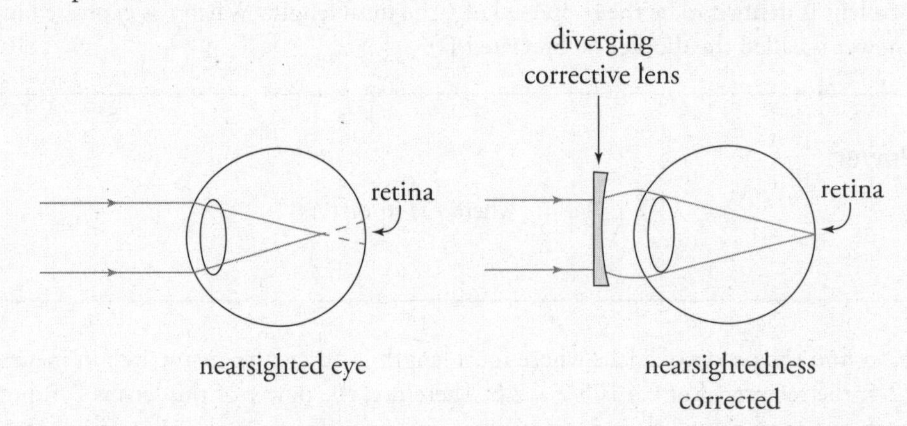

Correcting Hyperopia or Presbyopia. In these cases, light rays would be focused beyond the retina, either due to the diameter of the eye being smaller than the focal length of the lens of the eye or the inability of the ciliary muscles to decrease the focal length of the lens of the eye. To correct this defect, a lens that "accelerates" the focusing is required. In essence, what is needed is a lens to converge the rays before they enter the lens of the eye so that they will focus in front of the focal point of the unaided eye, specifically, on the retina. Because converging lenses have positive focal lengths, they have positive powers. (This follows from the definition $P = 1/f$.) The greater the distance between the focal point of the lens of the hyperopic eye and the retina, the more the auxiliary lens must converge the incoming rays, that is, the more powerful the corrective lens (and the more positive the lens power).

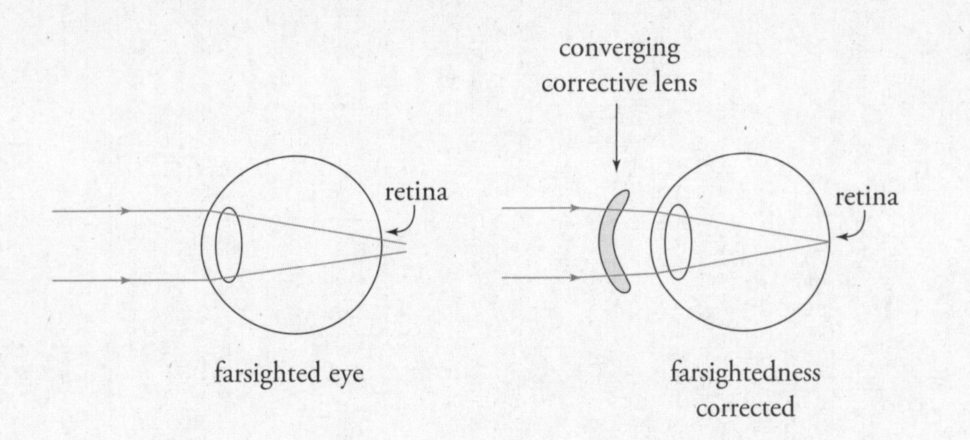

If you wear eyeglasses or contacts, check the prescription. If you have trouble seeing faraway objects, then you're nearsighted (myopic), and your corrective lenses are diverging and will have a negative power. On the other hand, if you have trouble seeing objects that are close-up, then you're farsighted (hyperopic), and your corrective lenses are converging and will have a positive power. Also, if the power of your left corrective lens is different from the power of your right corrective lens, the lens with the power of greater *magnitude* corresponds to the weaker eye. For example, if your left eye requires a lens of power –3.5 D while your right eye requires a lens of power –3.25 D, then your left eye is weaker because 3.5 > 3.25.

Summary of Formulas

Light acts as both a wave and a particle depending on the circumstance. In the former, energy is a function of amplitude; in the latter, energy is a function of frequency.

$c = 3 \times 10^8$ m/s for light in a vacuum

- All angles for reflection and refraction formulas are measured from the normal to the surface.

Photon energy: $E = hf = h\frac{c}{\lambda}$

Law of reflection: $\theta_1 = \theta_1'$

Index of refraction: $n = \frac{c}{v}, n \geq 1$

Law of refraction (Snell's law): $n_1 \sin\theta_1 = n_2 \sin\theta_2$

Total internal reflection: If $n_1 > n_2$ and $\theta_1 > \theta_{crit}$, where $\sin\theta_{crit} = \frac{n_2}{n_1}$

Total internal reflection (meaning no light is transmitted from the incident medium through the boundary) can occur for incident angles greater than θ_{crit} and only when the incident medium has a larger index of refraction (n) than that of the medium beyond the boundary.

Mirror/lens equation: $\frac{1}{o} + \frac{1}{i} = \frac{1}{f}$

Magnification: $m = -\frac{i}{o}$

Converging mirror or lens (concave mirror or convex lens) $\leftrightarrow$ f positive

Diverging mirror or lens (convex mirror or concave lens) $\leftrightarrow$ f negative

Note o is always positive; the sign for i corresponds to the sign conventions for f.

Real, inverted image $\leftrightarrow$ positive i

Virtual, upright image $\leftrightarrow$ negative i

Lens power: $P = \frac{1}{f}$ (P in diopters when f is expressed in meters)

Chapter 12
Modern Physics

The subject matter of the previous chapters was developed in the seventeenth, eighteenth, and nineteenth centuries, but as we delve into the physics of the very small, we enter the twentieth century. Let's first look at the structure of the atom, then travel into the nucleus itself. About 10 percent of the questions on the OAT will cover the field of modern physics.

12.1 THE RUTHERFORD MODEL OF THE ATOM

Around 1900, the atom was just considered a small bunch of positively charged "stuff" embedded with negatively charged electrons. This theoretical structure was known as the **raisin pudding model**; the pudding was the positively charged part of the atom and the raisins were the electrons. However, laboratory experiments in 1909 to 1911 led Ernest Rutherford to propose a radical revision of this model.

Rutherford fired **alpha particles** (α), which were known to be relatively massive and carry an electric charge of $+2e$, at an extremely thin sheet of gold foil. An alpha particle consists of two protons and two neutrons tightly bound together. If the atom is really just a glob of positive charge dotted with tiny negative electrons, then the heavy alpha particles should sail right through the target atoms, with little deviation.

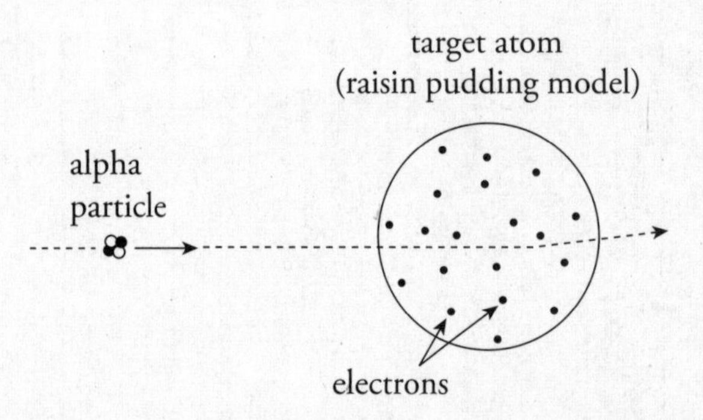

For the most part, this is what the experiments revealed. However, a small percentage of the alpha particles exhibited behavior that was completely unexpected: Some were deflected through very large angles (90° to 180°). This was explained by postulating that the positive charge of the atom was not spread throughout its volume, but was concentrated in a very tiny volume, at the atom's center. Alpha particles that came close to this concentration of positive charge experienced a strong Coulombic repulsive force and were deflected through large angles.

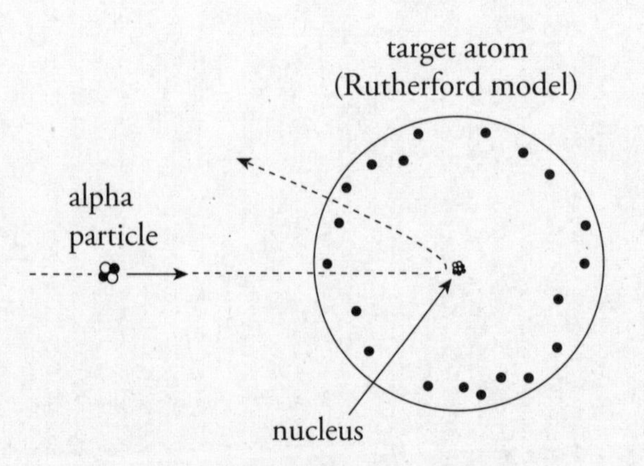

The tiny volume in which the positive charge is concentrated in an atom is known as the **nucleus**, and the nucleus is surrounded by a swarm of negatively charged electrons. This model is known as the **Rutherford nuclear model**.

12.2 PHOTONS AND THE PHOTOELECTRIC EFFECT

The particle-like nature of light was revealed and studied through the work of Max Planck in 1900, and later Albert Einstein (who won the 1921 Nobel Prize for work in this area). Electromagnetic radiation is emitted and absorbed by matter as though it existed in individual bundles called **quanta**. A quantum of electromagnetic energy is known as a **photon**. Light behaves like a stream of photons, and this is illustrated by the **photoelectric effect**.

When a piece of metal is illuminated by electromagnetic radiation (either visible light, ultraviolet light, or X-rays), the energy absorbed by electrons near the surface of the metal can liberate them from their bound state, and these electrons can fly off. The released electrons are known as **photoelectrons**. In this case, the classical, wave-only theory of light would predict the following three results:

1. There would be a significant time delay between the moment of illumination and the ejection of photoelectrons, as the electrons absorbed incident energy until their kinetic energy was sufficient to release them from the atoms' grip.
2. Increasing the intensity of the light would cause the electrons to leave the metal surface with greater kinetic energy.
3. Photoelectrons would be emitted regardless of the frequency of the incident energy, as long as the intensity was high enough.

Surprisingly, none of these predictions was observed. Photoelectrons were ejected within just a few billionths of a second after illumination, disproving prediction (1). Secondly, increasing the intensity of the light did not cause photoelectrons to leave the metal surface with greater kinetic energy. Although more electrons were ejected as the intensity was increased, there was a maximum photoelectron kinetic energy; prediction (2) was false. And, for each metal, there was a certain **threshold frequency,** f_0: If light of frequency lower than f_0 were used to illuminate the metal surface, *no* photoelectrons were ejected, regardless of how intense the incident radiation was; prediction (3) was also false. Clearly, something was wrong with the wave-only theory of light.

Einstein explained these observations by postulating that the energy of the incident electromagnetic wave was absorbed in individual bundles (photons).

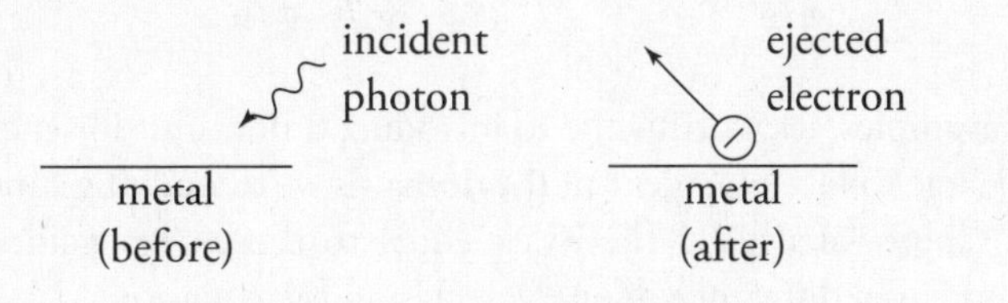

The energy of a photon is proportional to the frequency of the wave,

$$E = hf$$

where h is **Planck's constant** (about 6.63×10^{-34} J·s).

A certain amount of energy had to be imparted to an electron on the metal surface in order to liberate it; this was known as the metal's **work function**, or ϕ. If an electron absorbed a photon whose energy E was greater than ϕ, it would leave the metal with a maximum kinetic energy equal to $E - \phi$. This process could occur *very* quickly, which accounts for the rapidity with which photoelectrons are produced after illumination.

$$K_{max} = hf - \phi$$

Increasing the intensity of the incident energy means bombardment with more photons and results in the ejection of more photoelectrons—but since the energy of each incident photon is fixed by the equation $E = hf$, the value of K_{max} will still be $E - \phi$. This accounts for the observation that disproved prediction (2).

Finally, if the incident energy had a frequency that was less than ϕ/h, the incident photons would each have an energy that was less than ϕ; this would not be enough energy to liberate electrons. Blasting the metal surface with more photons (that is, increasing the intensity of the incident beam) would also do nothing; none of the photons would have enough energy to eject electrons, so whether there were one or one million wouldn't make any difference. This accounts for the observation of a threshold frequency, which we now know is ϕ/h.

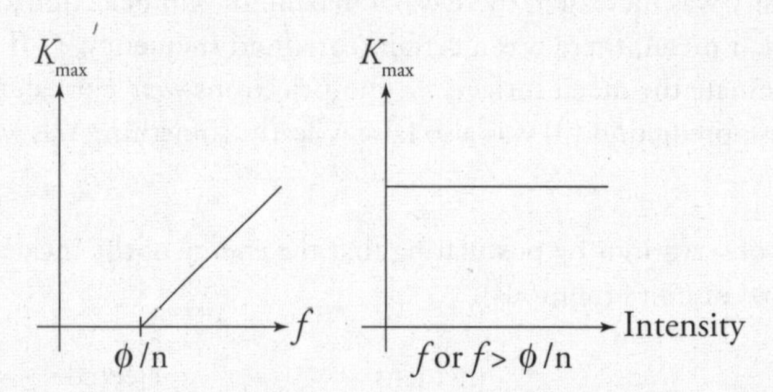

Before we get to some examples, it's worthwhile to introduce a new unit for energy. The SI unit for energy is the joule, but it's too large to be convenient in the domains we're studying now. We'll use a much smaller unit, the **electronvolt** (abbreviated eV). The eV is equal to the energy gained (or lost) by an electron accelerated through a potential difference of one volt. Using the equation $\Delta U_E = q\Delta V$, we find that

$$1 \text{ eV} = (1 \text{ e})(1 \text{ V}) = (1.6 \times 10^{-19} \text{ C})(1 \text{ V}) = 1.6 \times 10^{-19} \text{ J}$$

In terms of electronvolts, the value of Planck's constant is 4.14×10^{-15} eV•s.

Example: 12-1: The work function for a certain metal is 4.14 eV.

a) What is the threshold frequency required to produce photoelectrons from this metal?
b) To what wavelength does the frequency in Question 1 correspond?
c) Light with frequency 2×10^{15} Hz is directed onto the metal surface. Describe what would happen to the number of photoelectrons and their maximum kinetic energy if the intensity of this light were increased by a factor of 2.

Solution:

a) We know from the statement of the question that for a photon to be successful in liberating an electron from the surface of the metal, its energy cannot be less than 4.14 eV. Therefore, the minimum frequency of the incident light—the threshold frequency—must be

$$f_0 = \frac{\phi}{h} = \frac{4.14 \text{ eV}}{4.14 \times 10^{15} \text{ eV} \cdot \text{s}} = 1 \times 10^{15} \text{ Hz}$$

b) From the equation $\lambda f = c$, where c is the speed of light, we find that

$$\lambda = \frac{c}{f} = \frac{3 \times 10^{8} \text{ m/s}}{1 \times 10^{15} \text{ Hz}} = 3 \times 10^{-7} \text{ m}$$

c) Since the frequency of this light is higher than the threshold frequency, photoelectrons *will* be produced. If the intensity (brightness) of this light is then increased by a factor of 2, that means the metal surface will be hit with twice as many photons per second, so twice as many photoelectrons will be ejected per second. Thus, making the incident light brighter releases more photoelectrons. However, their maximum kinetic energy will not change. The only way to increase K_{max} is to increase the *frequency*—not the brightness—of the incident light.

12.3 THE BOHR MODEL OF THE ATOM

In the years immediately following Rutherford's announcement of his nuclear model of the atom, a young physicist, Niels Bohr, added an important piece to the atomic puzzle.

For fifty years it had been known that atoms in a gas discharge tube emitted and absorbed light only at specific wavelengths. The light from a glowing gas, passed through a prism to disperse the beam into its component wavelengths, produced patterns of sharp lines called **atomic spectra**. The visible wavelengths that appeared in the emission spectrum of hydrogen had been summarized by a simple formula. But *why* do atoms emit (or absorb) radiation only at certain discrete wavelengths?

Bohr's model of the atom explains. Using the simplest atom, hydrogen (which has one electron), Bohr postulated that the electron orbits the nucleus only at certain discrete radii. When the electron is in one of these special orbits, it does not lose energy (as the classical theory would predict). However, if the electron absorbs a certain amount of energy, it is **excited** to a higher orbit, one with a greater radius. After spending a short time in this excited state, it returns to a lower orbit, emitting a photon in the process. Since each allowed orbit—or **energy level**—has a specific radius (and corresponding specific energy), the photons emitted in each jump also have specific energies and wavelengths. We say that the electron's energy levels are **quantized**.

The energy levels within the hydrogen atom are given by the formula

$$E_n = \frac{1}{n^2}(-13.6 \text{ eV})$$

and for other one-electron atoms—ionized helium (Z = 2), doubly-ionized lithium (Z = 3), etc.—the energy levels are

$$E_n = \frac{Z^2}{n^2}(-13.6 \text{ eV})$$

where Z is the number of protons in the atom's nucleus.

When an excited electron drops from energy level $n = j$ to a lower one, $n = i$, the transition causes a photon of energy to be emitted, and the energy of a photon is the difference between the two energy levels:

$$E_{\text{emitted photon}} = |\Delta E| = E_j - E_i$$

Example 12-2: Refer to the diagram below.

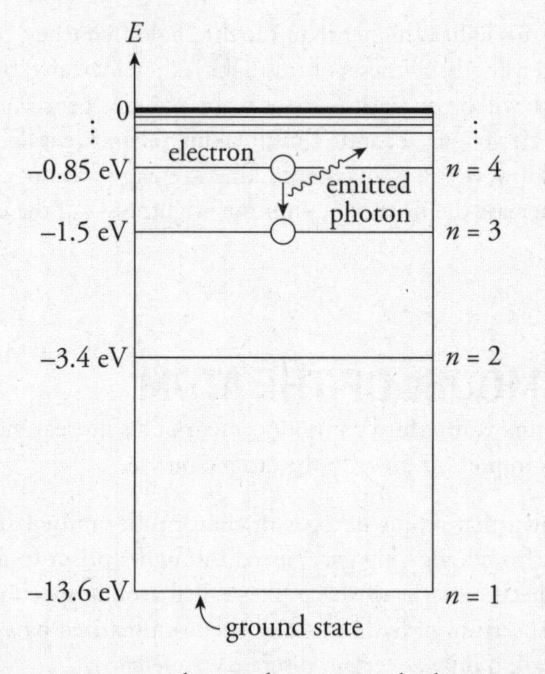

a) How much energy must a ground-state electron in a hydrogen atom absorb to be excited to the n = 4 energy level?

b) When the electron is in the n = 4 level, what energies are possible for the photon emitted when the electron drops to a lower energy level?

Solution:

a) For an electron to make the transition from E_1 to E_4, it must absorb energy in the amount $E_4 - E_1 = (-0.85\text{ eV}) - (-13.6\text{ eV}) = 12.8\text{ eV}$.

b) An electron in the $n = 4$ energy level can make several different transitions: It can drop to $n = 3$, $n = 2$, or all the way down to the ground state, $n = 1$.
So, there are three possible values for the energy of the emitted photon, $E_{4\to3}$, $E_{4\to2}$, or $E_{4\to1}$:

$$E_{4\to3} = E_4 - E_3 = (-0.85\text{ eV}) - (-1.5\text{ eV}) = 0.65\text{ eV}$$
$$E_{4\to2} = E_4 - E_2 = (-0.85\text{ eV}) - (-3.4\text{ eV}) = 2.55\text{ eV}$$
$$E_{4\to1} = E_4 - E_1 = (-0.85\text{ eV}) - (-13.6\text{ eV}) = 12.8\text{ eV}$$

12.4 WAVE–PARTICLE DUALITY

Light and other electromagnetic waves exhibit wave-like characteristics through interference and diffraction. However, as we saw in the photoelectric effect, light also behaves as if its energy were granular, composed of particles. This is **wave–particle duality**: *Electromagnetic radiation propagates like a wave but exchanges energy like a particle.*

Since an electromagnetic wave can behave like a particle, can a particle of matter behave like a wave? In 1923, the French physicist Louis de Broglie proposed that the answer is *yes*. His conjecture, which has since been supported by experiment, is that a particle of mass m and speed v—and thus with linear momentum $p = mv$—has an associated wavelength, which is called its **de Broglie wavelength**.

$$\lambda = \frac{h}{p}$$

Particles in motion can display wave characteristics, and behave as if they had a wavelength $\lambda = h/p$.

Since the value of h is so small, ordinary macroscopic objects do not display wave-like behavior. For example, a baseball (mass = 0.15 kg) thrown at a speed of 40 m/s has a de Broglie wavelength of

$$\lambda = \frac{h}{p} = \frac{h}{mv} = \frac{6.63\times10^{-34}\text{ J}\cdot\text{s}}{(0.15\text{ kg})(40\text{ m/s})} = 1.1\times10^{-34}\text{ m}$$

This is much too small to measure. However, with subatomic particles, the wave nature is clearly evident.

Example 12-3:

a) Name or describe an experiment that demonstrates that light behaves like a wave.

b) Name or describe an experiment that demonstrates that light behaves like a particle.

Solution:

a) Young's double-slit interference experiment shows that light behaves like a wave. Interference is a characteristic of waves, not of particles.

b) The photoelectric effect shows that light behaves like a particle, where the energy of the light is absorbed as photons: individual "particles" of light energy.

12.5 NUCLEAR PHYSICS

The nucleus of the atom is composed of particles called **protons** and **neutrons**, which are collectively called **nucleons.** The number of protons in a given nucleus is called the atom's **atomic number**, or Z, and the number of neutrons (the **neutron number**) is denoted N. The total number of nucleons, $Z + N$, is called the **mass number** (or **nucleon number**), and is denoted A. The number of protons in the nucleus of an atom defines the element. For example, the element chlorine (abbreviated Cl) is characterized by the fact that the nucleus of every chlorine atom contains 17 protons, so the atomic number of chlorine is 17; however, different chlorine atoms may contain different numbers of neutrons. In fact, about three-fourths of all naturally occurring chlorine atoms have 18 neutrons in their nuclei (mass number = 35), and most of the remaining one-fourth contain 20 neutrons (mass number = 37). Nuclei that contain the same numbers of protons but different numbers of neutrons are called **isotopes.**

> The notation for a **nuclide**—the term for a nucleus with specific numbers of protons and neutrons—is to write Z and A, one above the other, before the chemical symbol of the element.
>
> $${}^{A}_{Z}\mathrm{X}$$

The isotopes of chlorine mentioned earlier would be written as follows:

$${}^{35}_{17}\mathrm{Cl} \text{ and } {}^{37}_{17}\mathrm{Cl}$$

Example 12-4: How many protons and neutrons are contained in the nuclide ${}^{63}_{29}\mathrm{Cu}$?

Solution: The subscript (the atomic number, Z) gives the number of protons, which is 29. The superscript (the mass number, A) gives the total number of nucleons. Since $A = 63 = Z + N$, we find that $N = 63 - 29 = 34$.

Example 12-5: The element neon (abbreviated Ne, atomic number 10) has several isotopes. The most abundant isotope contains 10 neutrons, and two others contain 11 and 12. Write symbols for these three nuclides.

Solution: The mass numbers of these isotopes are 10 + 10 = 20, 10 + 11 = 21, and 10 + 12 = 22. So, we'd write them as follows:

$$^{20}_{10}\text{Ne}, \quad ^{21}_{10}\text{Ne}, \quad \text{and} \quad ^{22}_{10}\text{Ne}$$

Another common notation—which we also use—is to write the mass number after the name of the element. These three isotopes of neon would be written as neon-20, neon-21, and neon-22.

The Nuclear Force

Why wouldn't any nucleus that has more than one proton be unstable? After all, protons are positively charged and would therefore experience a repulsive Coulomb force from each other. Why don't these nuclei explode? And what holds neutrons—which have no electric charge—in the nucleus? These issues are resolved by the presence of another fundamental force, the **strong nuclear force**, which binds together neutrons and protons to form nuclei. Although the strength of the Coulomb force can be expressed by a simple mathematical formula (it's inversely proportional to the square of their separation), the nuclear force is much more complicated; no simple formula can be written for the strength of the nuclear force.

Binding Energy

The masses of the proton and neutron are listed below.

$$\text{proton: } m_p = 1.6726 \times 10^{-27} \text{ kg}$$

$$\text{neutron: } m_n = 1.6749 \times 10^{-27} \text{ kg}$$

Because these masses are so tiny, a much smaller mass unit is used. With the most abundant isotope of carbon (carbon-12) as a reference, the **atomic mass unit** (abbreviated **amu** or simply **u**) is defined as 1/12 the mass of a ^{12}C atom. The conversion between kg and u is 1 u = 1.6605×10^{-27} kg. In terms of atomic mass units

$$\text{proton: } m_p = 1.00728 \text{ u}$$

$$\text{neutron: } m_n = 1.00867 \text{ u}$$

Now consider the **deuteron**, the nucleus of **deuterium**, an isotope of hydrogen that contains 1 proton and 1 neutron. The mass of a deuteron is 2.01356 u, which is a little *less* than the sum of the individual masses of the proton and neutron. The difference between the mass of any bound nucleus and the sum of the masses of its constituent nucleons is called the **mass defect**, Δm. In the case of the deuteron (symbolized **d**), the mass defect is

$$\begin{aligned}\Delta m &= (m_p + m_n) - m_d \\ &= (1.00728\ \text{u} + 1.00867\ \text{u}) - (2.01356\ \text{u}) \\ &= 0.00239\ \text{u}\end{aligned}$$

What happened to this missing mass? It was converted to energy when the deuteron was formed. It also represents the amount of energy needed to break the deuteron into a separate proton and neutron. Since this tells us how strongly the nucleus is bound, it is called the **binding energy** of the nucleus.

The conversion between mass and energy is given by Einstein's **mass–energy equivalence** equation, $E = mc^2$ (where c is the speed of light); the binding energy, E_B, is equal to the mass defect, Δm

$$E_B = (\Delta m)c^2$$

Using $E = mc^2$, the energy equivalent of 1 atomic mass unit is about 931 MeV.

In terms of electronvolts, then, the binding energy of the deuteron is

$$E_B\ (\text{deuteron}) = 0.00239\ \text{u} \times \frac{931\ \text{MeV}}{1\ \text{u}} = 2.23\ \text{MeV}$$

Since the deuteron contains 2 nucleons, the **binding energy per nucleon** is

$$\frac{2.23\ \text{MeV}}{2\ \text{nucleons}} = 1.12\ \text{MeV/nucleon}.$$

This is the lowest value of all nuclides. The highest, 8.8 MeV/nucleon, is for an isotope of nickel, ^{62}Ni. Typically, when nuclei smaller than nickel are fused to form a single nucleus, the binding energy per nucleon increases, which tells us that energy is released in the process. On the other hand, when nuclei *larger* than nickel are *split*, binding energy per nucleon again increases, releasing energy.

12.6 RADIOACTIVITY

The stability of a nucleus depends on the ability of the nuclear force to balance the repulsive Coulomb forces between the protons. Many nuclides are ultimately unstable and will undergo spontaneous restructuring to become more stable. An unstable nucleus that will spontaneously change into a lower-energy configuration is said to be **radioactive**. Nuclei that are too large (A is too great) or ones in which the neutron-to-proton ratio is unfavorable are radioactive, and there are several different modes of radioactive decay. We'll look at the most important ones: **alpha** decay, **beta** decay (three forms), and **gamma** decay.

Alpha Decay

When a nucleus undergoes alpha decay, it emits an alpha particle, which consists of two protons and two neutrons and is the same as the nucleus of a helium-4 atom. An alpha particle can be represented as

$$\alpha,\ {}^{4}_{2}\alpha,\ \text{or}\ {}^{4}_{2}\text{He}$$

Very large nuclei can shed nucleons quickly by emitting one or more alpha particles, for example, radon-222 (${}^{222}_{86}\text{Rn}$) is radioactive and undergoes alpha decay.

$${}^{222}_{86}\text{Rn} \rightarrow {}^{218}_{84}\text{Po} + {}^{4}_{2}\alpha$$

This reaction illustrates two important features of any nuclear reaction.

(1) Mass number is conserved (in this case, 222 = 218 + 4).
(2) Charge is conserved (in this case, 86 = 84 + 2).

The decaying nuclide is known as the **parent**, and the resulting nuclide is known as the **daughter.** (Here, radon-222 is the parent nuclide and polonium-218 is the daughter.) Alpha decay decreases the mass number by 4 and the atomic number by 2. Therefore, alpha decay looks like the following:

$${}^{A}_{Z}\text{X} \rightarrow {}^{A-4}_{Z-2}\text{X}' + {}^{4}_{2}\alpha$$

Beta Decay

There are three subcategories of **beta** (**β**) decay, called **β^-**, **β^+**, and **electron capture** (EC).

β⁻ Decay

When the neutron-to-proton ratio is too large, the nucleus undergoes β^- decay, which is the most common form of beta decay. β^- decay occurs when a neutron transforms into a proton and an electron, and the electron is ejected from the nucleus. The expelled electron is called a **beta particle.** The transformation of a neutron into a proton and an electron (and another particle, the **electron-antineutrino,** $\bar{\nu}_e$) is caused by the action of the **weak nuclear force**, another of nature's fundamental forces. A common example of a nuclide that undergoes β^- decay is carbon-14, which is used to date archaeological artifacts.

$${}^{14}_{6}\text{C} \rightarrow {}^{14}_{7}\text{N} + {}^{0}_{-1}\text{e} + \bar{\nu}_e$$

Notice how the ejected electron is written: The superscript is its nucleon number (which is zero), and the subscript is its charge. The reaction is balanced, since 14 = 14 + 0 and 6 = 7 + (–1).

β^+ Decay

When the neutron-to-proton ratio is too small, the nucleus will undergo β^+ decay. In this form of beta decay, a proton is transformed into a neutron and a **positron**, ${}^{0}_{+1}e$ (the electron's **antiparticle**), plus another particle, the **electron-neutrino**, ν_e, which are then both ejected from the nucleus. An example of a positron emitter is fluorine-17.

12.6

$$ {}^{17}_{9}F \rightarrow {}^{17}_{8}O + {}^{0}_{+1}e + \nu_e $$

Electron Capture

Another way in which a nucleus can increase its neutron-to-proton ratio is to capture an orbiting electron and then cause the transformation of a proton into a neutron. Beryllium-7 undergoes this process.

$$ {}^{7}_{4}Be + {}^{0}_{-1}e \rightarrow {}^{7}_{3}Li + \nu_e $$

Gamma Decay

In each of the decay processes defined above, the daughter was a different element from the parent. Radon becomes polonium as a result of α decay, carbon becomes nitrogen as a result of β^- decay, fluorine becomes oxygen from β^+ decay, and beryllium becomes lithium from electron capture. By contrast, gamma decay does not alter the identity of the nucleus; it just allows the nucleus to relax and shed energy. Imagine that potassium-42 undergoes β^- decay to form calcium-42.

$$ {}^{42}_{19}K \rightarrow {}^{42}_{20}Ca^* + {}^{0}_{-1}e + \bar{\nu}_e $$

The asterisk indicates that the daughter calcium nucleus is left in a high-energy, excited state. For this excited nucleus to drop to its ground state, it must emit a photon of energy, a **gamma ray**, symbolized by γ.

$$ {}^{42}_{20}Ca^* \rightarrow {}^{42}_{20}Ca + \gamma $$

Example 12-6: What's the daughter nucleus in each of the following radioactive decays?

a) Strontium-90 (${}^{90}_{38}Sr$); $\beta-$ decay

b) Argon-37 (${}^{37}_{18}Ar$); electron capture

c) Plutonium-239 (${}^{239}_{94}Pu$); alpha decay

d) Cobalt-58 (${}^{58}_{27}Co$); $\beta+$ decay

Solution:

a) $^{90}_{38}\text{Sr} \rightarrow {}^{90}_{39}\text{Y} + {}^{0}_{-1}\text{e} + \bar{\nu}_e \Rightarrow$ daughter = yttrium-90

b) $^{37}_{18}\text{Ar} + {}^{0}_{-1}\text{e} \rightarrow {}^{37}_{17}\text{Cl} + \nu_e \Rightarrow$ daughter = chlorine-37

c) $^{239}_{94}\text{Pu} \rightarrow {}^{235}_{92}\text{U} + {}^{4}_{2}\alpha \Rightarrow$ daughter = uranium-235

d) $^{58}_{27}\text{Co} \rightarrow {}^{58}_{26}\text{Fe} + {}^{0}_{+1}\text{e}^{+} + \nu_e \Rightarrow$ daughter = iron-58

Radioactive Decay Rates

Although it's impossible to say precisely when a particular radioactive nuclide will decay, it *is* possible to predict the decay rates of a pure radioactive sample. As a radioactive sample disintegrates, the number of decays per second decreases, but the *fraction* of nuclei that decay per second—the **decay constant**—does not change. The decay constant is determined by the identity of the radioisotope. Boron-9 has a decay constant of 7.5×10^{17} s^{-1} (rapid), while uranium-238 has a decay constant of about 5×10^{-18} s^{-1} (slow).

The **activity** (A) of a radioactive sample is the number of disintegrations it undergoes per second; it decreases with time according to the equation

$$A = A_0 e^{-\lambda t}$$

where A_0 is the activity at time $t = 0$ and λ is the decay constant (not to be confused with wavelength).

Activity is expressed in disintegrations per second: 1 disintegration per second is one **becquerel (Bq)**. The greater the value of λ, the faster the sample decays. This equation also describes the number (N) of radioactive nuclei in a given sample, $N = N_0 e^{-\lambda t}$, or the mass (m) of the sample, $m = m_0 e^{-\lambda t}$.

The most common way to indicate the rapidity with which radioactive samples decay is to give their **half-life.** Just as the name suggests, the half-life is the time required for half of a given sample to decay.

Half-life, $T_{1/2}$, is inversely proportional to the decay constant, λ, and in terms of the half-life, the exponential decay of a sample's mass (or activity) can be written as

$$m = m_0 \left(\frac{1}{2}\right)^{t/T_{1/2}}$$

A sample's activity or mass can be graphed as a function of time; the result is the **exponential decay** curve, which you should study carefully.

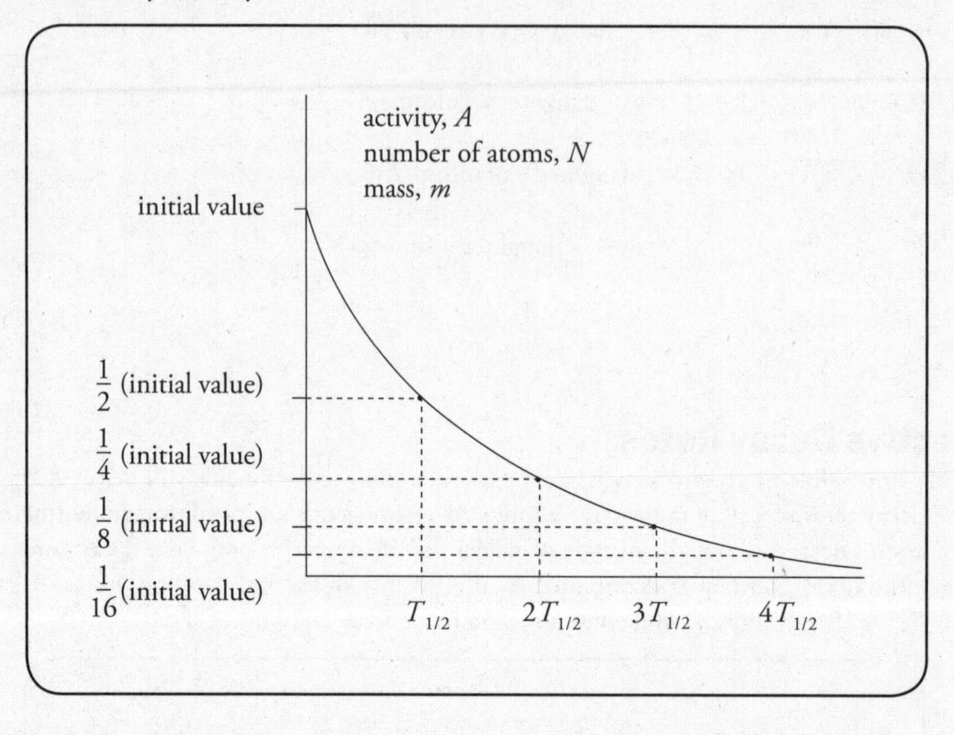

Example 12-7: The half-life of iodine-131 (a β^- emitter) is 8 days. If a sample of ^{131}I has a mass of 1 gram, what will the mass be 40 days later?

Solution: Every 8 days, the sample's mass decreases by a factor of 2. We can illustrate the decay in the following diagram:

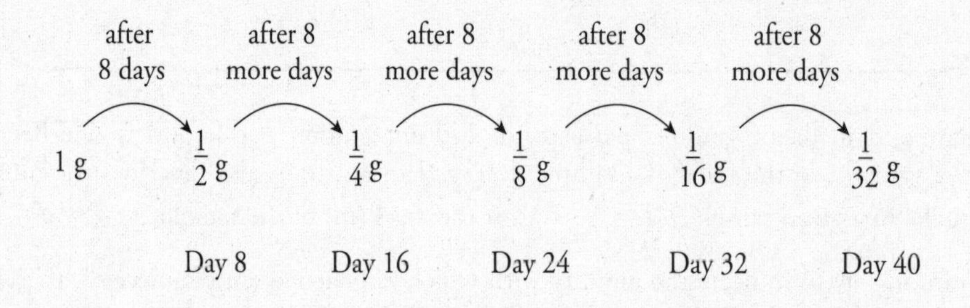

Example 12-8: Home smoke detectors contain a small radioactive sample of americium-241 ($^{241}_{95}Am$), an alpha-particle emitter that has a half-life of 430 years. What is the daughter nucleus of the decay?

Solution: $^{241}_{95}\text{Am} \rightarrow {}^{237}_{93}\text{Np} + {}^{4}_{2}\alpha \quad \Rightarrow$ daughter = neptunium-237

12.7 NUCLEAR REACTIONS

Natural radioactive decay provides one example of a nuclear reaction. Other examples of nuclear reactions include the bombardment of target nuclei with subatomic particles to artificially induce radioactivity (this is **nuclear fission**), and the **nuclear fusion** of small nuclei at extremely high temperatures. In all cases of nuclear reactions that we'll study, nucleon number and charge must be conserved. To balance nuclear reactions, we write ${}^{1}_{1}\text{p}$ or ${}^{1}_{1}\text{H}$ for a proton and ${}^{1}_{0}\text{n}$ for a neutron. Gamma-ray photons can also be produced in nuclear reactions; they have no charge or nucleon number and are represented as ${}^{0}_{0}\gamma$.

Example 12-9: A mercury-198 nucleus is bombarded by a neutron, which causes a nuclear reaction.

$$ {}^{1}_{0}\text{n} + {}^{198}_{80}\text{Hg} \rightarrow {}^{197}_{79}\text{Au} + {}^{?}_{?}\text{X} $$

What's the unknown product particle, X?

Solution: In order to balance the superscripts, we must have $1 + 198 = 197 + A$, so $A = 2$, and the subscripts are balanced if $0 + 80 = 79 + Z$, so $Z = 1$.

$$ {}^{1}_{0}\text{n} + {}^{198}_{80}\text{Hg} \rightarrow {}^{197}_{79}\text{Au} + {}^{2}_{1}\text{X} $$

Therefore, X must be a deuteron, ${}^{2}_{1}\text{H}$ (or just d).

Disintegration Energy

Nuclear reactions not only produce new nuclei and other subatomic particles, but also involve the absorption or emission of energy. Nuclear reactions must conserve total energy, so changes in mass are accompanied by changes in energy according to Einstein's equation $\Delta E = (\Delta m)c^2$.

A general nuclear reaction is written

$$ \text{A} + \text{B} \rightarrow \text{C} + \text{D} + Q $$

where Q is the **disintegration energy.**

If Q is positive, the reaction is **exothermic** and the reaction can occur spontaneously; if Q is negative, the reaction is **endothermic** and the reaction cannot occur spontaneously. The energy Q is calculated as follows:

$$ Q = [(m_A + m_B) - (m_C + m_D)]c^2 $$

For spontaneous reactions—ones that liberate energy—most of the energy is revealed as kinetic energy of the least massive product nuclei.

Summary of Formulas

For the test, be sure you are familiar with the following concepts from this chapter.

- Rutherford model of the atom
- Photons and the photoelectric effect
- The Bohr model of the atom
- Wave–particle duality
- Nuclear physics
- The nuclear force
- Binding energy
- Radioactivity
- Alpha decay
- Beta decay
- β^- decay
- β^+ decay
- Electron capture
- Radioactive decay rates
- Nuclear reactions
- Disintegration energy

Chapter 13
Thermodynamics

13.1 INTRODUCTION

Objects contain **thermal energy**, which is due to the random motion of its molecules. **Heat** is defined to be thermal energy transmitted from one body to another. Note that objects don't *contain* heat; heat is energy that's in *transit*. By contrast, **temperature** is a measure of the intensity of an object's internal thermal energy. The study of the energy transfers involving work and heat, and the resulting changes in internal energy, temperature, volume, and pressure is called **thermodynamics**.

The SI unit for temperature is the **Kelvin**, where *absolute zero* is defined as 0 K and the *triple point* of water (the point where the solid, liquid, and gas phase of water can coexist) is 273.16 K. A Kelvin is the same size as a Celsius degree, and the conversion between the **absolute temperature** T in kelvins and the temperature expressed in Celsius degrees is

$$T = T(\text{in }^\circ\text{C}) + 273.15$$

When a substance absorbs or gives off heat, one of two things can happen: (1) the temperature of the substance changes, *or* (2) the substance undergoes a phase change. If (1) occurs, then

$$Q = mc\Delta T$$

Where Q denotes the heat transferred, m is the mass of the sample, c is the specific heat, and ΔT is the resulting temperature change. Intuitively, a substance's specific heat measures its ability to absorb heat and resist changes in temperature; that is, the greater the value of c, the smaller ΔT will be for a given amount of heat, Q.

If (2) occurs, then the sample's temperature remains constant throughout the transformation (that is, $\Delta T = 0$, so the previous equation does not apply) and

$$Q = mL$$

Where L denotes the **latent heat of phase transformation.** This equation tells us how much heat must be transferred in order to cause a sample of mass m to completely undergo a phase change. In the case of a phase change from solid to liquid (or vice versa), L is called the **latent heat of fusion**. For a phase change between liquid and vapor, L is called the **latent heat of vaporization**. In general, more energy is required to break the intermolecular bonds in going from liquid to vapor than is required to loosen the intermolecular bonds to go from solid to liquid, so $L_{vaporization} > L_{fusion}$.

13.2 HEAT TRANSFER AND THERMAL EXPANSION

When a substance undergoes a temperature change, it changes in size. Steel beams that form bridges or railroad tracks elongate and can buckle on a hot day; a balloon filled with air shrinks when placed in a freezer. The change in the length of the steel beam or in the volume of the gas in the balloon depends on the amount of the temperature change and on the identity of the substance being affected.

Let's first consider changes in length (of a steel beam, for example). When its initial temperature is T_i, its length is L_i. Then, if the beam's temperature changes to T_f, the length changes to L_f, where

$$L_f - L_i = \alpha L_i(T_f - T_i)$$

Where α is the **coefficient of linear expansion** of the material. This equation is usually remembered in the simpler form

$$\Delta L = \alpha L_i \Delta T$$

Nearly all substances have a positive value of α, which means they expand upon heating. If α is negative, then the substance shrinks when heated.

Example 13-1: A steel beam used in the construction of a bridge has a length of 20 m when the ambient temperature is 10°C. On a very hot day, when the temperature is 35°C, by how much will the beam stretch? (The coefficient of linear expansion for structural steel is $+1.2 \times 10^{-5}$/°C.)

Solution: The change in length of the beam will be

$$\Delta L = \alpha L_1 \Delta T = \frac{1.2 \times 10^{-5}}{°\text{C}}(20\text{ m})(35°\text{C} - 10°\text{C}) = 6 \times 10^{-3}\text{ m} = 6\text{ mm}$$

Substances also undergo volume changes when heat is lost or absorbed. The change in volume, ΔV, corresponding to a temperature change, ΔT, is given by the equation

$$\Delta V = \beta V_i \Delta T$$

where V_i is the sample's initial volume and β is the **coefficient of volume expansion** of the substance. Nearly all substances have a positive value for β, which means they expand upon heating. If β is negative, then the substance shrinks when heated. An extremely important example of a substance with a negative value of β is liquid water between 0°C and 4°C. Unlike the vast majority of substances, liquid water *expands* as it nears its freezing point and solidifies (which is why ice floats in water).

Example 13-2: A driver fills up a spare tank with 12 gallons of gas near the top of a mountain where the temperature is 2°C. By how much will the volume of the gasoline expand when the temperature is 22°C at the bottom of the mountain? (The coefficient of volume expansion for gasoline is +9.5 × 10^{-4}/°C.)

Solution: The change in the volume of the gasoline will be

$$\Delta V = \beta V_1 \Delta T = \frac{9.5 \times 10^{-4}}{°\text{C}}(13 \text{ gal})(22°\text{C} - 2°\text{C}) = 0.25 \text{ gal}$$

13.3 THE KINETIC THEORY OF GASES

Unlike the condensed phases of matter–solid and liquid–the atoms or molecules that make up a gas do not oscillate around relatively fixed equilibrium positions. Rather, the motion is much more chaotic as the molecules zip around freely. As each gas molecule strikes a wall of its container, it exerts a force on the wall. The average force per unit area exerted by all the molecules is called the **pressure.**

The Ideal Gas Law

Three physical properties–pressure (P), volume (V), and temperature (T)–describe a gas. At low densities, all gases approach *ideal* or *perfect* behavior, which means that these three variables obey the equation

$$PV = nRT$$

where n is the number of moles of gas and R is the **universal gas constant** (equal to 8.31 J/mol·K). This equation is known as the **Ideal Gas Law.**

An important consequence of this equation is the observation that for a fixed volume of gas, an increase in P gives a proportional increase in T. The pressure increases when the gas molecules strike the walls of its container with more force, which occurs if they move more rapidly. We can make this more precise. Using Newton's Second Law (in the form *rate of change of momentum = force*) to find the average force–and, consequently, the pressure–that the gas molecules exert, it can be shown that the product of the pressure exerted by N molecules of gas in a container of volume V is related to the average kinetic energy of the molecules by the equation $PV = \frac{2}{3}NK_{avg}$. Comparing this to the Ideal Gas Law, we see that

$\frac{2}{3}NK_{avg} = nRT$. We can rewrite this equation in the form $\frac{2}{3}N_A K_{avg} = RT$, since, by definition, $N = nN_A$, where N_A is Avogadro's number. The ratio R/N_A is a fundamental constant of nature called **Boltzmann's constant** ($k_B = 1.38 \times 10^{-23}$ J/K), so our equation becomes

$$K_{avg} = \frac{3}{2}k_B T$$

This equation states that *the average translational kinetic energy of the gas molecules is directly proportional to the temperature of the sample.*

Since the average kinetic energy of the gas molecules is $K_{avg} = \frac{1}{2}m(v^2)_{avg}$, where m is the mass of each molecule, the equation above becomes $\frac{1}{2}m(v^2)_{avg} = \frac{3}{2}k_B T$, so

$$\sqrt{v^2_{avg}} = \sqrt{\frac{3k_B T}{m}}$$

The quantity on the left-hand side of this equation, the square root of the average of the square of v, is called the **root-mean-square** speed, v_{rms}, so

$$v_{rms} = \sqrt{\frac{3k_B T}{m}}$$

Because $k_B = R/N_A$ and $mN_A = M$ = the mass of one mole of the molecules (the **molar mass**), the equation for v_{rms} is also commonly written in the form

$$v_{rms} = \sqrt{\frac{3RT}{M}}$$

Notice that these last two displayed equations determine only v_{rms}, the molecules in the container have a wide range of speeds, some much slower and other much faster than v_{rms}. The importance of the root-mean-square speed is that it gives us an average speed that is easy to calculate directly from the temperature of the gas.

Example 13-3: Compare the average (root-mean-square) speeds of nitrogen molecules and oxygen molecules at room temperature (20 °C = 293 K).

Solution: First, since N_2 has a smaller molar mass than O_2 (28 g/mol for N_2 vs. 32 g/mol for O_2), the nitrogen molecules will move faster on average than the heavier oxygen molecules. The ratio of their root-mean-square speeds is

$$\frac{v_{\text{rms}}, N_2}{v_{\text{rms}}, O_2} = \sqrt{\frac{3RT / M_{N_2}}{3RT / M_{O_2}}} = \sqrt{\frac{M_{O_2}}{M_{N_2}}} = \sqrt{\frac{32 \text{ g/mol}}{28 \text{ g/mol}}} = \sqrt{\frac{8}{7}}$$

Example 13-4: A 0.2 mol sample of an ideal gas is confined to a container whose volume is 10 L. What will happen to the root-mean-square speed of its molecules if the sample is heated until the pressure doubles?

Solution: Since n and V are fixed, T is proportional to P (this follows from the Ideal Gas Law), therefore, if P doubles, then T doubles. Since v_{rms} is proportional to the square root of T, if T increases by a factor of 2, then v_{rms} will increase by a factor of $\sqrt{2} = 1.4$.

13.4 THE LAWS OF THERMODYNAMICS

The Zeroth Law of Thermodynamics

When two objects are brought into contact, heat will flow from the warmer object to the cooler one until they both reach **thermal equilibrium,** at which point their temperatures are the same. If Objects 1 and 2 are each in thermal equilibrium with Object 3, then Objects 1 and 2 are in thermal equilibrium with each other. The Zeroth Law assures us that the concept of temperature is well-defined and has a physical meaning.

The First Law of Thermodynamics

Simply put, the First Law of Thermodynamics is a statement of the Conservation of Energy that includes heat. To illustrate its use, we'll consider the following example of a system and its surroundings. It's the prototype that's studied extensively in thermodynamics.

An insulated, cylindrical container filled with an ideal gas rests on a heat reservoir that can serve as a heat source or a heat sink. The container is covered by a tight-fitting—but frictionless—weighted piston that can be raised or lowered. The confined gas is the *system*, and the piston and heat reservoir are the *surroundings.*

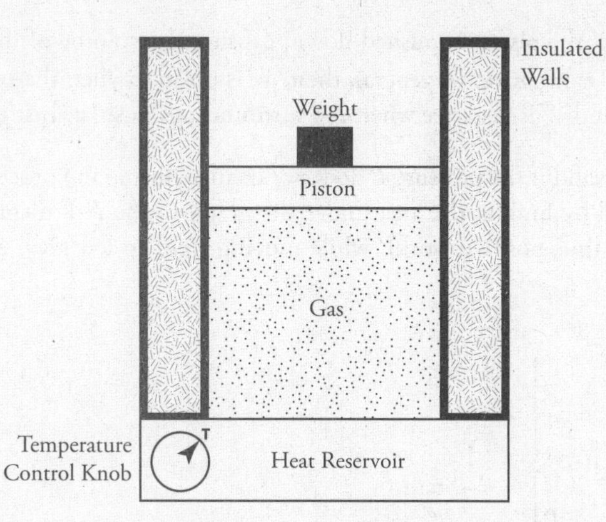

The **state** of the gas is given once the values of its pressure, volume, and temperature are known, and the equation that connects these state variables is the Ideal Gas Law, $PV = nRT$. Different experiments can be performed on the gas, such as heating it or allowing it to cool, increasing or decreasing the weight on the piston, etc., and we can determine not only the energy transfers (work and heat) but also how the state variables are affected. If each experiment is carried out slowly, so that at each moment, the system and its surroundings are in thermal equilibrium, we can plot the pressure (P) vs. the volume (V) on a **P-V diagram.** Each point in the diagram represents a particular value of P and V for the gas, and by following the graph, we can study how the system is affected as it moves from one state to another.

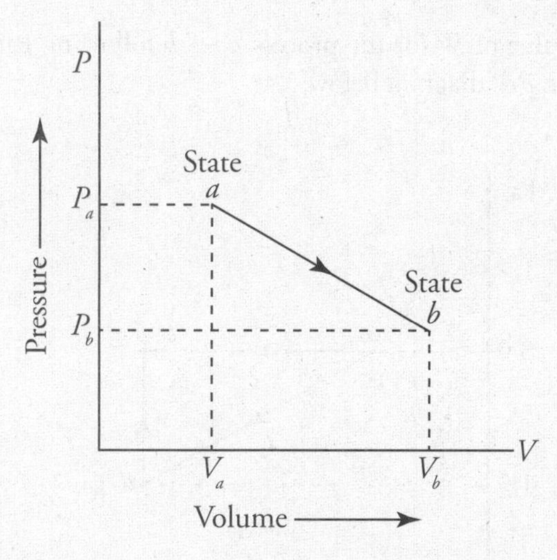

Work is done on or by the system when the piston is moved and the volume of the gas changes. For example, imagine that the gas pushes the piston upward, causing an increase in volume. The work done by the gas during its expansion is $W = F\Delta s$. But since $F = PA$, we have $W = PA\Delta s$, and because $A\Delta s = \Delta V$, we have, finally (assuming P is constant),

$$W = P\Delta V$$

This equation is also true if the piston is pushed down, causing the volume of the gas to decrease. In this case, ΔV is negative, so W is negative. In general, then, W is positive when the system does work pushing against its surroundings, and W is negative when the surroundings push against the system.

13.4

The equation $W = P\Delta V$ is valid if the pressure P does not change during the process. If P *does* change, then the work can be evaluated by finding the area under the graph in the P-V diagram; moving left to right gives a positive area (and thus positive work), while moving right to left gives a negative area (and thus negative work).

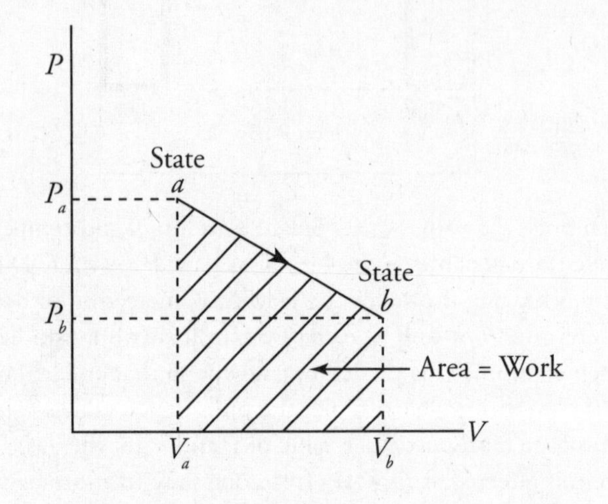

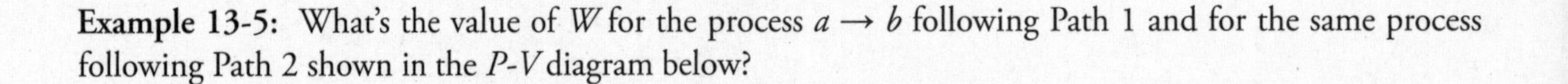

Example 13-5: What's the value of W for the process $a \to b$ following Path 1 and for the same process following Path 2 shown in the P-V diagram below?

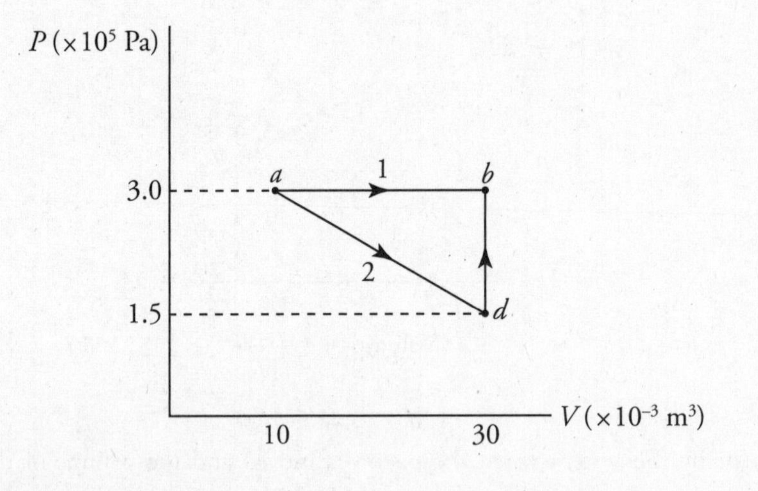

Solution: Along Path 1, P remains constant, so the work done is simply $P\Delta V$:

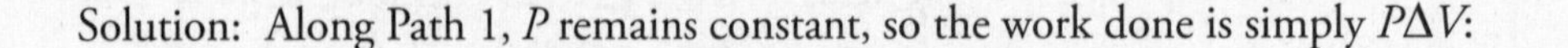

$$W = P\Delta V = (3 \times 10^5\ \text{Pa})[(30 \times 10^{-3}\ \text{m}^3) - (10 \times 10^{-3}\ \text{m}^3)] = 6000\ \text{J}$$

If the gas is brought from state *a* to state *b* along Path 2, then work is done only along the part from *a* to *d*. From *d* to *b*, the volume of the gas does not change, so no work can be performed. The area under the graph from *a* to *d* is the area of a trapezoid, so

$$W = \frac{1}{2}h(b_1 + b_2) = \frac{1}{2}(\Delta V)(P_a + P_d)$$

$$= \frac{1}{2}(20 \times 10^{-3}\text{ m}^3)[(3 \times 10^5\text{ Pa}) + (1.5 \times 10^5\text{ Pa})]$$

$$= 4500\text{ J}$$

Notice that $W_{a\to b} = 6000$ J along path 1, but $W_{a\to b} = 4500$ J along path 2.

As the preceding example shows, the value of *W* depends not only on the initial and final states of the system, but also on the path between the two. In general, different paths give different values for *W*. The value of *Q* is also path dependent. However, experiments have shown that the value of $Q - W$ is *not* path dependent; it depends *only* on the initial and final state of the system, so it must describe a change in some fundamental property. This fundamental property is called the system's **internal energy**, denoted *U*. Therefore, the change in the system's internal energy, ΔU, is equal to $Q - W$, regardless of the process that brought the system from its initial state to its final state. This statement is known as **The First Law of Thermodynamics:**

$$\Delta U = Q - W$$

Example 13-6: A 0.5 mol sample of an ideal gas is brought from state *a* to state *b* along the path shown in the *P-V* diagram below. [Since the pressure remains constant (as we can see since the graph in the *P-V* diagram is a horizontal line), the process is called *isobaric*.]

a) Compare the temperature at state *b* to the temperature at state *a*.
b) Calculate the work done during the process.
c) Given that the gas absorbed 10,000 J of heat from *a* to *b*, determine the change in its internal energy.

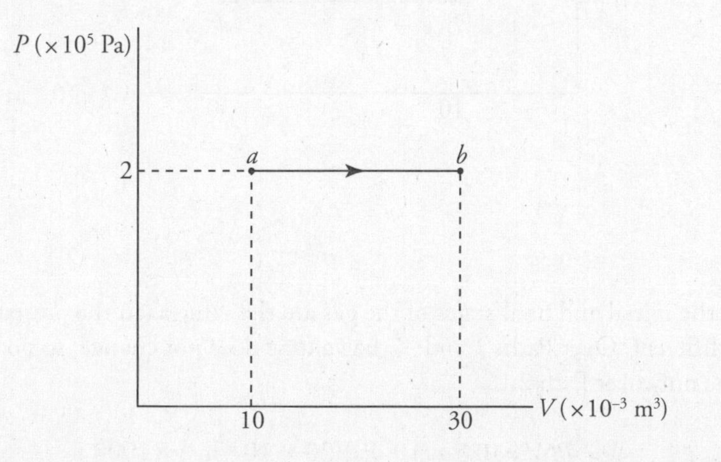

Solution:

a) The Ideal Gas Law tells us that if n and P are constant, then T is proportional to V. Since V increased by a factor of 3, so did the absolute temperature of the gas.
b) Since the pressure remains constant during the process, we can use the equation $W = P\Delta V$. Because $\Delta V = (30 - 10) \times 10^{-3}\ \text{m}^3 = 20 \times 10^{-3}\ \text{m}^3$, we find that

$$W = P\Delta V = (2 \times 10^5\ \text{Pa})(20 \times 10^{-3}\ \text{m}^3) = 4000\ \text{J}$$

The expanding gas did positive work against its surroundings, pushing the piston upward.

c) Since the gas *absorbed* heat, $Q = +10{,}000$ J, so by the First Law of Thermodynamics,

$$\Delta U = Q - W = 10{,}000\ \text{J} - 4000\ \text{J} = 6000\ \text{J}$$

We see that the internal energy increased is consistent with the fact that the temperature increased (part a).

Example 13-7: A 0.5 mol sample of an ideal gas is brought from state a to state b along the path shown in the P-V diagram below.

a) Calculate the work done during the process.
b) Determine the change in the internal energy of the gas.
c) How much heat was added to the gas?

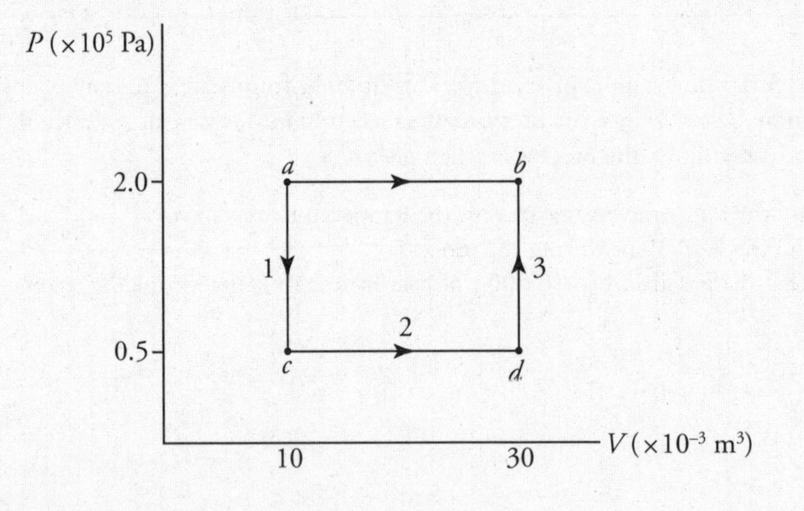

Solution:

a) Notice that the initial and final states of the gas are the same as in the preceding example, but the path is different. Over Paths 1 and 3, the volume does not change, so no work is done. Work is done only over Path 2:

$$W = P\Delta V = (0.5 \times 10^5\ \text{Pa})(20 \times 10^{-3}\ \text{m}^3) = 1000\ \text{J}$$

Once again, the expanding gas does positive work against its surroundings, pushing the piston upward.

b) Because the initial and final states of the gas are the same here as they were in the preceding example, the change in internal energy, ΔU, must be the same. Therefore $\Delta U = 6000$ J.
c) By the First Law of Thermodynamics, $\Delta U = Q - W$, so

$$Q = \Delta U + W = 6000 \text{ J} + 1000 \text{ J} = 7000 \text{ J}$$

Notice that neither Q nor W is the same as its value in the preceding example. Both Q and W are path dependent; change the path, and you will generally change the values of both these variables. But their difference $Q - W$, the change in internal energy (ΔU), depends on the initial state and the final state, not the choice of path.

Example 13-8: An *isochoric* process is one that takes place with no change in volume. What can you say about the change in internal energy of the gas if it undergoes an isochoric change of state?

Solution: An isochoric process appears as a vertical line in a *P-V* diagram. Since no change in volume occurs, $W = 0$. Then by the First Law of Thermodynamics, $\Delta U = Q - W = Q$. Therefore, the change in internal energy is entirely due (and equal to) to the heat transferred. If heat is transferred into the system (positive Q), then ΔU is positive; if heat is transferred out of the system (negative Q), then ΔU is negative.

Example 13-9: A 0.5 mol sample of an ideal gas is brought from state *a* back to state *a* along the path (cycle) shown in the *P-V* diagram below. Find

a) The change in the internal energy of the gas.
b) The work done on the gas during the cycle.
c) The heat added to (or removal from) the gas during the cycle.

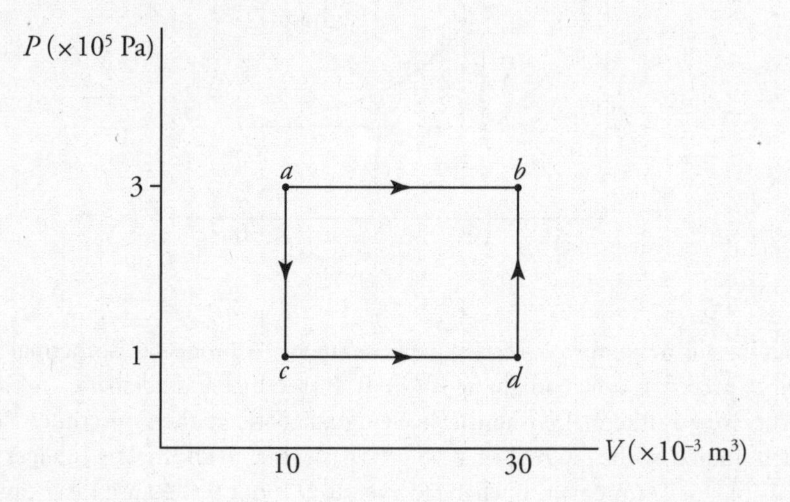

Solution: A process such as this, which begins and ends at the same state, is said to be cyclical.

a) Because the final state is the same as the initial state, the internal energy of the system cannot have changed; therefore, $\Delta U = 0$.

b) The total work involved in the process is equal to the work done from *c* to ***d*** plus the work done from *b* to *a,* because only along these paths does the volume change. Along these portions of the path, we find that

$$W_{cd} = P_{cd}\Delta V_{cd} = 1 \times 10^5 \text{ Pa})(+20 \times 10^{-3} \text{ m}^3) = +2000 \text{ J}$$
$$W_{ba} = P_{ba}\Delta V_{ba} = (3 \times 10^5 \text{ Pa})(-20 \times 10^{-3} \text{ m}^3) = -6000 \text{ J}$$

so the total work done is $W = -4000$ J. The fact that W is negative means that, overall, work was done *on* the gas by the surroundings. Notice that for a cyclical process, the total work done is equal to the area enclosed by the loop, with clockwise travel taken as positive and counterclockwise travel taken as a negative.

c) The First Law of Thermodynamics states that $\Delta U = Q - W$. Since $\Delta U = 0$, it must be true that $Q = W$ (which will always be the case for a cyclical process). Therefore, $Q = -4000$ J (and since Q is negative, heat was *removed* from the sample).

Example 13-10: A 0.5 mol sample of an ideal gas is brought from state ***a*** to state ***d*** along an isotherm, then isobarically to state *c* and isochorically back to state *a,* as shown in the *P-V* diagram below. By definition, the temperature remains constant along an *isotherm*, and a process that takes place with no variation in temperature is said to be *isothermal.* Given that the work done during the isothermal part of the cycle is 3300 J, how much heat is transferred during the isothermal process from ***a*** to ***d***?

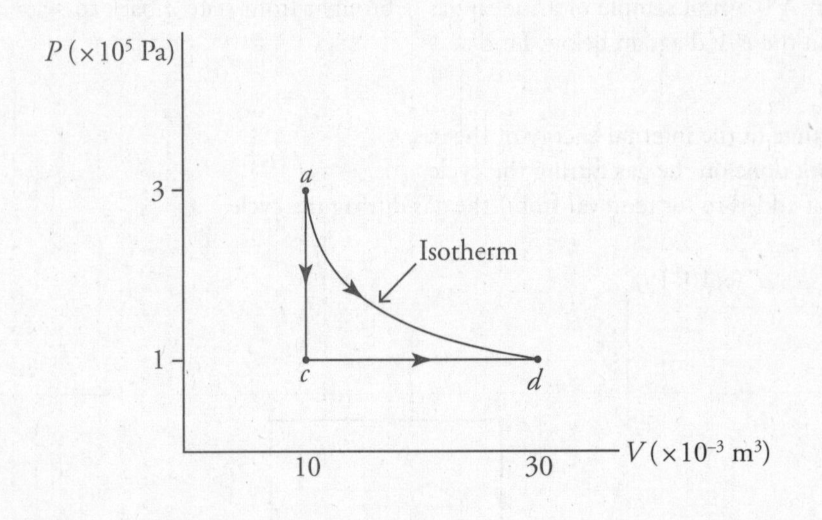

Solution: Be careful not to confuse *isothermal* with *adiabatic*. A process is isothermal if the temperature remains constant; a process is called **adiabatic** if $Q = 0$. Isothermal and adiabatic are two different things. How could a process be isothermal without also being adiabatic at the same time? Remember that the temperature is determined by the internal energy of the gas, which is affected by changes in Q or W or both. Therefore, it's possible for U to remain unchanged even if Q is not 0 (because there can be an equal W to cancel it out). In fact, this is the key to this problem. Since T doesn't change from *a* to *d,* neither can the internal energy, which depends entirely on T. Because $\Delta U = 0$, it must be true that $Q = W$. Since W equals 3300 J, so must Q. The gas absorbs heat from the reservoir and uses all this energy to do positive work as it expands and pushes the piston upward, leaving none to increase its internal energy.

The Second Law of Thermodynamics

The Second Law of Thermodynamics is called one of the grandest laws of physics, because in one of its many equivalent forms, it defines the direction of time. The form of the Second Law that we need sounds much less grandiose and deals with heat engines.

Converting work to heat is easy—slamming on your brakes. Even rubbing your hands together shows that work can be completely converted into heat. What we'll look at is the reverse process: How efficiently can heat be converted into work? A device that uses heat to produce useful work is called a **heat engine**. The internal-combustion engine in your car is an example. In particular, we're interested in engines that take its working substance (a mixture of air and fuel in the case of your car engine) through a cyclic process, so that the cycle can be repeated. The basic components of any cyclic heat engine are simple to describe: Energy in the form of heat comes into the engine from a high-temperature source, some of this energy is converted into useful work, the remainder is ejected as exhaust heat into a low-temperature sink, and the system returns to its original state to run through the cycle again.

Since we're looking at cyclic engines only, the system returns to its original state at the end of each cycle, so ΔU must be 0. Therefore, by the First Law of Thermodynamics, $Q_{net} = W$. That is, the net heat absorbed by the system is equal to the work performed by the system. The heat that is absorbed from the high-temperature source is denoted Q_H (H for *hot*), and the heat that is discharged into the low-temperature reservoir is denoted Q_C (C for *cold*). Because heat *in* is positive and heat *out* is negative, Q_H is positive and Q_C is negative, and the net heat absorbed is $Q_H + Q_C$. Instead of writing Q_{net} in this way, it's customary to write it as $Q_H - |Q_C|$, to show explicitly that Q_{net} is less than Q_H. The **thermal efficiency**, e, of the heat engine is equal to the ratio of what we get out – the work, W – to what we have to put in – the heat is absorbed, Q_H. Therefore, $e = W/Q_H$. Since $W = Q_{net} = Q_H - |Q_C|$, this gives

$$e = \frac{Q_H - |Q_C|}{Q_H} = 1 - \frac{|Q_C|}{Q_H}$$

Notice that unless $Q_C = 0$, the engine's efficiency is always less than 1. One of the forms of the **Second Law of Thermodynamics** states that for any cyclic heat engine, some exhaust heat is always produced. Because $Q_C \neq 0$, no cyclic heat engine can operate at 100% efficiency; it is impossible to completely convert heat into useful work.

Example 13-11: A heat engine draws 1000 J of heat from its high-temperature source and discards 600 J of exhaust heat into its cold-temperature reservoir each cycle. How much work does this engine perform per cycle, and what is its thermal efficiency?

Solution: The work output per cycle is equal to the difference between the heat energy drawn in and the heat energy discarded:

$$W = Q_H - |Q_C| = 1000 \text{ J} - 600 \text{ J} = 400 \text{ J}$$

Therefore, the efficiency of this engine is

$$e = \frac{W}{Q_H} = \frac{400\ \text{J}}{1000\ \text{J}} = 40\%$$

The Carnot Cycle

The Second Law of Thermodynamics tells us that there are no perfect heat engines. But how can we construct, in principle, the best possible heat engine—that is, one with the maximum possible efficiency that doesn't violate the Second Law? Such an engine is called a **Carnot engine**, and the cycle through which its working substance (gas) is carried is called a **Carnot cycle**, a specially-designed series of expansions and compressions. It can be shown that a heat engine utilizing the Carnot cycle has the highest possible efficiency consistent with the Second Law of Thermodynamics. The efficiency of a Carnot engine is given by the equation

$$e_C = \frac{T_H - T_C}{T_H} = 1 = \frac{T_C}{T_H}$$

Notice that the **Carnot efficiency** depends only on the absolute temperatures of the heat source and heat sink. The equation $e_C = 1 - (T_C/T_H)$ gives the maximum theoretical efficiency of any cyclic heat engine. It cannot equal 1 unless $T_C = 0$, that is, unless the temperature of the cold reservoir is absolute zero. But absolute zero can never be reached: the **Third Law of Thermodynamics**.

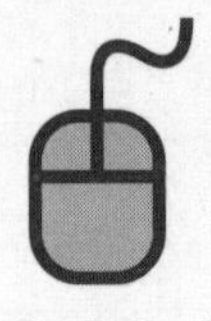

Go Online!

Summary of Formulas

Thermal Expansion: $\Delta L = \alpha L_i$ $\Delta V = \beta V_i \Delta T$

Ideal Gas Law: $PV = nRT$

Kinetic Theory of Gases: $K_{avg} = \frac{3}{2} k_B T$ $v_{rms} = \sqrt{\frac{3RT}{M}}$

Work Done during Isobaric Thermodynamic Process: $W = P\Delta V$

First Law of Thermodynamics: $\Delta U = Q - W$

Efficiency of Cyclic Heat Engine: $e = \frac{Q_H - |Q_C|}{Q_H} = 1 - \frac{|Q_C|}{Q_H}$

Math

Chapter 14
Math Overview

Section Format and Strategy

The Quantitative Reasoning Test (QRT) on the OAT contains 40 questions that you must complete in 45 minutes. The questions are not arranged in any useful order (for example, they are not in order of difficulty). Additionally, most students find that they do not have time to complete the section comfortably and must rush, at least to some extent, to complete the questions in the allotted time.

Two-Pass System

The above facts (time pressure and no order of difficulty) give rise to the first basic section strategy, the **Two-Pass System**. The Two-Pass System means to take two passes through a section. On the first pass, complete questions that you can answer quickly and easily. On the second pass, come back for questions that you know you can answer but are likely to take more time. By doing this, you will make sure that you get to all the questions that you definitely can answer; if you simply do the questions in the order that they are presented, you run the risk of putting too much time into an earlier but harder question (which you might get wrong anyway) and not getting to a question that you could have answered correctly if only you'd known it was there.

Generally, determining whether you know how to do a question quickly takes no more than a few seconds of reading, so skipping questions will not waste time; in fact, it will save you time. If you take the section in two passes, you'll get the easy questions right first, and then you'll have a very good idea how much time you have left for the harder questions. Thus, you will be able to allot your time more effectively.

The Two-Pass System takes some practice, so don't worry if it seems awkward at first. It will improve your score if you use it a few times.

Calculator

One change to the QRT in 2010 was the inclusion of an on-screen calculator that can be called up in the same way that you call up the periodic table in the Survey of the Natural Sciences. The calculator looks like this:

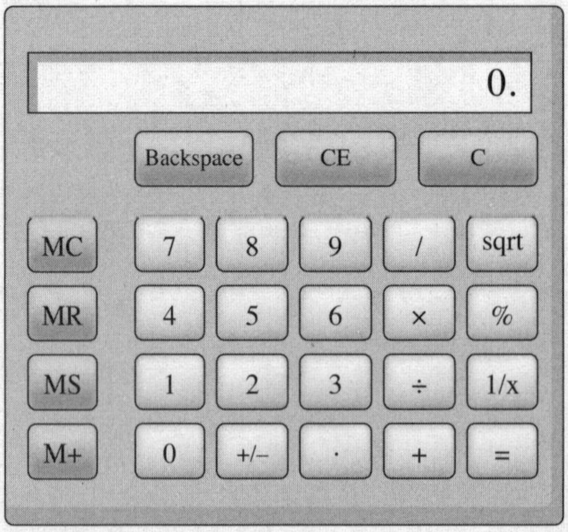

This is a basic four-function (not scientific or graphing) calculator. It can add, subtract, multiply, divide, take a square root, and take a reciprocal. However, it cannot do exponents, roots other than square roots, logs, or trig, and it does not know Order of Operations (it calculates as soon as you press buttons, rather than waiting for you to hit an "Enter" key).

Interestingly, this has not appeared to cause a major change in the test. The questions asked on the current QRT are not very different from the questions asked prior to the addition of the calculator.

Test Content

The questions cover arithmetic, algebra, geometry, and trigonometry. ADA describes the test content as follows:

I. **Mathematics Problems** (30)
   A. **Algebra** (12)
      1. Equations and expressions
      2. Inequalities
      3. Exponential notation and logarithms
      4. Absolute value
      5. Ratios and proportions
      6. Graphical analysis
   B. **Numerical calculations** (5)
      1. Fractions and decimals
      2. Percentages
      3. Approximations
      4. Scientific notation
   C. **Probability and statistics** (3)
   D. **Geometry** (5)
   E. **Trigonometry** (5)

II. **Applied Mathematics (Word) Problems** (10)

Note that this differs in emphasis from the content of the DAT. The OAT does not test Conversions. It also has more Algebra, slightly more Geometry and Trigonometry, and slightly fewer Numerical Calculations and Probability and Statistics. Also, the descriptions of the topics are rather vague. For example, "trigonometry" is tested, but what exactly that means is not specified. Does this just refer to the definitions of sine, cosine, and tangent? Does this also refer to more complex identities and laws? ADA is deliberately vague about this, which has provoked confusion and rumors among test-takers. We have carefully studied the test and determined what it tests regularly. Those topics are covered in the later chapters that cover the content of the test.

It is certainly true, as you might expect from the specifications above, that knowing the content of the test is extremely important in order to do well. Much of the rest of our discussion of the math on the test will focus on content. However, content is not the only aspect of the test that you should be familiar with. While it is certainly impossible to do well on the QRT without knowing certain mathematical facts and formulas, it is also important to make effective use of the knowledge that you already possess. We will discuss some of the most crucial techniques for doing this now.

Plugging In

Many questions on the test ask you to work with variables for everyday quantities. This is highly artificial and potentially confusing. In daily life, you probably don't walk around with d dollars in your pocket or travel f feet in t seconds. You probably have five dollars, or ten dollars, or travel four feet in two seconds, or some actual, constant number. Since these are the numbers that you use every day, you're probably quite familiar with them and make few mistakes with them. On the other hand, you probably do algebra only when you're asked to do algebra problems, which is not nearly as often. No matter how good you are at algebra, it's easier to know whether you've made a mistake when you use regular old numbers than when you use algebraic expressions. But how can you use regular numbers when the test gives you an algebra problem? That's the magic of Plugging In.

Plugging In Your Own Number

Let's say you're given the following problem.

1. If a, b, c, d, and e are nonzero numbers such that a is b percent of c and c percent of the square of d is e, then what percent of e is a, in terms of b and d ?

A. $\frac{100d^2}{b}$

B. $100b$

C. $\frac{d^2}{b}$

D. $\frac{d^2}{100b}$

E. $\frac{100b}{d^2}$

You might (if you weren't a savvy test-taker) panic and guess on this question. It looks pretty horrible, after all. You could set up a whole bunch of equations with a whole bunch of variables, and if you make one little mistake anywhere, the whole problem is shot. However, take heart: You don't need to do any of that to solve this.

The whole point of algebraic formulas is that they relate variables that can have whatever value you could dream up. If the right answer is really right, it should work for *any* values of a, b, c, d, and e that fit the requirements they mention. Thus, you can just make up some values and run through the problem with those. If the answer doesn't work with the values that you chose, eliminate it.

Let's do that here. Since we're taking b percent of c to find a, let's make $b = 10$ and $c = 50$. This is easy enough: 10% of 50 is one-tenth of 50, which just removes the zero from the 50, so it's 5. With these numbers, then, $a = 5$.

The next portion of the problem says that c percent of the square of d is e. Now, c is already 50. Next, let's choose an easy square near these numbers, such as $d = 4$, so the square of d is 16. Thus, the question says that 50 percent of 16 is e. That means $e = 8$.

Now, the question is asking what percent of e is a, which might as well be saying what percent of 8 is 5. This is $\frac{5}{8}$, which you plug into the on-screen calculator to find that it is 62.5%. Thus, the answer to the question should be 62.5, if $a = 5$, $b = 10$, $c = 50$, $d = 4$, and $e = 8$.

At this point, the problem becomes pure calculation: Plug these numbers into answer A and see if you get out 62.5. You don't. Answer A gives $\frac{100 \times 4^2}{10} = 160$. Likewise, B gives 1000, C gives 1.6, D gives 0.016, and E gives 62.5, so E is the right answer.

Okay, now for the bottom line. The point of this question is that on just about any question that asks for an algebraic expression, uses variables or unknown quantities, or uses the phrase "in terms of" (which, frankly, is meaningless here anyway—all of the answers are in terms of the right variables, so feel free to ignore that phrase entirely), you can make up your own numbers instead of working with their variables. The right answer should be right no matter what numbers you're using, so feel free to use the simplest, easiest numbers you can. Using regular numbers (constants) instead of variables is called Plugging In, and in this case, you're **Plugging In Your Own Number** (a number that you made up).

Notice, by the way, that this question is pretty darn hard unless you plug in. If you were to try to solve this with algebra, your first step would be to write down three equations: $a = \frac{b}{100}c$, $\frac{c}{100}d^2 = e$, and $\frac{x}{100}e = a$ (where x is the value you're actually solving for). From there, you would have to solve for x in terms of b and d by eliminating the other variables. This is challenging algebra. The only thing challenging about the plugging in solution is making sure that you use numbers that are easy enough to manipulate that you keep the problem from becoming even more unwieldy than it has to be.

On some other questions, it's not necessarily *hard* (in the sense of being complicated) to get the right answer, even if you don't plug in. However, such questions can be extremely *tricky*, since it's difficult to tell whether $\frac{x^2}{y}$ is okay or wildly wrong, whereas if you know that the answer should be about 20 and you get that the answer is 0.2, you know you've forgotten to multiply by 100 somewhere. The second crucial point is this: Plugging In will make some questions easier to *work*, but its true significance is that it makes most questions easier to *check*. You're less likely to get wrong answers—or more likely to catch wrong answers if you get them—if you plug in.

Plugging In More Than Once

In general, when you make up numbers, it's possible to choose numbers such that more than one answer works. You must check all five answer choices when Plugging In Your Own Number, because you have to make sure that the answer that works is the *only* answer that works. If more than one answer works, try another number. A few tips to avoid having more than one answer work:

- Do plug in numbers that fit the constraints in the question (if it says "even" numbers, use an even number).
- Do plug in numbers that make the math easy. On most problems, this means 2, 3, 5, 10, or 100.
- Don't plug in 0 or 1. These numbers have strange properties and tend to break things.
- Don't plug in numbers that appear in the question.
- Don't plug in the same number for more than one variable.

Bear in mind that these only apply to the first number you plug in. You may need to break several of these rules if you have to plug in again (discussed below).

Let's consider another example.

2. If x is an integer, which of the following must be an odd integer?

   A. $x + 2$
   B. $x - 3$
   C. $2x$
   D. $3x$
   E. $2x - 3$

To solve this, you might plug in. The only constraint on x is that it be an integer (not a fraction or a decimal), so let's try $x = 2$. In that case, A would be 4, which is not odd, so eliminate it. B would be –1, which is odd, so keep it. C would be 4, which is not odd, so eliminate it. D would be 6, which is also not odd, so eliminate it. E would be 1, which is odd, so keep that as well. With $x = 2$, both B and E work. They're not both correct; it's just that while both of them *could* be an odd integer, only one of them *must* be an odd integer, as the question stem says.

So try a different number, and since we're talking about odd and even and tried an even number before, try an odd number. Let's say $x = 3$. In that case, we don't have to check A, C, or D again; we know that they don't *have* to be odd. Just check B and E. B is 0, which is not odd (it's even), so eliminate it. E is 3, which is still odd, so it must be the right answer.

There are two points to this question. First, check all five answers when you're Plugging In Your Own Number! If you had just gone with the first answer that worked, you would've chosen B and gotten the question wrong.

Second, notice (and take seriously) words like "must" or "could." If a question asks what "must" be the case, then it's likely that many of the answers *could* work, given the right values of x, but only one of them *must* work with all values of x. On the other hand, if a question asks what "could" be the case, then it's likely that you need very particular values of x to make anything work at all, and with most values of x that you could choose, none of the answers will be right. You're just looking for an answer that *could ever* be right, which means that there might only be one value of x that ever makes it right, and your job is to find it. There's a pretty good chance you'll have to Plug In more than once on questions that ask what *must* or *could* be true, and there's nothing worse than Plugging In repeatedly but getting that B and E always work. You need to try different, weird numbers in order to differentiate between answers.

What are different, weird numbers? Well, for your second try at Plugging In on the same question, everything that we just said about not choosing numbers that break the question goes completely out the window. In fact, 0, 1, numbers in the question, and the same number for more than one variable are among the first things that you should try if you're working a question on which you have to Plug In a second time. The acronym **ZONE-F** may be useful: try zero, one, negatives, extremes (very large and very small), and fractions, if you're trying to find different numbers to Plug In that don't just give the same results as what you've already done.

Remember, this only applies when you're plugging in a second time on the same question, which you should only do if more than one answer worked on your first try.

Plugging In a Given Value

Sometimes questions will ask what the value of an expression is if a variable equals something (also known as **substitution**). For example, "What is the value of $x + 4$ when $x = 6$?" We substitute 6 for the x in the expression $x + 4$ and get $6 + 4$, which equals 10. This is plugging in, but the test has already given you the value to use. Consider the following examples.

3. Evaluate $2x + 7$ when $x = -3$.

A. -13
B. -1
C. 1
D. 8
E. 13

Once we substitute -3 for x, we get $2(-3) + 7 = -6 + 7 = 1$. Thus, the answer is C.

4. If $f(x) = 3x^2 - x - 1$, what is $f(2)$?

A. 9
B. 11
C. 13
D. 15
E. 33

Once we substitute 2 for x, we get $f(2) = 3(2^2) - 2 - 1 = 12 - 2 - 1 = 9$. Thus, the answer is A.

5. What is the value of $(3x)^2 - x - 1$ when $x = 2$?

A. 9
B. 11
C. 13
D. 15
E. 33

Be sure to notice the difference between this expression and the one in the previous example. Substitute 2 for x and evaluate: $(3 \cdot 2)^2 - 2 - 1 = 6^2 - 2 - 1 = 33$. Thus, the answer is E.

6. Evaluate $2x + 3y$ when $x = 1$ and $y = -4$.

A. –14
B. –10
C. –5
D. 6
E. 14

We substitute 1 for x and –4 for y, then simplify: $2(1) + 3(-4) = 2 + (-12) = -10$. Thus, the answer is B.

Plugging In Points

On a graphical question, sometimes you can choose points from the graph to plug into an equation, and this will help you eliminate answers. Consider the following example.

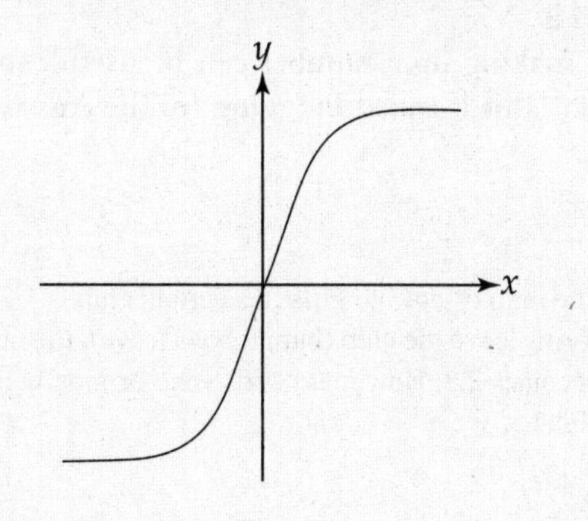

7. Which of the following equations represents the graph above?

A. $y = \dfrac{10x-1}{\sqrt{x^2+1}}$

B. $y = \dfrac{10x^2+2}{\sqrt{x^4+1}}$

C. $y = \dfrac{x^2+1}{\sqrt{x^2+2}}$

D. $y = \dfrac{10x+1}{\sqrt{x^2+1}}$

E. $y = \dfrac{10x}{\sqrt{x^2+1}}$

Okay, these are not normal equations. There is no way you're supposed to know, off the top of your head, the shapes of the graphs of these equations. However, there is one point on the graph that you know: The origin. When $x = 0$ on this graph, $y = 0$. Thus, plug in this point! In A, when $x = 0$, $y = \frac{-1}{1}$, which is definitely not 0. Eliminate A. In B, when $x = 0$, $y = \frac{2}{1}$, which is also not 0, so eliminate B. In C, when $x = 0$, $y = \frac{1}{\sqrt{2}}$, which is still not 0, so eliminate C. In D, when $x = 0$, $y = \frac{1}{1}$, which continues to not be 0, so eliminate D. Presumably it's E, and when you plug in $x = 0$, you get that $y = \frac{0}{1}$, which is indeed equal to 0, so E must be the answer. It's the only option that contains the one identifiable point in the graph.

Whenever you have any question that involves a graph, remember that you can plug in points.

Plugging In The Answers

For much the same reasons as making up a number can be useful, sometimes it can be useful to test answers to see if they are correct. This is called **Plugging In The Answers**. For example, consider the following problem.

8. The ratio of boys to girls in a certain club is 1:2. When 5 girls leave the club (but no boys leave), the ratio becomes 2:3. How many girls were originally in the club?

A. 2
B. 5
C. 10
D. 15
E. 20

Notice that the answer choices are arranged in order. This is typically the case. Thus, start in the middle (for reasons that will become apparent in a moment if they are not already). The question is how many girls were originally in the club, and if there were 10 originally in the club (as answer C indicates), then the 1:2 ratio says that there would have been 5 boys in the club. So there were 5 boys and 10 girls, and then 5 girls left. That means that there are now 5 boys and 5 girls. That's a 1:1 ratio, not a 2:3 ratio, so C is not the right answer.

Next, we can tell that C is too small. A 2:3 ratio means that there are more girls than boys, so because 10 girls gave a 1:1 ratio, there are not enough girls. Go for a larger number. If there were 15 girls originally, then the 1:2 ratio says that there would have been 7.5 boys. This seems pretty unlikely, but if you want to follow it all the way through, then after the 5 girls left, there would have been 7.5 boys and 10 girls; this is 3:4 ratio, which is still not right (but is closer than 1:1 was).

So presumably the answer is E, if C is too small and D is unlikely. If you want to be sure, you can run this one through as well: 20 girls would mean 10 boys originally, and then after the 5 girls leave, there would be 10 boys and 15 girls, which is a 2:3 ratio. So E is in fact the right answer.

In general, regular numbers (not variables) in the answer choices are an indication that you can likely Plug In The Answers. That is, when you see variables in the answer, you can probably Plug In Your Own Number, and when you don't, you can probably Plug In The Answers.

Estimation

Answer choices on the test are often substantially different, so that even if you don't know exactly what the answer is, you can eliminate several that are not even close. A reasonable estimate is sometimes as good as an exact answer, so **estimation** is another major technique. Some questions explicitly ask for an estimate, as in the following.

9. Which of the following is the best approximation of the value of $\left(\sqrt{80}+\dfrac{11}{9}\right)^{3.01}$?

    A. 1
    B. 11
    C. 108
    D. 1075

To solve this, note first that the square root of 81 should be pretty close to the square root of 80, and the square root of 81 is an integer, so use that instead. That is, simplify $\sqrt{80} \approx \sqrt{81} = 9$. Also, 11 divided by 9 is going to be only slightly more than 9 divided by 9, and 9 divided by 9 is an integer, so use that instead. That is, $\dfrac{11}{9} \approx \dfrac{9}{9} = 1$. Thus, $\sqrt{80}+\dfrac{11}{9} \approx 9+1=10$, so the expression inside the parentheses should be pretty close to 10. (Since the square root of 80 is only *barely* less than the square root of 81, whereas 11 divided by 9 is somewhat more than 9 divided by 9, we can even say that it should be a little more than 10, although it makes no difference in this particular problem.) Now, that exponent is not a friendly one, but it is quite close to an integer, so just say that $3.01 \approx 3$, and you're left with $10^3 = 1000$. The only answer that is even close is D.

In general, when approximating, try to make expressions into integers by changing as little as possible. The square root of 80 is almost exactly equal to the square root of 81 (it differs by less than 1%), but it's not nearly as close to the square roots of 64 or 100, so using those to approximate would be substantially less accurate.

In addition to questions that specifically ask for an estimate, some questions that don't mention approximating in any way can still be solved by this method. Consider the following example.

10. If log 2 = 0.301, log 3 = 0.477, and log 5 = 0.699, then what is the value of log 900 ?

    A. 0.010
    B. 0.100
    C. 1.477
    D. 2.186
    E. 2.954

Okay, this looks like a monster. This is some sort of "rules of logarithms" question. Set that aside for a second, and focus on the end of the question, where it actually asks the important part. What is the value of log 900? That's the bit you have to answer.

Now, remember that a log is asking, "What power do I need to raise 10 to in order to get this number?" In other words, log 900 will be whatever the exponent has to be on a 10 to get 900. That is, if log 900 = x, then $10^x = 900$. So what do you have to raise 10 to in order to get 900? Well, to get 1000, you need to raise 10 to the 3. To get 900, you should raise 10 to somewhat less than 3 (not much less, since $10^2 = 100$, which is nowhere near 900). There's only one answer that's even close anyway: E. If you're curious how to get an exact answer (why is it 2.954, not 2.955 or some other number that is somewhat less than 3?), we'll cover that in the section on logs. The point for right now is that an estimate can get you the answer just as well as anything else, and this will frequently be true on the test.

14.1 ARITHMETIC

Properties of Numbers Vocabulary

Integer: Not a fraction or decimal, including positives (1, 2, 3, …), negatives (–1, –2, –3, …), and zero.

Positive: Greater than zero.

Negative: Less than zero.

Sum: Result of addition.

Difference: Result of subtraction.

Product: Result of multiplication.

Quotient: Result of division.

Remainder: Amount left over after division (for example, when 5 is divided by 2, the remainder is 1).

Factor: An integer that divides into another integer with no remainder.

Multiple: The result of multiplying a number by an integer.

Distinct: Different. Not equal.

Prime: Having exactly two distinct factors.

Sum and Product Properties

positive × positive = positive

negative × negative = positive

negative × positive = positive × negative = negative

anything × 0 = 0

even + even = even

odd + odd = even

even + odd = odd + even = odd

even × even = even

odd × odd = odd

even × odd = odd × even = even

Fractions

Multiply fractions as follows:

$$\frac{a}{c} \times \frac{b}{d} = \frac{ab}{cd}$$

Divide fractions by multiplying by the reciprocal:

$$\frac{a}{c} \div \frac{b}{d} = \frac{a}{c} \times \frac{d}{b} = \frac{ad}{cb}$$

Add or subtract fractions as follows:

$$\frac{a}{c} + \frac{b}{d} = \frac{ad + bc}{cd}$$

Decimals

Use the calculator whenever possible for decimals.

To add or subtract decimals, line up the decimal points.

To multiply decimals, multiply without the decimal points and then count the number of spaces after each decimal point.

To divide decimals, convert to integers by multiplying by 10 and then divide normally.

Percents

Percent means "divide by 100." You may also use the following table for problems involving fractions, decimals, and percents.

Verbal statement	Equivalent algebraic expression/symbol
two-thirds of a number	$\frac{2}{3}x$ ("of" means multiply)
two out of three	$\frac{2}{3}$ ("out of" means divide)
five percent	$\frac{5}{100}$ or 0.05
is	=
what	x, y, or any other variable

Exponents and Roots

Exponents indicate repeated multiplication (for example, $2 \times 2 \times 2 = 2^3$).

A root undoes an exponent (for example, $2^2 = 4$, so $\sqrt{4} = 2$).

To multiply with the same base, add the exponents.

To divide with the same base, subtract the exponents.

To raise to another power, multiply the exponents.

Exponents distribute to multiplied or divided terms (e.g. $(4 \times 5)^2 = 4^2 \times 5^2$).

Anything to the zero is 1 (except 0^0, which is undefined).

Negative exponents are reciprocals (e.g. $2^{-3} = \frac{1}{2^3}$).

Fractional exponents are roots (e.g. $2^{\frac{1}{3}} = \sqrt[3]{2}$).

Scientific notation writes numbers in the form $a \times 10^b$, where $1 \leq a < 10$ and b is an integer.

Logarithms

A logarithm expresses an exponent differently, as follows:

If $a^b = c$, then $b = \log_a c$.

A log asks to what power (*b*) you raise the base (*a*) in order to get the number (*c*). Hence, the log (base 10) of 100 is 2, because you raise 10 to the 2 in order to get 100.

$\log(a) + \log(b) = \log(ab)$

$\log(a) - \log(b) = \log\left(\frac{a}{b}\right)$

$\log(a)^b = b\log(a)$

Order of Operations

Perform arithmetic operations in the following order (PEMDAS, or Please Excuse My Dear Aunt Sally):

- Parentheses
- Exponents
- Multiplication and Division
- Addition and Subtraction

Read from left to right to avoid ambiguity.

14.2 ALGEBRA

Solving Equations

To solve an algebraic equation, if you want to do something to one side of an equation, you must do it to the other as well.

The Distributive Law says that $a(b + c) = ab + ac$. In the same way, to multiply sums, multiply each term in one sum by each term in the other sum. For example, FOIL (Firsts Outsides Insides Lasts): $(a + b)(c + d) = ac + ad + bc + bd$.

Factoring is undoing distribution. That is, divide a common factor out of each part of a sum. You can simplify algebraic fractions or solve quadratics by factoring, too.

$(x + y)(x + y) = x^2 + 2xy + y^2$

$(x - y)(x - y) = x^2 - 2xy + y^2$

$(x + y)(x - y) = (x - y)(x + y) = x^2 - y^2$

Solve simultaneous equations (multiple equations with multiple variables, such as x and y) by multiplying equations by integers (if necessary) and then adding or subtracting them from each other.

Absolute Value and Inequalities

The absolute value of a number is its distance from 0 (always a positive number).

An inequality is a relation that does not involve an equals sign. For example, $4 > 3$, $6 \leq 7$, or $1 \neq 2$.

Solve inequalities by the same means as you would solve equations, except that if you multiply or divide by a negative number, you must switch the direction of the inequality.

Functions

A function is a set of instructions for operations to perform on a number, often in function $f(x)$ notation, but sometimes with funny symbols.

Solve functions by plugging the given numbers into the equation defining the function.

14.3 WORD PROBLEMS

Translating a Verbal Statement into an Algebraic Expression

Verbal statement	Equivalent algebraic expression
a number increased by 2	$x + 2$
a number decreased by 5	$x - 5$
5 less than a number	$x - 5$
5 decreased by a number	$5 - x$ [*not* $x - 5$]
3 more than twice a number	$2x + 3$ [*not* $2(x + 3)$, which is "twice the sum of a number and 3"]
7 less than three times a number	$3x - 7$ [*not* $7 - 3x$, which is "7 decreased by three times a number"]
the square of 1 more than a number	$(x + 1)^2$ [*not* $x^2 + 1$, which is "1 more than the square of a number"]
two consecutive integers	n and $n + 1$
two consecutive even integers	n and $n + 2$ (where n is an even integer)
two consecutive odd integers	n and $n + 2$ (where n is an odd integer)
the sum of three consecutive integers	$n + (n + 1) + (n + 2)$
8 more than four times the cube of a number	$4x^3 + 8$

The following are common types of word problems:

- Counting and ratios
- Age
- Money
- Averages and rates
- Mixtures and weighted averages
- Groups

14.4 ADVANCED ARITHMETIC

Statistics, Probability, and Arrangements

Mean: Average.

Median: The middle of a list of numbers arranged in order.

Mode: The most frequently occurring number in a list of numbers.

Standard deviation and variance: Expressions of the spread of data. The higher the standard deviation or variance, the farther the data points are from the mean value.

Normal distribution: A bell curve.

$$\text{Probability} = \frac{\text{Number of outcomes you want}}{\text{Number of outcomes possible}}$$

Factorial: The product of all the integers from the starting down to 1. For example, $3! = 3 \times 2 \times 1$.

The number of ways of doing a series of things is the product of the number of ways of doing each thing.

If you are choosing things from the same set of options without replacement, the number of ways of choosing decreases by one with each decision.

If order doesn't matter, you must divide by the factorial of the number of choices you had.

14.5 PLANE GEOMETRY

Vocabulary

Acute angle: Less than 90°.

Right angle: Equal to 90°.

Obtuse angle: Greater than 90°.

Straight angle: Equal to 180°.

Complementary: Angles that add up to 90°.

Supplementary: Angles that add up to 180°.

When two lines cross (and are not perpendicular), they create two kinds of angles: big angles and small angles. All the big angles are equal, all the small angles are equal, and any big angles plus any small angles equals 180°. The same applies when parallel lines are added.

Polygons

Polygon: A closed figure with straight sides.

The sum of the interior angles of an n-sided polygon is $(n + 2)180$.

Perimeter: The sum of the lengths of the sides.

Area: The size of the region enclosed by the sides.

Congruent: Same size and same shape. The angles of one polygon are equal to the angles of the congruent polygon, and the sides of one are equal to the sides of the other as well.

Similar: Same shape, but not necessarily the same size. The angles of one polygon are equal to the angles of the similar polygon, and their sides are proportional.

Triangles

Triangle: A 3-sided polygon.

The sum of the interior angles is 180°.

$$A = \frac{1}{2}bh$$

Equilateral: Three equal sides and three equal angles.

Isosceles: Two equal sides and two equal angles.

Scalene: No equal sides and no equal angles.

Obtuse triangle: A triangle containing an obtuse angle.

Right triangle: A triangle containing a right angle.

Acute triangle: A training containing only acute angles.

Pythagorean Theorem: $a^2 + b^2 = c^2$ in a right triangle, where c is the length of the longest side (the hypotenuse) and a and b are the lengths of the shorter sides (the legs).

Quadrilaterals

Quadrilateral: A 4-sided polygon.

The sum of the interior angles is 360°.

Parallelogram: Opposite sides are parallel and equal. The perimeter is $2b + 2c$, if b and c are the side lengths, and the area is bh, if b is the base and h is the height.

Rectangle: All angles are 90°, and opposite sides are equal. The perimeter is $2b + 2h$, and the area is bh, if b and h are the side lengths.

Square: All angles are 90°, and all sides are equal. The perimeter is $4b$ and the area is b^2, if the side length is b.

Circles

Circle: The set of points in a plane that are a fixed distance from a center point.

Radius: The distance from the center to the outer rim of the circle.

Diameter: Twice the radius. A line segment with endpoints on the circle and passing through the center.

Tangent: A line that touches a circle at a single point. It is perpendicular to the radius at that point.

$A = \pi r^2$

Circumference: Like perimeter, the distance around the outside of the circle, given by $C = 2\pi r$.

Arc: A portion of the circumference. Proportional to the central angle defining the arc and also to the sector bounded by the arc.

Semicircle: Half a circle.

Solve geometric word problems by drawing diagrams of the situations they describe.

14.6 SOLID AND COORDINATE GEOMETRY

Solid Geometry

Volume is the amount of space enclosed in a 3D shape.

Surface area is the sum of the areas of its faces.

Box (rectangular prism): $V = l \times w \times h$ and $SA = 2lw + 2lh + 2wh$

Cube: $V = l^3$ and $SA = 6l^2$

Any prism: $V = Bh$, where B is the area of the base

Any cone or pyramid: $V = \frac{1}{3}Bh$

Coordinate Geometry

Find the distance between two points in the coordinate plane by making a right triangle. The general formula is $d = \sqrt{(x_2 - x_1)^2 + (y_2 - y_1)^2}$.

The slope m of a line passing through (x_1,y_1) and (x_2,y_2) is $m = \frac{y_2 - y_1}{x_2 - x_1}$.

The equation of a line is $y = mx + b$.

Inequalities are represented with shading and sometimes dashed lines.

14.7 TRIGONOMETRY

SOHCAHTOA

$$\sin\theta = \frac{\text{opposite}}{\text{hypotenuse}} \qquad \cos\theta = \frac{\text{adjacent}}{\text{hypotenuse}} \qquad \tan\theta = \frac{\text{opposite}}{\text{adjacent}}$$

Reciprocal Trigonometry Functions

$$\csc\theta = \frac{1}{\sin\theta} = \frac{\text{hypotenuse}}{\text{opposite}} \qquad \sec\theta = \frac{1}{\cos\theta} = \frac{\text{hypotenuse}}{\text{adjacent}} \qquad \cot\theta = \frac{1}{\tan\theta} = \frac{\text{adjacent}}{\text{opposite}}$$

θ	**sin** θ	**cos** θ
0°	$\frac{\sqrt{0}}{2} = 0$	$\frac{\sqrt{4}}{2} = 1$
30°	$\frac{\sqrt{1}}{2} = \frac{1}{2}$	$\frac{\sqrt{3}}{2}$
45°	$\frac{\sqrt{2}}{2}$	$\frac{\sqrt{2}}{2}$
60°	$\frac{\sqrt{3}}{2}$	$\frac{\sqrt{1}}{2} = \frac{1}{2}$
90°	$\frac{\sqrt{4}}{2} = 1$	$\frac{\sqrt{0}}{2} = 0$

θ	**tan** θ	**csc** θ	**sec** θ	**cot** θ
0°	0	undefined	1	undefined
30°	$\frac{\sqrt{3}}{3}$	2	$\frac{2\sqrt{3}}{3}$	$\sqrt{3}$
45°	1	$\sqrt{2}$	$\sqrt{2}$	1
60°	$\sqrt{3}$	$\frac{2\sqrt{3}}{3}$	2	$\frac{\sqrt{3}}{3}$
90°	undefined	1	undefined	0

$A = \frac{1}{2}ab\sin\theta$ in a triangle with sides of a and b and θ the angle between them.

Inverse trig functions undo trig functions. For example, if $\sin\theta = a$, then $\theta = \sin^{-1}a$.

π radians = 180°

Use the unit circle to find values of trig functions of angles greater than 90°.

$\sin^2\theta + \cos^2\theta = 1$

If given other identities in the text of a problem, use those identities, even if they are unfamiliar.

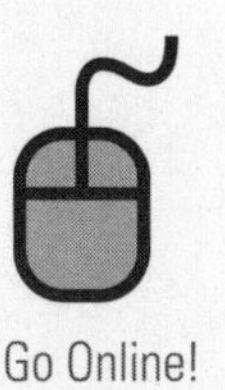

Go Online!

- For a reaction at equilibrium under standard state conditions, $\Delta G° = -RTlnK_{eq}$.
- For a reaction under nonequilibrium conditions, ΔG can be calculated using $\Delta G = \Delta G° + RTlnQ$.

XI. **Electrochemistry**
   A. **Oxidation-Reduction Reactions**
   B. **Galvanic Cells**
   C. **Standard Reduction Potentials**
   D. **Electrolytic Cells**
   E. **Faraday's Law of Electrolysis**
   F. **Nonstandard Conditions and Concentration Cells**

Summary of Key Concepts:

- Oxidation is electron loss; reduction is electron gain (remember "OIL RIG").
- A species that is oxidized is a reducing agent, and a species that is reduced is an oxidizing agent.
- In all electrochemical cells, oxidation occurs at the anode and reduction occurs at the cathode.
- Electrons always flow from the anode to the cathode.
- Salt bridge anions always migrate toward the anode, and cations always migrate toward the cathode.
- The free energy of an electrochemical cell can be calculated from its potential based on $\Delta G = -nFE$.
- A galvanic cell spontaneously generates electrical power ($-\Delta G$, $+E$).
- An electrolytic cell consists of nonspontaneous reactions and requires an external electrical power source ($+\Delta G$, $-E$).
- In a galvanic cell, electrons spontaneously flow from the negative (–) terminal to the positive (+) terminal. Therefore, it follows that in a galvanic cell the anode is negatively charged (–) and the cathode is positively charged (+).
- In an electrolytic cell, electrons are forced from the positive (+) terminal to the negative (–) terminal, and therefore the anode is positively charged (+) and the cathode is negatively charged (–).
- Standard reduction and potentials are intrinsic values and therefore should not be multiplied by molar coefficients in balanced half reactions.
- For a given reduction potential, the reverse reaction, or oxidation potential, has the same magnitude of E but the opposite sign.
- Faraday's law of electrolysis states that the amount of chemical change is proportional to the amount of electricity that flows through the cell.
- Under nonstandard conditions, the potential of an electrochemical cell can be calculated using the Nernst equation: $E = E° - (RT\ nF)\mathrm{In}Q$.

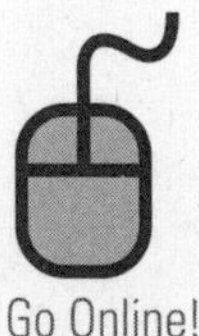

Go Online!

Organic Chemistry

18.1 ORGANIC CHEMISTRY OVERVIEW

The material in the OAT Organic Chemistry section is not designed to be a comprehensive review, but rather is a set of outlines to help you guide your studying. Comprehensive Organic Chemistry review for the OAT can be found in *Cracking the DAT.*

I. **Organic Chemistry Basics**
   A. **Basic Nomenclature and Functional Groups**
      1. Common Functional Groups
      2. Line Structures
      3. Nomenclature of Alkanes
      4. Nomenclature of Haloalkanes
      5. Nomenclature of Alcohols

Summary of Key Concepts:

- Hydrocarbons are named according to the longest continuous chain of carbon atoms.
- A number of common functional groups are common to organic structures, and nomenclature is modified to reflect the number and position of functional groups.
- Line structures involve connection of non-hydrogen atoms and labeling of heteroatoms with the number of lines reflecting the number of bonds between atoms.
- Haloalkanes are named according to the position of the halogen substituent and are described according to a prefix for each atom (e.g. fluoro-).
- Alcohols are named by position and the suffix "-ol" is added to the end of the name of compound to reflect the hydroxyl group.

II. **Structure and Bonding**
  A. **Bonding and Hybridization**
    1. Hybridization
    2. Sigma (σ) Bonds
    3. Pi (π) Bonds
  B. **Structure**
    1. Degrees of Unsaturation
    2. Bond Length and Bond Dissociation Energy
    3. Constitutional Isomers
    4. Conformational Isomers
    5. Stereoisomers and Chirality
    6. Enantiomers
    7. Diastereomers
    8. Optical Activity
    9. Meso Compounds
    10. Geometric Isomers
  C. **Physical Properties of Hydrocarbons**
    1. Melting and Boiling Points
    2. Solubility
    3. Carbocations, Alkyl Radicals, and Carbanions
    4. Inductive Effects
    5. Resonance Stabilization
    6. Acidity
    7. Ring Strain

Summary of Key Concepts:

- Sigma (σ) bonds generally form through the end-on-end overlap of hybrid orbitals; pi (π) bonds form through the side-to-side overlap of unhybridized *p* orbitals.
- Saturated compounds have the general formula C_nH_{2n+2}; unsaturated molecules contain rings or π bonds.
- Compounds with the same molecular formula are known as *isomers*; structural, or constitutional isomers differ by the connectivity of atoms in the molecule.
- Conformational isomers differ by rotation around an σ bond.
- Stereoisomers have the same atom connectivity, but different spatial orientation of atoms.
- Chiral molecules have chiral centers (carbon with four different substituents), are not superimposable on their mirror image, and rotate plane-polarized light.
- Enantiomers are non-superimposable mirror images and have opposite absolute configuration at all chiral centers.
- Enantiomers rotate plane-polarized light an equal magnitude, but in opposite direction, therefore a 50:50 mixture of enantiomers, or a racemic mixture, is not optically active.
- Diastereomers are stereoisomers that are not mirror images; they differ in absolute configuration for at least one, but not all carbons.

- Epimers are diastereomers that differ in absolute configuration at only one stereocenter.
- Geometric isomers are diastereomers that are *cis*/*trans* (or *Z*/*E*) pairs on a ring or double bond. When highest priority groups are on the same side of a ring or bond the molecule is *cis* (or *Z*); when they're on opposite sides, the compound is *trans* (or *E*).
- Meso compounds are achiral molecules with chiral centers and an internal mirror plane.
- As the substitution of carbocations and radicals increases, so does their stability due to the inductive effect; carbanions are more stable when they are less substituted.
- Resonance stabilization results from the ability of π electrons or charge to move and delocalize through a system of conjugated π bonds or unhybridized *p* orbitals.

III. **Substitution and Elimination Reactions**
   A. **Free Radical Halogenation**
      1. Initiation
      2. Propagation
      3. Termination
      4. Inhibition of Free Radical Halogenation
      5. Stereochemistry
      6. Stability of Radicals
      7. Selectivity
   B. **Nucleophilic Substitutions**
      1. Nucleophiles and Electrophiles
      2. S_N2 Reactions
      3. S_N1 Reactions
      4. Substitution Reactions of Ethers and Amines
   C. **Elimination Reactions**
      1. E1 Reactions
      2. E2 Reactions
   D. **Properties of Alcohols**
      1. Hydrogen Bonding
      2. Acidity
   E. **Formation of Alkyl Halides**
      1. Reactions of Alcohols with Phosphorus Halides
      2. Reactions of Alcohols with Thionyl Chloride

Summary of Key Concepts:

- Radical brominations are regioselective for tertiary bromides, while chlorinations yield mixtures of substitution products.
- All free radical halogenations are non-stereoselective, giving racemic mixtures of products when one new stereocenter is formed.
- Radical selectivity = product distribution/# of identical hydrogens.
- Nucleophiles are Lewis bases and are electron rich, while electrophiles are Lewis acids and are electron deficient.

- Nucleophiles are stronger when negatively charged, less electronegative, or larger in size.
- Leaving groups are more likely to leave as their stability in solution increases (uncharged and/or larger groups are usually better LGs).
- More substituted substrates and protic solvents favor S_N1 over S_N2.
- Carbocation intermediates formed in either S_N1 or E1 reactions will rearrange if possible to form a more stable carbocation.
- Second order reactions (S_N2 or E2) require specific spatial orientations of the reacting species (S_N2 = backside attack of Nuc-; E2 = antiperiplanar conformation of H and LG).
- First order reactions (S_N1 or E1) do not depend on the concentration of the Nuc- or base.
- Eliminations break two σ bonds and form one π bond.
- Non-nucleophilic bases and heat favor eliminations over substitutions, and strong bases favor E2 over E1.
- Zaitsev's rule favors the formation of the more substituted bond in elimination reactions (E2 reactions must use small bases), and trans double bonds are favored over cis.

IV. **Electrophilic Addition Reactions**
   A. **Markovnikov Additions**
      1. Electrophilic Additions and the Pi bond
      2. H-X Addition Across a Bond
      3. Acid-catalyzed Hydration of Alkenes
      4. Oxymercuration-demercuration Reactions
   B. **Anti-markovnikov Additions**
      1. Hydroboration
      2. HBr Addition in the Presence of Peroxides
   C. **Other Electrophilic Additions**
      1. Addition of Halogens to a π Bond
      2. Epoxide Formation and Hydrolysis
      3. Oxidation of π Bonds with Dilute $KMnO_4$
      4. Hydrogenation of Alkenes and Alkynes
      5. Ozonolysis
   D. **Aromatic Compounds**
      1. Hückel Numbers and Aromaticity
      2. Electrophilic Aromatic Substitution

Summary of Key Concepts:

- The loosely held electrons in C=C π bonds can act as nucleophiles in addition reactions, which replace one π bond with two σ bonds.
- When p electrons attack electrophiles, the resulting carbocation will be on the more substituted carbon and yield the Markovnikov (more substituted) product.
- Addition reactions that put the new, non-hydrogen group on the less substituted carbon are termed anti-Markovnikov additions.

- Anti-addition puts two new substituents on opposite sides of the planar double bond, while syn-addition puts two new substituents on the same side of the planar double bond.
- Addition reactions are usually not stereospecific since the alkene is planar. Electrophiles will add with equal frequency to both faces of the bond, giving mixtures of enantiomers.
- Double bonds are split by ozonolysis, yielding two carbonyl-bearing compounds.
- Alkenes and alkynes can be hydrogenated by use of H_2 and metal catalysts.
- Aromatic compounds are cyclic, planar, conjugated (all sp^2 hybridized atoms), have $4^{n+2\pi}$ electrons, and are exceptionally stable.
- Under the influence of very strong electrophiles, aromatic electrons can be nucleophilic, resulting in aromatic substitution.
- Substituents that add electron density to a benzene ring are activating for substitution chemistry, and favor reaction at *ortho* and *para* positions.
- Substituents that withdraw electron density from benzene are ring deactivating, and all but the halogens favor substitution at *meta* positions.

V. **Nucleophilic Addition and Cycloaddition Reactions**
   A. **Aldehydes and Ketones**
      1. Addition of Oxidizing Agent to Primary and Secondary Alcohols
      2. Acidity and Enolization
      3. Keto-enol Tautomerism
   B. **Nucleophilic Addition Reactions**
      1. Addition of Reducing Agent to Ketones and Aldehydes
      2. Organometallic Reagents
      3. Wittig Reaction
      4. Acetals and Hemiacetals
      5. Imine Formation
      6. Aldol Condensation
      7. Conjugate Addition to α,β-Unsaturated Carbonyl Compounds
   C. **Carboxylic Acids**
      1. Acidity and Hydrogen Bonding
      2. Inductive Effects on Carboxylic Acid Acidity
      3. Decarboxylation Reactions of β-Keto Acids
      4. Carboxylic Acid Derivatives
      5. Esterification Reactions
   D. **Cycloaddition Reactions**

Summary of Key Concepts:

- The C=O bond is very polarized due to the high electronegativity of oxygen, resulting in the carbon of the carbonyl group being electrophilic.
- Protons α to a carbonyl are acidic and can be removed by a strong base to yield a nucleophilic carbanion, or enolate.

- Keto-enol tautomerism is the rapid equilibration of the more stable keto form of a carbonyl and the less stable enol form where the a-proton shifts to the carbonyl oxygen.
- Nucleophilic additions involve the attack of a nucleophile on the carbon of an aldehyde or ketone; these reactions break one π bond to form two σ bonds.
- Hydride reduction, a type of nucleophilic addition, can convert ketones or aldehydes into alcohols; alcohols can be converted back to carbonyl compounds using oxidizing agents.
- An aldol condensation is a C—C bond forming reaction where the carbonyl carbon of one molecule is the electrophile, while the a-carbon of another carbonyl is the nucleophile.
- α,β-Unsaturated carbonyl compounds are electrophilic at the β-carbon and undergo Michael, or conjugate addition reactions.
- Acidity of carboxylic acids results from the resonance stability of the carboxylate anion.
- Electron withdrawing groups increase the acidity of carboxylic acids by stabilizing the negative charge of the carboxylate anion via the inductive effect.
- The reactivity of carboxylic acid derivatives decreases as follows: acid halide > acid anhydride > ester > amide
- Nucleophilic addition to the carbonyl carbon in a carboxylic acid derivative is usually followed by elimination due to the presence of a good electronegative leaving group.

VI. **Laboratory Techniques and Spectroscopy**

A. **Separations**
1. Extractions
2. Crystallization and Precipitation
3. Thin-layer (TLC) and Flash Chromatography
4. Gas Chromatography
5. Distillations

B. **Spectroscopy**
1. Infrared (IR) Spectroscopy
2. UV/Vis Spectroscopy
3. Proton (^{1}H) Nuclear Magnetic Resonance (NMR) Spectroscopy
4. Carbon (^{13}C) NMR

Summary of Key Concepts:

- Organic compounds are separated via extraction based on their differing solubility in polar (aqueous) or nonpolar (organic) solvents.
- Organic acids (COOHs and PhOHs) and bases (amines) can undergo acid-base reactions to generate ions, which preferentially dissolve in the aqueous layer during an extraction.
- Thin layer chromatography (TLC) separates molecules based on polarity; the more polar compound travels the least distance up the plate and has the lowest R_f value.
- Distillation and gas chromatography separate compounds based on boiling point.

- IR spectroscopy identifies the functional groups present in molecules.
- The most common IR resonances tested on the DAT are the C=O bond (~1700 cm^{-1}), the C=C bond (~1650 cm^{-1}) and the O–H bond (~3600 cm^{-1}).
- The number of resonances in a ^{1}H NMR spectrum indicates the number of non-equivalent hydrogens present in a molecule.
- The number of Hs each signal represents is determined by the integration of the peak.
- Protons that are more deshielded (near electronegative groups) will be further downfield (at higher ppm), and protons that are more shielded (near electron donating groups) will be more upfield (at lower ppm).
- Splitting in a ^{1}H NMR spectrum occurs when one H has non-equivalent protons located on an adjacent atom (signal will be split into $n + 1$ lines; n = # of nonequivalent adjacent hydrogens).
- The number of resonances in a ^{13}C NMR spectrum indicates the number of non-equivalent carbons present in a molecule.

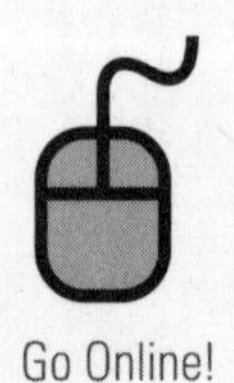

Go Online!

Practice

PHYSICS DRILL

Mechanics III

1. An automobile with a certain shape experiences a drag force due to air resistance that is, in Newtons, equal to one-third the square of the car's speed, in meters per second. How much power would the engine have to supply to the wheels to balance this drag force when the car is moving at a constant speed of 30 m/s ?

(A) 10 W
(B) 300 W
(C) 9 kW
(D) 27 kW

2. A young child is sliding down a hill at an incline of 30 degrees on a sled with total combined mass of 10 kg. If the coefficient of friction between the hill and the sled is 0.3 m and the length of the hill is 50 m, how much work has been done by gravity when the child reaches the bottom of the hill?

(A) 1000 J
(B) 2500 J
(C) 3535 J
(D) 4330 J

3. An experiment is conducted where a cue ball (mass 0.25 kg) moves at 10 m/s towards an adjacent numbered ball (mass 0.25 kg) at rest. In Trial 1, the collision is elastic. In Trial 2, the collision is perfectly inelastic. What is the speed of the cue ball immediately after the collision in Trial 1 and Trial 2 respectively?

(A) 0 m/s and 5 m/s
(B) 0 m/s and 10 m/s
(C) 5 m/s and 0 m/s
(D) 5 m/s and 5 m/s

4. A 200 kg roller coaster starts from rest 50 m above the ground. It falls toward the ground without any friction, then once it reaches ground level, the brakes are applied over 30 m in order to bring the coaster to a complete stop. How much work is done by the brakes?

(A) 10×10^4 J
(B) 10×10^5 J
(C) -10×10^4 J
(D) -10×10^5 J

5. A 1000 kg car traveling at 60 km/h hits a stationary truck weighing 20,000 N. If the truck has a velocity of 1 m/s after the crash, what is the velocity of the car after the crash?

(A) 14.5 m/s in the same direction it was initially traveling
(B) 14.5 m/s in the opposite direction it was initially traveling
(C) 19 m/s in the same direction it was initially traveling
(D) 19 m/s in the opposite direction it was initially traveling

6. A 7 kg ball is dropped from 20 m. If the speed just before it hits the ground is 18 m/s, what is the work done by air resistance?

(A) 266 J
(B) 13 J
(C) –13 J
(D) –266 J

Fluids and Elasticity of Solids

7. A person is leaning on his elbow on a table. If the amount of force the table must exert to keep the person upright is *F*, the area of contact between the person and the table is *A*, and the angle that the person's arm makes with the table's surface is θ, how much pressure is exerted by the person on the table?

(A) $\frac{F}{A}$

(B) $\frac{F\sin\theta}{A}$

(C) $\frac{F\cos\theta}{A}$

(D) Since the force exerted by the person on the table is not given, the pressure exerted by the person on the table cannot be determined.

8. If the density of a person is approximately the density of water, and the density of air is approximately 1 kg/m^3, how many times greater is the weight of the person than the buoyant force from the air on the person?

   (A) 10
   (B) 100
   (C) 1000
   (D) 10000

9. Will an object with more mass but the same volume as another object sink faster in a non-viscous fluid?

   (A) No, because acceleration due to gravity is independent of the mass of the object being accelerated.
   (B) No, because the buoyant force is greater on an object with more mass.
   (C) Yes, because it weighs more, and the weight itself induces greater acceleration for the heavier object than for the lighter.
   (D) Yes, because the buoyant force impedes the downward acceleration of a greater mass less than it does a lesser mass.

10. A particular eucalyptus tree has a density of 667 kg/m^3 and a mass of 6000 kg. What volume of the tree would float above the surface of water?

   (A) 3 m^3
   (B) 5 m^3
   (C) 6 m^3
   (D) 9 m^3

Electricity and Magnetism

11. Determine the total power dissipated through the circuit shown below in terms of V, R_1, R_2, and R_3.

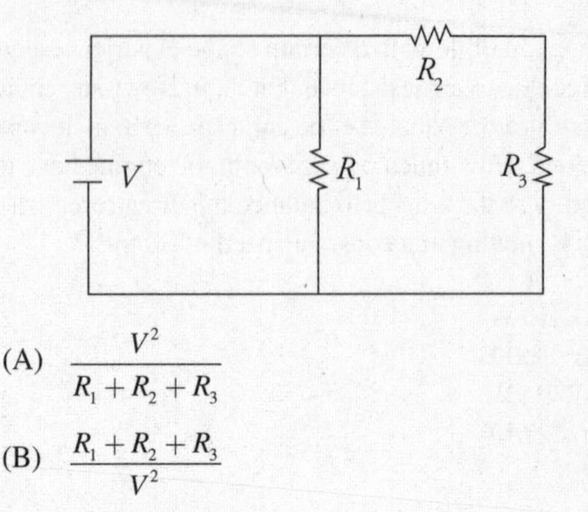

   (A) $\frac{V^2}{R_1 + R_2 + R_3}$
   (B) $\frac{R_1 + R_2 + R_3}{V^2}$
   (C) $\frac{R_1(R_2 + R_3)}{V^2(R_1 + R_2 + R_3)}$
   (D) $\frac{V^2(R_1 + R_2 + R_3)}{R_1(R_2 + R_3)}$

12. Lightning is an atmospheric discharge of electricity that can propagate at speeds of up to 60,000 m/s and can reach temperatures of up to 30,000 C. A single lightning strike lasts for approximately 250 ms and can transfer up to 500 MJ of energy across a potential difference of 2×10^7 volts. Estimate the total amount of charge transferred and average current of a single lightning strike.

   (A) 6.25×10^{-4} coulombs, 8×10^7 amps
   (B) 6.25×10^{-4} coulombs, 2.5×10^{-3} amps
   (C) 25 coulombs, 100 amps
   (D) 25 coulombs, 8×10^7 amps

13. Which of the following statements will increase the resistance of a closed circuit system?

   I. Replacing the wire with one that has a smaller cross sectional area
   II. Adding a voltmeter to the wire
   III. Doubling the wire length in the closed circuit

   (A) III only
   (B) I and III only
   (C) II and III only
   (D) I, II and III

14. If the resistance of a wire in a household appliance becomes 4 times its original value, which of the following statements is/are correct?

    I. The voltage of the wire becomes quadrupled.
    II. The current through the wire becomes 1/4th the original value.
    III. The power consumed by the appliance becomes quadrupled.

    (A) I only
    (B) II only
    (C) I and III only
    (D) II and III only

Modern Physics

15. A metal whose work function is 6.0 eV is struck with light of frequency 7.2×10^{15} Hz. What is the maximum kinetic energy of photoelectrons ejected from the metal's surface?

    (A) 7 eV
    (B) 13 eV
    (C) 19 eV
    (D) 24 eV
    (E) No photoelectrons will be produced.

16. An atom with one electron has an ionization energy of 25 eV. How much energy will be released when the electron makes the transition from an excited energy level, where $E = -16$ eV, to the ground state?

    (A) 9 eV
    (B) 11 eV
    (C) 16 eV
    (D) 25 eV
    (E) 41 eV

17. The single electron in an atom has an energy of –40 eV when it's in the ground state, and the first excited state for the electron is at –10 eV. What will happen to this electron if the atom is struck by a stream of photons, each of energy 15 eV ?

    (A) The electron will absorb the energy of one photon and become excited halfway to the first excited state, then quickly return to the ground state, without emitting a photon.
    (B) The electron will absorb the energy of one photon and become excited halfway to the first excited state, then quickly return to the ground state, emitting a 15 eV photon in the process.
    (C) The electron will absorb the energy of one photon and become excited halfway to the first excited state, then quickly absorb the energy of another photon to reach the first excited state.
    (D) The electron will absorb two photons and be excited to the first excited state.
    (E) Nothing will happen.

18. What is the de Broglie wavelength of a proton whose linear momentum has a magnitude of 3.3×10^{-23} kg•m/s ?

    (A) 0.0002 nm
    (B) 0.002 nm
    (C) 0.02 nm
    (D) 0.2 nm
    (E) 2 nm

19. Compared to the parent nucleus, the daughter of a β^- decay has

    (A) the same mass number but a greater atomic number.
    (B) the same mass number but a smaller atomic number.
    (C) a smaller mass number but the same atomic number.
    (D) a greater mass number but the same atomic number.
    (E) None of the above

20. The reaction ${}^{218}_{85}\text{At} \rightarrow {}^{214}_{83}\text{Bi}$ is an example of what type of radioactive decay?

    (A) alpha
    (B) β^-
    (C) β^+
    (D) electron capture
    (E) gamma

21. Tungsten-176 has a half-life of 2.5 hours. After how many hours will the disintegration rate of a tungsten-176 sample drop to $\frac{1}{10}$ its initial value?

(A) 5
(B) 8.3
(C) 10
(D) 12.5
(E) 25

22. What's the missing particle in the following nuclear reaction?

$^{2}_{1}H + ^{63}_{29}Cu \rightarrow ^{64}_{30}Zn + (?)$

(A) Proton
(B) Neutron
(C) Electron
(D) Positron
(E) Deuteron

23. What's the missing particle in the following nuclear reaction?

$^{196}_{78}Pt + ^{1}_{0}n \rightarrow ^{197}_{78}Pt + (?)$

(A) Proton
(B) Neutron
(C) Electron
(D) Positron
(E) Gamma

24. The impossibility of making simultaneous, arbitrarily precise measurements of the momentum and the position of an electron is accounted for in

(A) thermodynamics.
(B) quantum mechanics.
(C) classical electrodynamics.
(D) special relativity.
(E) general relativity.

Vectors

25. Two vectors are added together and the resulting vector has a magnitude of 10 units. Which of the following must be true about the two vectors?

(A) The sum of their magnitudes is less than 10 units.
(B) The sum of their magnitudes is equal to 10 units.
(C) The sum of their magnitudes is greater than 10 units, but the difference of their magnitudes is less than 10 units.
(D) The sum of their magnitudes is greater than10 units, but the difference of their magnitudes is equal to 10 units.
(E) None of the above can be determined about them unless their relative directions are known.

26. Each of the following contains at least one scalar quantity EXCEPT one. Which one is the EXCEPTION?

(A) Velocity, mass, power
(B) Momentum, displacement, speed
(C) Electric field, torque, impulse
(D) Acceleration, force, kinetic energy

27. A vector has a length of 4 and makes a 30° angle with the *x*-axis. Which of the following best expresses the *x*-component of the vector?

(A) 0.86
(B) 1
(C) 1.7
(D) 2
(E) 3.4

28. A vector and its equivalent scalar quantity have:

(A) The same magnitude and direction
(B) The same magnitude and units
(C) The same direction only
(D) The same magnitude only
(E) The same units only

29. A vector has a magnitude of 5, and another vector has a magnitude of 2. The sum of the two vectors has a magnitude of 3. Which of the following must be true of the two vectors?

(A) They are parallel.
(B) They are antiparallel.
(C) They are perpendicular.
(D) They form an acute angle when put tip-to-tail.
(E) They form an obtuse angle when put tip-to-tail.

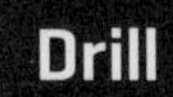

Thermodynamics

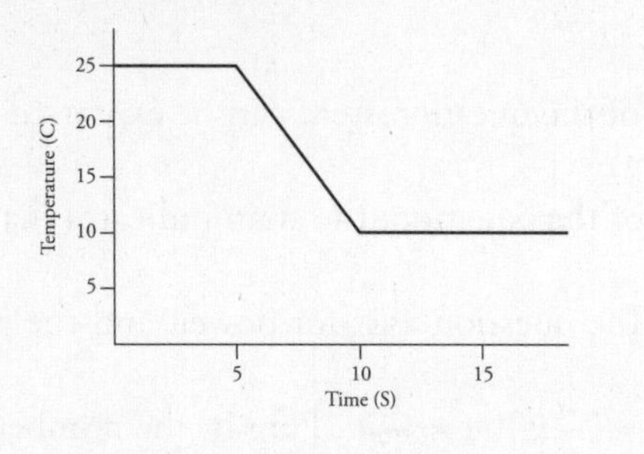

30. When a certain copper object is heated to 10 degrees Celsius, it gains 3,850 joules of energy. The graph above shows the temperature of the copper object as a function of time. How much heat was lost in the time from $t = 5$ seconds to $t = 10$ seconds?

(A) 1925 J
(B) 3850 J
(C) 5775 J
(D) 7700 J
(E) It cannot be determined, because the mass of the object is not known.

31. The melting point of mercury is –39°C. Which of the following is most nearly the heat that must be added to a 1-kilogram block of solid mercury at –39°C to melt it and to raise its temperature to 1°C? (Heat of fusion of mercury = 1.2×10^4 joules per kilogram; specific heat of mercury = 140 joules per kilogram • °C)

(A) 1.8×10^4 J
(B) 1.3×10^4 J
(C) 1.2×10^4 J
(D) 6.8×10^3 J
(E) 5.6×10^3 J

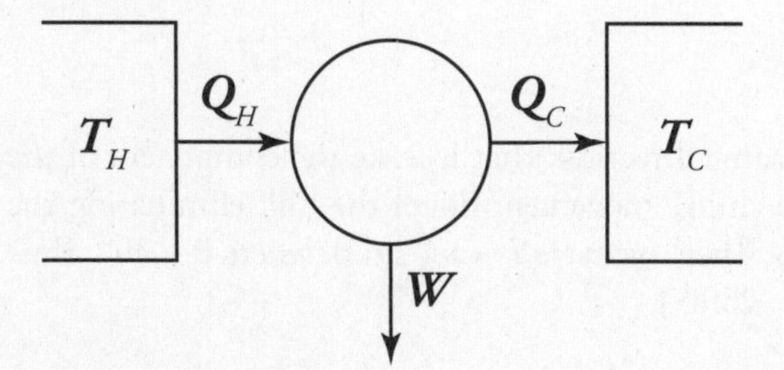

32. A heat engine draws thermal energy from a hot reservoir that is kept at a temperature of 400 Kelvins and exhausts thermal energy into a cold reservoir kept at a temperature of 200 Kelvins, as shown. If the heat engine takes in 4800 joules of thermal energy and does 1200 joules of work, which of the following is most nearly the efficiency of the heat engine?

(A) 0.25
(B) 0.33
(C) 0.50
(D) 0.75
(E) 1.00

33. Which of the following properties must increase as the temperature of a gas increases, no matter the circumstances?

(A) Average kinetic energy of the gas molecules
(B) Molecular weight of the gas
(C) Density of the gas
(D) Pressure exerted by the gas
(E) Volume of the gas

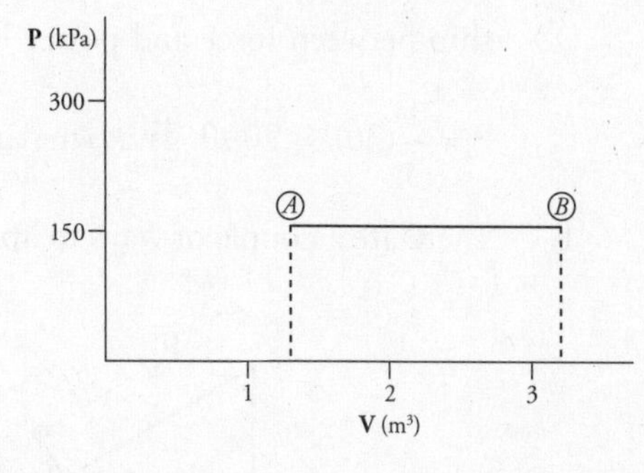

34. The pressure as a function of the volume of an ideal gas in a closed container is shown. The gas goes from state A, a pressure of 300 kilopascals at a volume of 1 cubic meters, to state B, a pressure of 300 kilopascals at a volume of 3 cubic meters. How much work is done by the expanding gas?

(A) 1×10^5 J
(B) 2×10^5 J
(C) 3×10^5 J
(D) 6×10^5 J
(E) 9×10^5 J

35. An aluminum bar of length 2 meters is heated from –10° Celsius to 40° Celsius. If the coefficient of linear expansion of aluminum is 2.5×10^{-5}/°C, by how much will the bar lengthen?

(A) 0.25 mm
(B) 1.25 mm
(C) 2.5 mm
(D) 1.25 cm
(E) 2.5 cm

Answers and Explanations

1. C The word-equation given in the first sentence of the question stem can be expressed as $F_{drag} = \frac{1}{3}v^2$. (Ignore the dimensional incorrectness of the equation; the stem indicates that speed units of m/s will give force units of N here.) The question asks for power, and the relationship between force and power is $P = Fv$, so $P = (\frac{1}{3}v^2)(v) = \frac{1}{3}v^3$. Plug in the number given: $P = \frac{1}{3}(30)^3 = 9000$. Thus, the answer is 9 kW.

2. B There are a couple of ways to approach this problem:

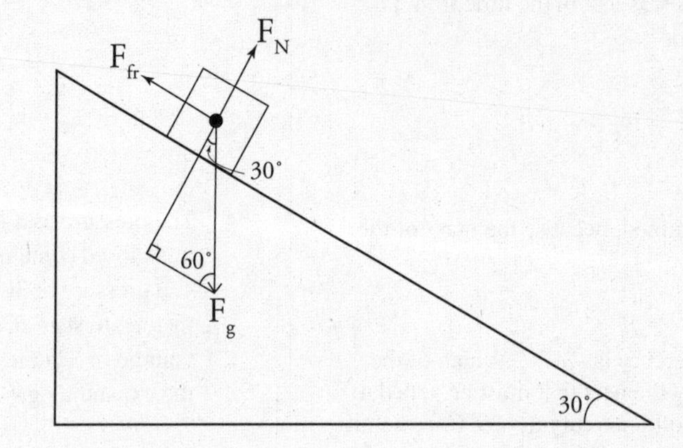

Number 1:

The formula for work is $W = Fd \cos \theta$, where W is the work, F is the force, d is the displacement, and θ is the angle between the force and displacement vectors. To determine the work done by gravity, we use gravitational force and length of the hill to get: $W = (mg)(d) \cos 60°$, where 60° is from the direction of gravitational force vertically down and d is along the ramp. Thus, $W = (10)(10)(50)(0.5) = 2500$ J.

Number 2:

We can resolve the F and d to be in the same direction, that is, take the component of the force acting in the same direction as the child's movement down the hill, eliminating the $\cos \theta$ (since $\cos 0° = 1$) from the equation. Then, we have $F = mg \sin \theta$, where $\theta = 30°$. Thus, $W = Fd = (mg \sin \theta)d = (10)(10)(0.5)(50) = 2500$ J.

3. A In a perfectly inelastic collision, recall that total momentum is conserved but not total kinetic energy, and that the balls all stick together. Initial momentum must be equal to final momentum. $p_{\text{initial}} = p_{\text{final}} = m_1v_1 = (m_1 + m_2)v' \rightarrow v' = m_1v_1 / (m_1 + m_2) = (0.25)(10) / (0.25 + 0.25) = 5$ m/s. This is the value for Trial 2, eliminating choices B and C. For the elastic collision, kinetic energy must be conserved in addition to total momentum, and both objects can move at different velocities after the collision. Since momentum is conserved, $p_{\text{initial}} = p_{\text{final}} = m_1v_1 = m_1v_{1f} + m_2v_{2f}$. Since $m_1 = m_2$, we have that $v_{2f} = v_1 - v_{1f}$. Similarly, if kinetic energy is conserved, then $KE_{\text{initial}} = KE_{\text{final}} = \frac{1}{2}m_1v_1^2 = \frac{1}{2}m_1v_{2f}^2 + \frac{1}{2}m_2v_{2f}^2$. Therefore, $v^2_{2f} = v_1^2 - v^2_{1f}$. In order for these two equations to hold true, v_{1f} must equal either 0 m/s or 10 m/s. Since 10 m/s would indicate the two balls did not collide at all (and 10 m/s for Trial 1 is not an option), the cue ball must have velocity of 0 m/s immediately following the elastic collision, transferring all kinetic energy to the numbered ball.

4. C This question requires you to use the work-kinetic energy theorem, which states that $W = \Delta KE$. The kinetic energy at the bottom is equal to the potential energy at the top, by conservation of energy, which is $mgh = (200)(10)(50) = 10^5$ J. The change in kinetic energy is the final kinetic energy minus the initial. Therefore, the work done by friction to bring the roller coaster to a stop is equal to $\Delta KE = -10^5 \text{ J} = -10 \times 10^4$ J.

5. A For collisions, you must use conservation of momentum. Initially, the momentum is just of the car, and is equal to m_cv_c = (1000 kg)(60 km/h) = (1000 kg)(16.5 m/s) = 16500 kg·m/s. This is equal to the momentum after, which is $m_cv_f + m_tv_t$. Solving for v_f gives 14.5 m/s, and since it is a positive number, the car is traveling in the same direction as it was at the beginning.

6. D The initial energy is $mgh = (7)(10)(20) = 1400$ J. The final energy is completely kinetic, $1/2(mv^2) = 1134$ J. The equation for conservation of energy with frictional is $E_i + W_{\text{by friction}} = E_f$. Thus, the work done by friction is negative and equal to 1134 – 1400 = –266 J.

7. B First, eliminate D because the force exerted by the table on the person, given as F, is equal in magnitude to the force exerted by the person on the table, according to Newton's third law. Next, the way that pressure, force, and area are related is $P = \frac{F_\perp}{A}$. Since the given angle is between the arm and the table, the vertical component of the force will be related to the

sine of that angle. Thus, $P = \frac{F \sin\theta}{A}$. Choice A is wrong because it would be the pressure if the force were not at an angle, and choice C is wrong because it would be the pressure if the angle given were between the arm and a line perpendicular to the table's surface.

8. C The weight of a person, in terms of density, is $w_p = \rho_p V_g$, where V is the volume of the person. The buoyant force from air on the person is $F_B = \rho_{air} V_g$, where V is again the volume of the person because the whole person is submerged in air. This means that the only difference is the density of the person as compared to the density of air, and since we are told that the density of the person is approximately the density of water (1000 kg/m^3), and air has a density of approximately 1 kg/m^3, the relevant factor is 1000.

9. D Begin by setting up the forces and finding the acceleration. $F_{net} = ma$, as always, so (defining the sinking direction as positive) $w - F_B = ma$. Next, specify weight and the buoyant force: $mg - \rho_f V_{sub} g = ma$. Divide by m, which yields $a = g - \frac{\rho_f V_{sub} g}{m}$. For a larger mass, the subtracted buoyant force will be less, and subtracting less means ending up with a greater number. So, the acceleration is greater for an object with greater mass, provided that the compared objects are sinking in the same fluid on the same planet (that is, ρ_f and g are the same for the two objects), and they have the same volume (as the stem indicates they do). Notice that it is the buoyant force term that makes the difference here: mass canceled in the weight term. Objects fall at the same rate in vacuum, so it can't be the weight itself that is causing this effect, which is the reason that choice C is wrong. It is the buoyant force that is responsible for the difference in accelerations. Choices A and B are wrong for their "No" answers; choice A gives a true justification (acceleration due to gravity is independent of the mass of the object being accelerated), but it neglects the effect of the buoyant force, and choice B gives an incorrect reason, since equal volumes mean that the magnitude of the buoyant force on each object is the same.

10. A Recall that for floating objects $\frac{\rho_o}{\rho_f} = \frac{V_{sub}}{V}$. Since the density of the object is 667 kg/m^3 and the density of water is 1000 kg/m^3, two-thirds of the object will be submerged and one-third will be above the surface of the water. Since $\rho = \frac{m}{V}$, then $V = \frac{m}{\rho} = \frac{6000}{667} = 9\ \text{m}^3$. The total volume of the object is 9 m^3, and one-third of that is 3 m^3.

11. D Power can be expressed as $P = V^2 / R$. Therefore, begin by determining total resistance of the circuit, R_{TOT}. In this circuit, R_2 and R_3 are connected in series, and are connected in parallel to R_1. R_2 and R_3 can be reduced to $R_{EQ} = R_2 + R_3$. This equivalent resistor connects in parallel to R_1, and can be further reduced to $R_{TOT} = R_1 (R_2 + R_3) / (R_1 + R_2 + R_3)$. Use this equation for total resistance in the equation for power to yield $P = V^2 / R_{TOT}$, or choice D.

12. C Change in electrical potential energy is given by the equation $\Delta PE = qV$. The problem states that there is an energy transfer of 500 megajoules across a potential difference of 20 megavolts. Solving for q yields a charge transfer of 500 MJ / 20 MV, or 25 coulombs. The problem states that the time over which the charge is transferred is 250 msec, or 0.25 seconds. Using the equation $I = Q/t$, the average current can be calculated as 25 coulombs / 0.25 seconds, or 100 amps.

13. D Item I is correct because the electrical resistance of a metal wire is inversely proportional to its cross sectional area (choices A and C can be eliminated). Note that since both remaining choices include Item III, Item III must be correct and we only need to evaluate Item II. Item II is also correct. The internal resistance of a voltmeter is very high, and thus adding a voltmeter will increase the resistance of the whole system (choice B can be eliminated and choice D is correct). Item III is in fact correct. According to the formula $R = \rho L / A$, the resistance of the wire R, is directly proportional to its length L. Therefore, as the length of the wire increases, so does the overall resistance of the system.

14. B Item I is false. The voltage is the electromotive force that drives the current through the wire. Therefore, it remains constant and unaffected by the increase in resistance (choices A and C can be eliminated). Note that the remaining choices both include Item II so Item II must be true: according to the equation $V = IR$, when V is constant, the current I is inversely proportional to the resistance R. Item III is false. The power P is expressed by the equation $P = IV$, where I is the current through the wire and V is the voltage that drives the current. Since V stays constant, and I becomes 1/4 of the original value, the power P would be $1/4\ I \times V = 1/4\ IV$, which is 1/4 the original power output (choice D is wrong and choice B is correct).

15. D The energy of the incident photons is

$$E = hf = (4.14 \times 10^{-15}\ \text{eV} \cdot \text{s})(7.2 \times 10^{15}\ \text{Hz}) = 30\ \text{eV}$$

Since $E > \phi$, photoelectrons will be produced, with maximum kinetic energy

$$K_{max} = E - \phi = 30\ \text{eV} - 6\ \text{eV} = 24\ \text{eV}$$

16. A If the atom's ionization energy is 25 eV, then the electron's ground-state energy must be –25 eV. Making a transition from the –16 eV energy level to the ground state will cause the emission of a photon of energy.

$$\Delta E = (-16 \text{ eV}) - (-25\text{eV}) = 9 \text{ eV}$$

17. E The gap between the ground-state and the first excited state is

$$-10 \text{ eV} - (-40 \text{ eV}) = 30 \text{ eV}$$

Therefore, the electron must absorb the energy of a 30 eV photon (at least) to move even to the first excited state. Since the incident photons have only 15 eV of energy, the electron will be unaffected.

18. C The de Broglie wavelength of a particle whose momentum is p is $\lambda = h/p$. For this proton, we find that

$$\lambda = \frac{h}{p} = \frac{6.63 \times 10^{-34} \text{ J} \bullet \text{s}}{3.3 \times 10^{-23} \text{ kg} \bullet \text{m/s}} = 2.0 \times 10^{-11} \text{ m} = 0.02 \text{ nm}$$

19. A In β^- decay, a neutron is transformed into a proton and an electron. Therefore, the total nucleon number (mass number) doesn't change, but the number of protons (the atomic number) increases by one.

20. A Since the mass number decreased by 4 and the atomic number decreased by 2, this is an alpha decay.

21. B After 3 half-lives, the activity will drop to $(1/2)^3 = 1/8$ its initial value, and after 4 half-lives, it will drop to $(1/2)^4 = 1/16$ its initial value. Since 1/10 is between 1/8 and 1/16, the time interval in this case is between 3 and 4 half-lives, that is, between 3(2.5 h) = 7.5 h and 4(2.5 h) = 10 h. Only B is in this range.

22. B In order to balance the mass number (the superscripts), we must have 2 + 63 = 64 + A, so A = 1. In order to balance the charge (the subscripts), we need 1 + 29 = 30 + Z, so Z = 0. A particle with a mass number of 1 and no charge is a neutron, ${}^{1}_{0}\text{n}$.

23. **E** To balance the mass number (the superscripts), we must have 196 + 1 = 197 + *A*, so *A* = 0.

To balance the charge (the subscripts), we need 78 + 0 = 78 + *Z*, so *Z* = 0. The only particle listed that has zero mass number and zero charge is a gamma-ray photon, ${}^{0}_{0}\gamma$.

24. **B** Making simultaneous measurements of position and momentum is limited by the Uncertainty Principle, a quantum mechanical law.

25. **E** If one of the vectors had a magnitude of 9 and the other had a magnitude of 1, and they pointed in the same direction, then they would add to 10. In that case, B would be true. However, if one had a magnitude of 11 and the other had a magnitude of 1, but they pointed in opposite directions, their sum would still have a magnitude of 10 (as the stem describes), but the sum of their magnitudes would be 12. That would make D true. This makes the answer E, since either B or D could be true and the other false. (A is impossible, but C could be true: imagine perpendicular vectors with magnitudes of 6 and 8.)

26. **C** This previews some of the content that you'll see in later chapters, but this is a typical vector question on the OAT. Mass and power in A are scalars. Speed in B is a scalar. Kinetic energy in D is a scalar. All the quantities in C are vectors, however.

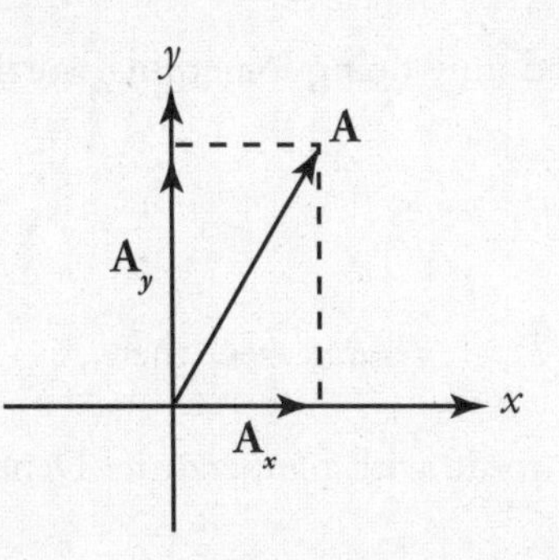

27. **D** Draw it! From the picture, you want 4 sin 30°, which is 2. That's D.

28. **E** Direction is the easiest to get rid of; scalars don't even have direction, so eliminate A and C. Vector and scalar equivalents don't always have the same magnitude, which you can see if you consider distance and displacement. Imagine moving to the left one meter and then back to the right one meter. Your net displacement is zero meters, but your total distance is two meters. Those are different magnitudes. Eliminate B and D. The answer must be E, as you can see from the above example (both displacement and distance have units of meters).

29. **B** Since 5 – 2 = 3, the only way for the two vectors to sum to 3 is for them to be in opposite directions. B expresses that. If they were parallel, as in A, they would add to 7. If they were perpendicular, as in C, they would add to approximately 5.4. If they formed an acute angle, they would add to something between 3 and 5.4, and if they formed an obtuse angle, they would add to something between 5.4 and 7.

30. C The figure shows that from time $t = 5$ seconds to $t = 10$ seconds, the object drops from a temperature of 25°C to 10°C. This is a drop of 15°C. The question also mentions that when the object is heated 10°C, it gains 3850 J. To relate these, use $q = mc\Delta T$: since it's the same object in both the temperature increase and decrease, m and c are held fixed, so q is directly proportional to ΔT. A drop of 1.5 times as much in temperature (that is, 1.5 times as much ΔT) should release 1.5 times as much energy (that is, 1.5 times as much q). Take 3850 and multiply by 1.5, and you get C.

31. A First, to melt the mercury, use $q = mL$. In this case, that's $q = (1)(1.2 \times 10^4)$. Next, to raise the temperature from –39°C to 1°C, use $q = mc\Delta T$. In this case, that's $q = (1)(140)(40) =$ 5600 J. Add the two together, and 12000 + 5600 = 17600 J. Round, and you get answer choice A.

32. A The actual efficiency of a heat engine is $e = \frac{W}{Q_H}$ (not to be confused with the Carnot efficiency, the maximum possible efficiency). In this case, that's $e = \frac{1200}{4800} = 0.25$. That's A. (It's taking 4800 J and only doing something worthwhile with 25% of them, hence an efficiency of 0.25.)

33. A Given that $K_{avg} = \frac{3}{2}k_B T$, if T increases, then K_{avg} has to increase. Molecular weight shouldn't have anything to do with temperature. Density would most likely decrease with an increase in temperature, from $PV = nRT$ (an increase in T can increase V, decreasing density). Pressure and volume could increase with increasing temperature, but neither has to.

34. D This is $W = P\Delta V$. Since P is fixed at 300,000 and V changes from 1 to 3, $W = (300{,}000)(2) =$ 600,000 J. That's D.

35. C Apply $\Delta L = \alpha L_i \Delta T$. Here, that comes to $\Delta L = (2.5 \times 10^{-5})(2)(50) = 2.5 \times 10^{-3}$. Convert to millimeters, and you get C.

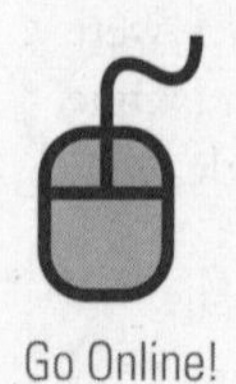

Go Online!

NATURAL SCIENCES DRILL

What follows is a small sample of problems that surveys some of the content that you will see in the Survey of Natural Sciences portion of the OAT. If, after reading the topic outlines in this book, you feel fairly confident that you know the stuff tested on the SNS, complete these problems to test your knowledge. If you get most of them right, great! You probably need only a light review of the science topics, and some combination of going over your old class notes and taking practice tests probably will suffice. If you get a sizable number wrong, or if you feel unsure about this content, you should review these topics in more detail. One way to do that is to purchase *Cracking the DAT,* which covers in detail the topics that the DAT and the OAT share.

Bear in mind, also, that what follows is not completely comprehensive. It's a sample of a few representative topics, not a survey of all possible topics. However, it covers Biology, General Chemistry, and Organic Chemistry, which are the three subjects on the SNS, and it covers a number of different topics within each subject, so you should be able to get a sense of where you are from working these problems.

Biology

1. Which of the following statements is NOT true?

   (A) Lipids are frequently found in the interior, hydrophobic regions of globular proteins.
   (B) Cholesterol is the precursor to steroid hormones.
   (C) Unsaturated fats have one or more double bonds.
   (D) Lipids are hydrophobic and lipophilic.
   (E) The cell membrane is made up of amphipathic phospholipids.

2. A nucleotide made of which of the following would be found in DNA?

   (A) Ribose, phosphate, and uracil
   (B) Ribose, phosphate, and thymine
   (C) Deoxyribose, ribose, and thymine
   (D) Deoxyribose, phosphate, and uracil
   (E) Deoxyribose, phosphate, and thymine

3. A red blood cell in a hypertonic salt solution will

   (A) swell up and explode.
   (B) shrivel up.
   (C) absorb the salt and explode.
   (D) absorb the salt and shrivel up.
   (E) remain the same.

4. During which phase of the cell cycle are the sister chromatids separated?

   (A) S phase
   (B) Telophase
   (C) Prophase
   (D) Metaphase
   (E) Anaphase

5. Which of the following statements about prokaryotes and eukaryotes is true?

   (A) Both prokaryotes and eukaryotes translate proteins in the cytosol.
   (B) Both prokaryotes and eukaryotes transcribe RNA in the nucleus.
   (C) Prokaryotes have a cell wall and eukaryotes have only a cell membrane.
   (D) Prokaryotes rely only on glycolysis for energy, while eukaryotes can get energy from the electron transport chain and oxidative phosphorylation (aerobic respiration).
   (E) Prokaryotes can exchange plasmids by conjugation, while eukaryotes exchange plasmids during sexual reproduction.

6. A reaction that would proceed quickly and spontaneously would have a

   (A) positive ΔG and a low energy of activation.
   (B) negative ΔG and a low energy of activation.
   (C) positive ΔG and a high energy of activation.
   (D) negative ΔG and a high energy of activation.
   (E) positive ΔG and a high ΔS.

7. Catalysts

   I. stabilize the transition state of a reaction.
   II. can drive a non-spontaneous reaction forward.
   III. reduce the energy of activation of a reaction.

   (A) I only
   (B) III only
   (C) I and II
   (D) I and III
   (E) I, II, and III

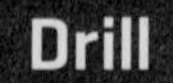

8. In fermentation, why is pyruvate reduced to ethanol or lactic acid?

(A) To prepare pyruvate to enter the Krebs cycle
(B) To oxidize NADH, so that glycolysis can continue to run in the absence of oxygen
(C) So that yeast can produce the alcohol in wine and beer
(D) So that the resulting drop in pH can increase the activity of the glycolytic enzymes
(E) So that muscle cells can continue the Krebs cycle in the absence of oxygen

9. Which of the following is NOT true about DNA replication?

(A) DNA gyrase unwinds the helix at the origin.
(B) It is semiconservative.
(C) The leading strand is polymerized in the same direction as the DNA is unwinding.
(D) It occurs in the 5′ to 3′ direction.
(E) It requires an RNA primer.

10. Which of the following is NOT a difference between replication and transcription?

I. In replication, the new DNA is edited to correct mistakes, while in transcription there is no proofreading.
II. In replication, DNA is synthesized in the 5′ to 3′ direction, while in transcription, RNA is synthesized in the 3′ to 5′ direction.
III. Both strands of the DNA are replicated, while typically only one strand of the DNA is transcribed.

(A) I only
(B) I and II only
(C) II only
(D) II and III only
(E) I, II, and III

11. If the frequency of the allele causing a dominant disorder is 0.1, what is the frequency of affected individuals in the population?

(A) 0.01
(B) 0.09
(C) 0.19
(D) 0.81
(E) 0.90

12. A woman with blood type B– marries a man with blood type A+. They have a child with blood type O+. Which of the following is true?

(A) The man is homozygous for blood type A (genotype I^AI^A).
(B) The child is homozygous for the Rh factor (genotype *RR*).
(C) The man must be the father of the child.
(D) The man is not the father of the child.
(E) The man might be the father of the child.

13. A pure-breeding white mouse is crossed with a pure-breeding black mouse. All offspring are grey. This is an example of

(A) codominance.
(B) incomplete dominance.
(C) epistasis.
(D) classical dominance.
(E) recombination.

14. A man who is colorblind marries a woman who does not carry the colorblindness allele. His daughter marries a man with normal vision. What is the probability that the man's grandson is colorblind?

(A) 0
(B) $\frac{1}{4}$
(C) $\frac{1}{2}$
(D) $\frac{3}{4}$
(E) 1

15. All chordates have several features in common. Which of the following is NOT a shared feature of chordates?

(A) Notochord
(B) Postanal tail
(C) Pharyngeal gill slits
(D) Bony skeletons
(E) Dorsal hollow nerve cord

16. Which of the following is NOT an example of a prezygotic barrier to speciation?

(A) The sperm of a hamster cannot fertilize the egg of a rabbit.
(B) A mule, the offspring of a horse and a donkey, is sterile.
(C) Birds have different mating seasons; some mate in the spring and some mate in the fall.
(D) Elephants and mice are physically incompatible and cannot mate.
(E) Swans do not know the mating rituals of geese.

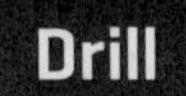

17. Large evergreen trees that use cones as reproductive structures, and whose dominant life stage is the sporophyte are classified as

(A) monocots.
(B) dicots.
(C) ferns.
(D) gymnosperms.
(E) angiosperms.

18. Which of the following is true of a cardiac muscle cell action potential but NOT a neuronal action potential?

(A) The initial depolarization is caused by the influx of sodium.
(B) Na^+/K^+ ATPases maintain resting potential for the cell.
(C) Repolarization in a cardiac muscle cell is caused by the efflux of calcium.
(D) Cardiac muscle action potentials have a plateau phase caused by the influx of calcium.
(E) Repolarization is caused by the efflux of potassium.

19. Which of the following hormones is NOT made by the pituitary gland?

(A) Thyroid stimulating hormone (TSH)
(B) Prolactin
(C) Oxytocin
(D) Adrenocorticotropic hormone (ACTH)
(E) Growth hormone

20. The kidney uses three main processes to make urine: filtration, reabsorption, and secretion. When compared to plasma concentration, the urine concentration of a secreted substance is

(A) higher, because secretion moves substances from the blood to the filtrate.
(B) lower, because secretion moves substances from the blood to the filtrate.
(C) higher, because secretion moves substances from the filtrate to the blood.
(D) lower, because secretion moves substances from the filtrate to the blood.
(E) equal, because secretion is the process that originally filters substances out of the blood.

21. Each of the following are functions of the pancreas EXCEPT

(A) secrete bicarbonate.
(B) produce bile.
(C) release insulin.
(D) secrete digestive enzymes.
(E) release glucagon.

22. Which of the following would be expected to occur if blood pressure was too low?

I. Aldosterone secretion would be increased
II. Antidiuretic hormone would be inhibited
III. Renin would be released

(A) I and II only
(B) II only
(C) I and III only
(D) II and III only
(E) I, II, and III

23. During which step of the sliding filament theory is ATP hydrolyzed?

(A) Myosin pulls actin toward the center of the sarcomere (power stroke).
(B) Myosin releases actin.
(C) Myosin binding sites on actin are exposed.
(D) Myosin binds to actin (crossbridge formation).
(E) Myosin is reset to its high-energy conformation.

24. All of the following are characteristics of protostomes EXCEPT

(A) They are all coelomates.
(B) They undergo spiral and determinate cleavage.
(C) The first opening (blastopore) develops into the mouth and the second opening into the anus.
(D) The fates of the embryonic cells are decided very early in development.
(E) The group includes echinoderms and chordates.

General Chemistry

1. What is the correct electron configuration for Zn^{2+}?

(A) $[Ar]3d^8$
(B) $[Ar]3d^{10}$
(C) $[Ar]4s^2 3d^8$
(D) $[Ar]4s^2 3d^9$
(E) $[Ar]4s^1 3d^{10}$

2. Bismuth-212 undergoes α decay followed by β decay. What is the resultant nucleus?

(A) ^{210}Po
(B) ^{208}Tl
(C) ^{208}Bi
(D) ^{208}Pb
(E) ^{207}Hg

3. Which of the following atoms will have the smallest atomic radius?

(A) Oxygen
(B) Sodium
(C) Carbon
(D) Sulfur
(E) Iron

4. What is the shape of chlorine trifluoride?

(A) T-shaped
(B) Square planar
(C) Trigonal bipyramid
(D) Trigonal pyramid
(E) Bent

5. Which of the following best describes why the temperature of a pot of boiling water remains constant despite the continual addition of heat?

(A) The heat is increasing the internal kinetic energy of the water rather than increasing the temperature.
(B) The heat is decreasing the internal kinetic energy of the water rather than increasing the temperature.
(C) The heat is used to break hydrogen bonds between water molecules rather than increasing the temperature.
(D) The heat is used to form hydrogen bonds between water molecules rather than increasing the temperature.
(E) None of the above

6. There are an unknown number of moles of Argon in a steel container. A chemist injects two moles of nitrogen into the container. The temperature and volume do not change, but the pressure increases by ten percent. Originally the container held:

(A) 16 moles of Ar.
(B) 18 moles of Ar.
(C) 20 moles of Ar.
(D) 22 moles of Ar.
(E) 24 moles of Ar.

7. Air is a mixture of many gases. Yet, N_2 (78%) and O_2 (21%) comprise 99% of its composition. If the pressure of air at sea level is 760 torr, what are the approximate partial pressures of N_2 and O_2, respectively?

(A) 590 torr, 160 torr
(B) 590 torr, 380 torr
(C) 160 torr, 590 torr
(D) 160 torr, 380 torr
(E) 380 torr, 380 torr

8. The packaging and storage of carbonated liquids (such as soda) is largely predicated on the properties of gas solubility in liquids. Which of the following best describes the relationship between solubility, pressure, and temperature for gases in liquids?

(A) Gases (such as CO_2) are most soluble in liquids at high pressures and high temperatures.
(B) Gases (such as CO_2) are most soluble in liquids at low pressures and low temperatures.
(C) Gases (such as CO_2) are most soluble in liquids at low pressures and high temperatures.
(D) Gases (such as CO_2) are most soluble in liquids at high pressures and low temperatures.
(E) Gases (such as CO_2) are not soluble unless combined with other compounds.

9. A chemist is attempting to identify an unknown salt. When she adds a solution of silver nitrate, a white precipitate forms. Which of the following may be the identity of the unknown salt?

I. Li_2CO_3
II. $Ba(CH_3COO)_2$
III. NaCl

(A) I only
(B) II only
(C) III only
(D) I and II
(E) I and III

10. Which of the following statements is always true about the kinetics of a chemical reaction?

(A) The rate law includes all reactants in the balanced overall equation.
(B) The overall order equals the sum of the reactant coefficients in the overall reaction.
(C) The overall order equals the sum of the reactant coefficients in the slow step of the reaction.
(D) The structure of the catalyst remains unchanged throughout the reaction progress.
(E) The units of the rate constant are $M^{-1}s^{-1}$.

11. Based on the reaction mechanism shown below, which of the following statements is correct?

$$2\,NO + O_2 \rightarrow 2\,NO_2$$

1) $2\,NO \rightarrow N_2O_2$ (*fast*)
2) $N_2O_2 + O_2 \rightarrow 2\,NO_2$ (*slow*)

(A) Step 1 is the rate-determining step and the rate of the overall reaction is $k[N_2O_2]$.
(B) Step 1 is the rate-determining step and the rate of the overall reaction is $k[NO]^2$.
(C) Step 2 is the rate-determining step and the rate of the overall reaction is $k[NO_2]^2$.
(D) Step 2 is the rate-determining step and the rate of the overall reaction is $k[N_2O_2][O_2]$.
(E) The rate-determining step cannot be determined from the data provided.

12. Given the following equilibrium:

$$N_2(g) + 3H_2(g) \rightleftharpoons 2NH_3(g) \quad \Delta H = -91.8\text{kJ}$$

How would an increase in temperature affect the concentration of N_2 at equilibrium?

(A) The concentration of N_2 will increase because of an increase in K_{eq}.
(B) The concentration of N_2 will decrease because of an increase in K_{eq}.
(C) The concentration of N_2 will increase because of a decrease in K_{eq}.
(D) The concentration of N_2 will decrease because of a decrease in K_{eq}.
(E) The concentration of N_2 will remain unchanged.

13. Which of the following salts is least soluble in water?

(A) PbI_2 ($K_{sp} = 7.9 \times 10^{-9}$)
(B) $Mg(OH)_2$ ($K_{sp} = 6.3 \times 10^{10}$)
(C) $Zn(IO_3)_2$ ($K_{sp} = 3.9 \times 10^{6}$)
(D) SrF_2 ($K_{sp} = 2.6 \times 10^{-9}$)
(E) Ag_2CrO_4 ($K_{sp} = 1.1 \times 10^{-12}$)

14. A graph depicting a titration of a weak acid with a strong base will start at a

(A) high pH and slope downwards with an equivalence pH equal to 7.
(B) high pH and slope downwards with an equivalence pH below 7.
(C) low pH and slope upwards with an equivalence pH equal to 7.
(D) low pH and slope upwards with an equivalence pH above 7.
(E) neutral pH and slope upwards with an equivalence pH above 7.

15. List the following compounds by increasing pK_a:

I. H_2SO_4
II. NH_3
III. CH_3CH_2COOH
IV. HF

(A) I < III < II < IV
(B) I < IV < III < II
(C) III < I < IV < II
(D) II < III < IV < I
(E) I < II < III < IV

16. Which of the following best explains why disorder tends to favor spontaneity?

(A) First Law of Thermodynamics
(B) Second Law of Thermodynamics
(C) Third Law of Thermodynamics
(D) Hess' Law
(E) None of the above

17. Which of the following should have the highest enthalpy of vaporization?

(A) N_2
(B) Br_2
(C) Hg
(D) Al
(E) He

Organic Chemistry

1. In the molecule below, what are the hybridizations of C_1, C_2, C_3, and C_4 respectively?

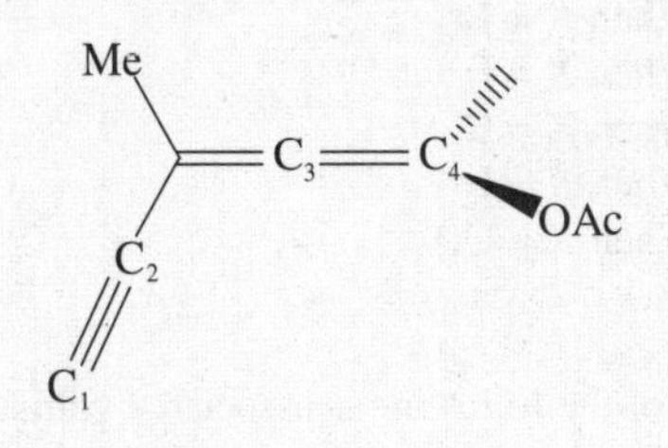

(A) *sp*, *sp*, *sp*^{2}, *sp*^{2}
(B) *sp*, *sp*, *sp*, *sp*^{2}
(C) *sp*^{2}, *sp*^{2}, *sp*, *sp*
(D) *sp*^{2}, *sp*, *sp*, *sp*
(E) *sp*^{2}, *sp*^{3}, *sp*^{3}, *sp*

2. Which of the following describes epimeric compounds?

   I. Contain multiple chiral centers
   II. Are non-superimposable, mirror images
   III. Differ in absolute configuration at a single chiral center.

   (A) I only
   (B) II only
   (C) I and III
   (D) I, II, and III
   (E) I and II

3. Rank the conformations of 2-aminoethanol by increasing stability.

   (A) anti < gauche < eclipsed
   (B) eclipsed < anti < gauche
   (C) gauche < anti < eclipsed
   (D) eclipsed < gauche < anti
   (E) anti < eclipsed < gauche

4. Which of the following is the strongest nucleophile?

   (A) CN^-
   (B) OH^-
   (C) CH_3OH
   (D) NH_3
   (E) NH_4^+

5. Which reaction proceeds the fastest?

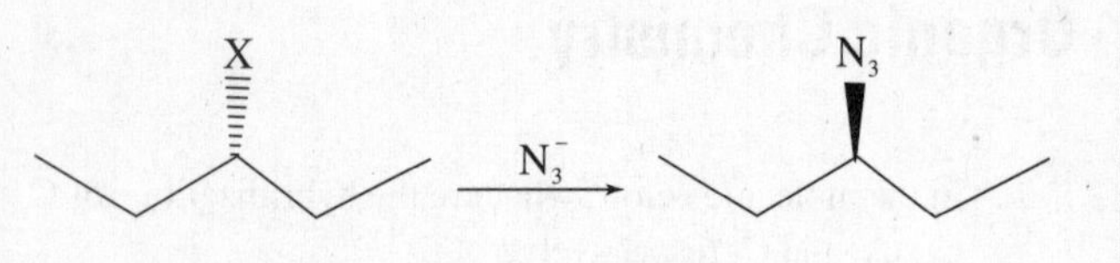

   (A) When X = Br
   (B) When X = F
   (C) When X = Cl
   (D) When X = I
   (E) When X = CH_3

6. Which of the following is associated with an S_N2 reaction?

   (A) sp^2 hybridized intermediate
   (B) A unimolecular rate law
   (C) An antiperiplanar conformation
   (D) Inversion of configuration
   (E) Formation of a carbocation

7. Which step of the radical process does the following reaction represent?

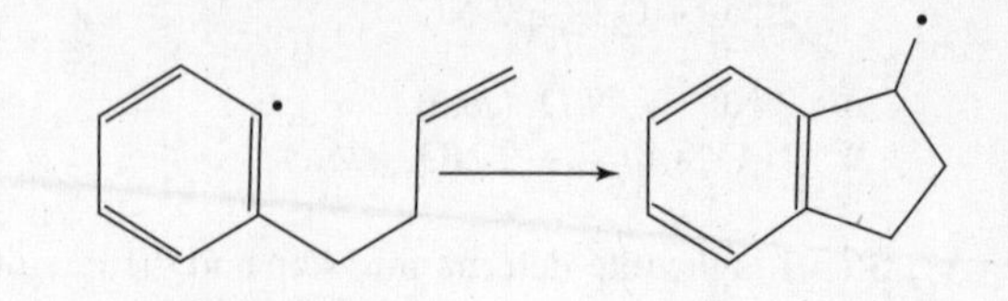

   (A) Initiation
   (B) Propagation
   (C) Termination
   (D) Elimination
   (E) Substitution

8. Which of the following reactions may involve a carbocation rearrangement?

   (A) S_N1 only
   (B) S_N2 only
   (C) S_N1 and E1 only
   (D) S_N2 and E2 only
   (E) S_N1, S_N2, and E1

9. If an alkyne is treated with two equivalents of hydrogen in the presence of platinum, what is the net change in bonds?

   (A) – 1 pi bond, + 4 sigma bonds
   (B) – 2 pi bonds, + 2 sigma bonds
   (C) – 2 pi bonds, + 4 sigma bonds
   (D) – 2 pi bonds, + 6 sigma bonds
   (E) – 4 pi bonds, + 6 sigma bonds

10. If benzene is treated with two equivalents of bromine in the presence of a $FeBr_3$ catalyst and elevated temperatures, what is the maximum number of disubstituted isomeric products that could be produced?

   (A) 1
   (B) 2
   (C) 3
   (D) 4
   (E) 5

11. The acid-catalyzed Markovnikov addition of H_2O to 1-butene should give a(n):

   (A) primary alcohol.
   (B) secondary alcohol.
   (C) tertiary alcohol.
   (D) *cis*-diol.
   (E) aldehyde

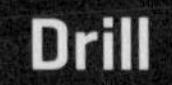

12. Which of the following of the following substituents is most likely to be meta directing?

(A) –OH
(B) $-OCH_3$
(C) –Cl
(D) $-NO_2$
(E) $-CH_2CH_3$

14. Rank the protons from least acidic to most acidic.

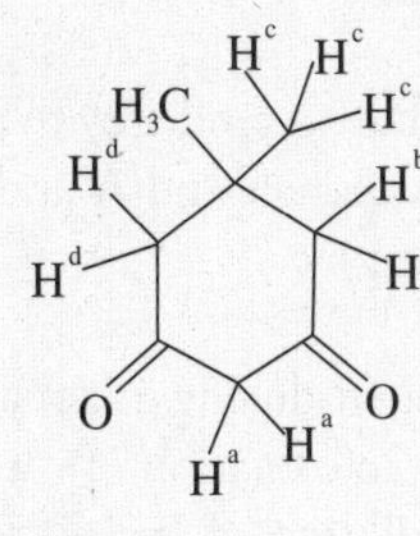

(A) $H_a < H_b = H_d < H_c$
(B) $H_c < H_d < H_b < H_a$
(C) $H_c < H_b = H_d < H_a$
(D) $H_c < H_b < H_d < H_a$
(E) $H_a = H_b < H_c < H_d$

15. Which of the following carbonyl compounds cannot undergo a symmetrical aldol condensation?

(A) 2,2,4,4-tetramethylpentan-3-one
(B) 1,2,2-triphenylethanone
(C) tert-butyl acetate
(D) pentan-2-one
(E) 2-methylpentan-3-one

16. The ^{13}C NMR spectrum for Compound X shows one peak at 128 ppm. If elemental analysis shows that the compound has an empirical formula of CH, how many possible stereoisomers could Compound X have?

(A) 0
(B) 1
(C) 2
(D) 4
(E) 8

17. For the following reaction, how would the R_f value of the product compare to that of the starting material if monitored by TLC on a normal silica gel plate?

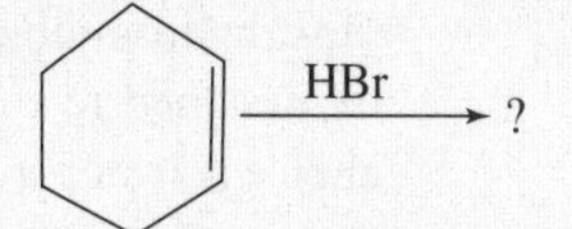

(A) The R_f value of the product would be greater than that of the reactant because the product is more polar.
(B) The R_f value of the product would be greater than that of the reactant because the product is less polar.
(C) The R_f value of the product would be smaller than that of the reactant because the product is more polar.
(D) The R_f value of the product would be smaller than that of the reactant because the product is less polar.
(E) The R_f values of the reactants and products would be the same, because their polarities are similar.

18. What will the 1H NMR spectrum of isobutane show?

(A) One 6 H triplet and one 4 H quartet
(B) Two 3 H triplets and two 2 H quartets
(C) One 9 H doublet and one 1 H multiplet
(D) One 6 H triplet, one 2 H multiplet, and one 2 H triplet
(E) Two 3 H triplets and one 4 H multiplet

ANSWERS AND EXPLANATIONS

1. A While lipids are hydrophobic, they are not frequently found in the interior of globular proteins, hydrophobic or not. They could be—for example, some carrier proteins in the blood are designed to transport lipids (the lipoproteins)—but they are not *frequently* found there (choice A is not true and the correct answer choice). All other statements are true.

2. E Nucleotides contain only one sugar, either deoxyribose or ribose (C is wrong), and for DNA, the sugar is deoxyribose (A and B are wrong). Uracil is a base found in RNA (D is wrong), while thymine is a base found in DNA (E is correct).

3. B A salt solution that is hypertonic to the red blood cell will have a tendency to draw water out of the cell by osmosis, causing the cell to shrivel up (B is correct and A and E are wrong). The salt cannot cross the cell membrane (C and D are wrong).

4. E The replicated chromosomes (sister chromatids) are separated during anaphase. DNA replication occurs in S phase (A is wrong), cytokinesis and the reformation of the nucleus occur in telophase (B is wrong), creation of a spindle and dissolution of the nuclear membrane occur in prophase (C is wrong), and alignment of the replicated chromosomes at cell center occurs during metaphase (D is wrong).

5. A Protein synthesis (translation) occurs in the cytosol in both prokaryotes and eukaryotes. However, only eukaryotes transcribe RNA in the nucleus because prokaryotes lack cellular organelles. Prokaryotic transcription takes place in the cytosol as well (B is wrong). Prokaryotes do have a cell wall, but eukaryotes do not have ONLY a cell membrane; some have cell walls also (plant cells, fungi; C is wrong). Prokaryotes can also participate in aerobic respiration (and eukaryotes can perform glycolysis; D is wrong). Eukaryotes do not usually carry plasmids, and if they do, do not exchange them during sexual reproduction. Sexual reproduction in eukaryotes involves the fusion of egg and sperm (E is wrong).

6. B A spontaneous reaction must have a negative DG (choices A, C, and E are wrong). A reaction with a low energy of activation will proceed more quickly than one with a high energy of activation (B is correct and D is wrong).

7. D Statement I is true: catalysts stabilize the transition state of a reaction (B can be eliminated). By stabilizing the transition state, the energy of activation (energy required to produce the transition state) is lowered, so Statement III is also true (A and C can be eliminated). However, Statement III is false: catalysts cannot make a non-spontaneous reaction spontaneous. All they can do is make an already spontaneous reaction go faster (E can be eliminated and D is correct).

8. B Fermentation occurs in the absence of oxygen, when the PDC and the Krebs cycle are shut down (A and E are wrong). In order to continue running glycolysis, NADH must be oxidized back to NAD^+, and the reduction of pyruvate, to either ethanol or lactic acid, allows the oxidation of NADH. Fermentation in yeast does produce the alcohol in wine and beer, but this is not the reason that fermentation occurs (C is wrong). A drop in pH would reduce enzyme activity, not increase it (D is wrong).

9. A The enzyme that unwinds DNA at the origin to begin replication is called helicase. DNA gyrase is the enzyme that supercoils prokaryotic DNA (A is not true and is the correct answer). All of the other statements are true.

10. C Statement I is a valid difference: there is no proofreading or editing of newly made RNA transcripts (A, B, and E can be eliminated). Statement II is NOT a difference: both DNA and RNA are synthesized 5′ to 3′. Statement III is a valid difference: replication strives to produce two identical DNA strands from a single parent molecule, while the goal of transcription is to create a single RNA molecule from the DNA. Because the two strands of DNA are complementary, each DNA strand would produce a different strand of RNA, thus, typically only one of the DNA strands is transcribed (called the template strand, D can be eliminated and C is correct).

11. C The Hardy-Weinberg equation for allele frequency is $p + q = 1$. If the frequency of the dominant allele (p) is 0.1, then the frequency of the recessive allele (q) must be 0.9. Plugging these values into the equation for genotype frequency ($p^2 + 2pq + q^2 = 1$), we find that the frequency of homozygous dominant individuals (p^2) is 0.01, the frequency of heterozygous individual ($2pq$) is 0.18, and the frequency of homozygous recessive individuals (q^2) is 0.81. Individuals affected by the dominant allele include homozygous dominants and heterozygotes; $0.01 + 0.18 = 0.19$.

12. E The child with blood type O must be homozygous ii, thus, both the man and woman must be heterozygous; the woman $I^B i$ and the man $I^A i$ (A is wrong). Since the child is Rh+, it could be either homozygous *RR* or heterozygous *Rr;* however, since the mother is Rh–, she must have the genotype rr. Thus all she could donate to the child is r, and the child must be heterozygous *Rr* (B is wrong). The man could be the father of the child, his genotype could be $I^A iRR$ and could have donated *i* and *R* to the child (D is wrong). However, this does not absolutely establish paternity, as other men could also have the necessary blood types to produce an O+ child with this woman (for example, men with blood types O+ and B+, C is wrong and E is correct).

13. B If a pure-breeding (homozygous) white mouse (WW) is crossed with a pure-breeding (homozygous) black mouse (BB), then all offspring mice will be heterozygous (WB). If their phenotype is a blended version of the parental phenotypes, then this is an example of incomplete dominance. Codominance is when both alleles are expressed, but independently of each other (i.e., not blended, like blood typing; A is wrong). Epistasis is when the expression of one gene prevents the expression of another (e.g., the gene for baldness prevents the expression of hair shape genes; C is wrong). Classical dominance is when one allele is expressed and one is silent; if this were the case all the heterozygous offspring would look like one of the parents (the one expressing the dominant phenotype; D is wrong). Recombination occurs between two different genes on the same chromosome, e.g., fur color and whisker length. Since only one gene is involved here, it cannot be recombination (E is wrong).

14. C Colorblindness is an X-linked disorder, so the man's genotype must be $X^C Y$. His daughter inherits X^C from him and X^N (the normal allele) from her mother (the man's wife does not carry the colorblindness allele). The daughter's husband's genotype is $X^N Y$. For the daughter to have a boy, her husband had to donate the Y chromosome. The probability that the boy is colorblind depends on what the daughter donates, either X^C (colorblind) or X^N (normal), one-half.

15. D Not all chordates have bony skeletons, some are cartilaginous as in sharks (D is not a shared feature and is the correct answer choice). All other choices list shared features.

16. B Prezygotic barriers to speciation prevent the union of sperm and egg into a zygote. They include species-specific sperm recognition (A is a prezygotic barrier and can be eliminated), temporal barriers such as different mating seasons (C is a prezygotic barrier and can be eliminated), mechanical barriers such as size differences (D is a prezygotic barrier and can be eliminated), and behavioral barriers, such as mating rituals (E is a prezygotic barrier and can be eliminated). Only B describes a postzygotic barrier; in this situation the sperm and egg fuse, and the hybrid develops, but is sterile and the line cannot continue (B is not a prezygotic barrier and the correct answer choice).

17. D The question describes conifers, tall pine trees that produce pinecones for reproduction. The seeds are not enclosed, and the plants are described as "naked seed" plants, or gymnosperms. Angiosperms are flowering plants and have enclosed seeds; monocots and dicots are subclasses of angiosperms (A, B, and E are wrong). Ferns are short, shrubby plants, not tall trees (their dominant stage is the sporophyte, however). C is wrong.

18. D Cardiac muscle cells have voltage-gated calcium channels that open shortly after the action potential is initiated. The resulting influx of calcium greatly prolongs the cardiac action potential (200–300 msec), producing the characteristic plateau phase seen in these cells. Neuronal action potentials are about 100 times shorter (only 2–3 msec) and are not dependent on the influx of calcium. In both cardiac muscle cells and neurons the initial depolarization is caused by the influx of sodium, Na^+/K^+ ATPases maintain resting potential, and repolarization is caused by the efflux of potassium (A, B, and E are true of both and can be eliminated, and C is not true of either and can be eliminated).

19. C Oxytocin is released by the posterior pituitary, but is actually made by neuron cell bodies the hypothalamus and transported into the posterior pituitary for release. This is also true of ADH, the other posterior pituitary hormone. All other hormones listed are synthesized and released by the anterior pituitary.

20. A Secretion is the process used to move substances from the blood into the filtrate (C, D, and E are wrong). This helps eliminate substances faster than by filtration alone, because not only is the substance filtered, additional molecules of the substance are added to the filtrate as it is processed into urine. The concentration of the substance in the initial filtrate will be equal to plasma concentration of that substance, but as the substance is secreted, its concentration in the plasma will fall and its concentration in the filtrate will rise. Thus, the final urine concentration of the substances will be higher than plasma concentration (A is correct and B is wrong). Substances that are typically secreted include drugs and toxins.

21. B The pancreas is a major source of digestive enzymes for the GI tract (D is a function and can be eliminated). It also secretes bicarbonate along with those enzymes; this helps neutralize acidic chyme coming from the stomach and keeps the intestines at a more neutral pH of about 6–7 (A is a function and can be eliminated). The pancreas is also an endocrine organ, releasing insulin or glucagon to help regulate blood glucose levels (C and E are functions and can be eliminated). Bile, however, is made by the liver, not the pancreas (B is not a function and is the correct answer).

22. **C** Statement I would occur: aldosterone acts to increase sodium reabsorption at the distal tubule of the nephron. The resulting increase in blood osmolarity triggers the release of antidiuretic hormone that causes increased reabsorption of water, an increase in blood volume, and an increase in blood pressure (B and D can be eliminated). Statement II is false: the inhibition of antidiuretic hormone would lead to increased loss of water through the urine with a subsequent drop in blood volume and blood pressure (A and E can be eliminated and C is correct). Statement III is true: renin is released by the kidney when blood pressure falls. It catalyzes the conversion of angiotensinogen into angiotensin I, which is further converted to angiotensin II. Angiotensin II is a powerful vasoconstrictor that increases blood pressure.

23. **E** Returning myosin to its high-energy state (also referred to as "cocking" the myosin head) requires the hydrolysis of ATP. The power stroke, where myosin pulls actin toward the center of the sarcomere is simply myosin returning to its low-energy state, and does not require ATP hydrolysis (A is wrong). The release of actin by myosin requires the binding of ATP, but not ATP hydrolysis (B is wrong). Exposing the myosin binding sites requires calcium, but not ATP (C is wrong) and the actual binding of actin to myosin does not require anything special (D is wrong).

24. **E** "Proto" means "first" and "stoma" means "mouth," so in protostomes the first opening (the blastopore) develops into the mouth, and the second opening into the anus (C is true and can be eliminated). They are all coelomates (have a fluid-filled cavity separating their digestive tract from their body wall, A is true and can be eliminated). They undergo spiral (smaller cells lie in grooves between larger cells) and determinate cleavage (the fate of the embryonic cells is decided early in development (B and D are true and can be eliminated). However, the group includes annelids, mollusks, and arthropods; echinoderms and chordates are classified as deuterostomes (E is not true and is the correct answer).

General Chemistry

1. **B** The electron configuration for Zn (non-ionized) is $[Ar]4s^2\ 3d^{10}$. Transition (*d*-block) elements always lose electrons from their highest energy *s* orbital first, meaning that the correct answer takes two electrons away from the 4*s* orbital.

2. **D** The only type of decay that changes the mass number of an atom is α decay, which results in the loss of two protons and two neutrons, meaning that the mass number is decreased by 4. Thus, the daughter nucleus must have a mass number of $212 - 4 = 208$, eliminating A and E. The atomic number is affected by both α and β (which when present without a modifier refers to β^- decay) decay, with α decay decreasing the atomic number by 2, and β decay increasing it by 1. The atomic number of bismuth is 83, so $83 - 2 + 1 = 82$, which is the atomic number for lead, Pb.

3. **A** Remember that atomic radius increases as you go from right to left (since you decrease the number of protons in the nucleus providing an attractive force on the valence electrons) and as you go from up to down (since you increase the number of filled shells which provide a repulsive force on the valence electrons). Thus, the trend for smallest is the opposite; the smallest elements are found the upper right of the periodic table. Of the elements listed, oxygen is the one that is furthest towards the upper right hand corner, and thus is the smallest.

4. A To determine the shape of a molecule (which takes into account the number of lone pairs), we must first determine the geometry (which takes into account the total number of electron groups around the central atom, including both lone pairs and bonds). First, count the number of valence electrons on each atom. Since all are halogens, each will have seven valence electrons. With the chlorine as the central atom, there is a single bond between it and each of the fluorine atoms. Thus, each of the fluorine atoms has its valences satisfied. This leaves two lone pairs on the central chlorine, making a total of five electron groups. Five electron groups gives a geometric family of trigonal bipyramid. Since the geometry is trigonal bipyramid, but there are two lone pairs, the shape is T-shaped.

5. C During a phase transition such as boiling, the temperature of the substance does not change because the heat provided is used to disrupt the intermolecular forces between molecules (eliminating D). Since the temperature of a substance is a measure of its internal kinetic energy and is not changing, A and B may also be eliminated.

6. C At constant V and T, the pressure of an ideal gas reflects the number of particles (regardless of their identity). It is a simplification of the ideal gas law from $PV = nRT$ to $P \propto n$. So, if the addition of two moles of N_2 into the chamber results in an increase in P of 10 percent, then the moles added must be 10 percent of the initial number of Ar moles. Two moles are 10 percent of 20 moles.

7. A According to Dalton's law, the sum of the partial pressures of gases must equal to the total pressure of the system. Therefore, B and D may be eliminated, as they do not add up to approximately 760 torr. In addition, since the mole fractions of the two gases are not equal, E may also be eliminated. Therefore, since the proportion of nitrogen greatly exceeds that of oxygen, A must be correct.

8. D Based upon phase solubility rules, the solubility of gases increases with increasing pressure and decreases with increasing temperature. This is why carbonated beverages are maintained under pressure and are best stored at lower temperatures.

9. E Silver salts are generally insoluble unless they contain nitrate, perchlorate, or acetate ions. Since nitrate salts are always soluble, there is no cation among the items that would result in precipitation. Therefore, at least one of the anions must result in an insoluble salt. Based upon the solubility rules of silver salts, only the acetate ion (item II) would result in a soluble salt, therefore both items I and III would make insoluble salts.

10. C A is incorrect because rate laws are dependent on the slowest step. If a reactant does not participate in the slow step, it will not be included in the overall rate law. B is incorrect because rate laws of overall reactions can only be determined experimentally. D is incorrect because while it is true that a catalyst comes out of a reaction unchanged, it can undergo temporary transformations during the reaction and revert back into its original form at the end. E may be eliminated because the units of the rate constant are dependent upon the order of the reaction. Therefore, C is the best option because rate laws can be determined from elementary steps of a reaction mechanism by simply raising the reactants to their respective coefficients.

11. D The rate-determining step of a reaction mechanism is the slowest step of that mechanism, eliminating A and B. The rate law of an elementary step can be determined from the coefficients of the reactants in the elementary step. Because Step 2 is the rate determining step, the overall rate law will be equivalent to the rate law for the step. Therefore, rate = $k[N_2O_2]\,[O_2]$.

12. C Since the reaction is exothermic, an increase in temperature will shift the equilibrium to the left, and the concentration of N_2 will increase, eliminating B, D, and E. For exothermic reactions, an increase in temperature will decrease the K_{eq}, eliminating A and making C the correct answer.

13. E All of the compounds are composed of three ions, so comparing K_{sp} values will give relative solubility. Since the question asks for an extreme, the middle values of the variable cannot be correct, eliminating A, B, and D. The compound with the lowest K_{sp} value will have the lowest solubility according to the K_{sp} expression, K_{sp} = [cation]*x*[anion]*y*, where *x* and *y* represent the coefficients and total 3. Therefore, E is correct.

14. D A graph showing the titration of a weak acid will start at a low pH and slope upward as the titrant (in this case, a strong base) is added. Therefore, A and B cannot be true. As the weak acid and titrant strong base react, water and salt are formed as products. The salt will determine the pH at the equivalence point. The conjugate acid of a strong base has no acidic properties and will be neutral in solution. However, the conjugate base of the weak acid will be weakly basic. Because of this, the pH at the equivalence point will be above 7.

15. B A higher pK_a means a weaker acid, while a lower pK_a means a stronger acid. Since this is a ranking question, start with the extremes. Compound I is a strong acid and will have the lowest pK_a, eliminating C and D. Compound II is the only base so it will have the largest pK_a and A and E can be eliminated.

16. B The Second Law explains that the entropy of the universe must increase for a spontaneous reaction or that disorder favors spontaneity, making B the best answer. Hess' Law (D) relates to the enthalpy of the reaction rather than the entropy and may be eliminated. The First Law explains that energy can neither be created nor destroyed, but does not explain the impact of disorder eliminating A. The Third Law relates to the entropy of a substance rather than its impact on spontaneity, eliminating C.

17. D Enthalpy of vaporization is the heat energy required per mole to change from the liquid to gas phase. He and N_2 are gases at room temperature, Br_2 and Hg are both liquids at room temperature, and Al is a solid at room temperature. Therefore, it is expected that Al will have the highest enthalpy of vaporization, making D correct.

Organic Chemistry

1. B Both C_1 and C_2 make up the triple bond. They are both *sp* hybridized so you can eliminate C, D, and E. C_3 is part of an allene. The bonds that it forms with its neighbors are linear (180°), so it is also *sp*. You can eliminate A, which leaves B as the correct answer. C_4 has a double bond and two single bonds so it is sp^2.

2. C Epimeric compounds are diasteromers that differ in configuration at a single chiral center (recall the relationship between sugar molecules). Subsequently, Items I and III are correct. Item II may be eliminated because diasteromers are non-superimposable AND non-mirror images of one another.

3. B Since this is a ranking question, look for obvious extremes and eliminate answers. A, C, and E should be eliminated because the eclipsed conformation is always the least stable due to sterics and electron repulsions in aligned bonds. D is the more enticing answer of the remaining two because the general rule of thumb is that the anti conformation is the most stable because the bulky groups are farthest apart, while they are 60° apart in a *gauche* conformation. This question is tricky, however, because in this case there is intramolecular hydrogen bonding which can occur in the *gauche* conformation, making it the most stable one (eliminate D).

4. A Nucleophiles are electron dense, since E is positively charged it would make a poor nucleophile. While neutral compounds that have lone pairs can be nucleophilic, negatively charged nucleophiles tend to be stronger (eliminate C and D). The stronger nucleophile is the more reactive nucleophile; more reactive corresponds to less stable. Therefore, the nucleophile that is less able to stabilize a negative charge will be the stronger nucleophile. For A and B, the negative charge resides on the C and O, respectively. Since carbon is less electronegative than oxygen, it is therefore less able to stabilize a negative charge, making cyanide the best nucleophile (eliminate B).

5. D This is an S_N2 reaction, since it occurs with inversion of stereochemistry. Therefore the rate of the reaction is determined by both the nucleophile and the haloalkane. Since alkyl groups are not able to stabalize a negative charge well, E may be eliminated. The halogen that can best stabilize a negative charge will be the best leaving group and give the fastest reaction. Acidity of HX acids increases going down the periodic table because the larger halogens can spread the negative charge over a larger surface area to stabilize it. Because iodine is the largest of the halogens, it is also the best leaving group.

6. D In an S_N2 reaction, the starting substrate undergoes a backside attack where the nucleophile attacks opposite the leaving group, causing a complete stereochemical inversion. A can be eliminated because the there is no intermediate in this reaction. B can be eliminated because S_N2 is a bimolecular process, as the name implies. C can be eliminated because the conformation of the groups is not an important factor for the S_N2 reaction. E may be eliminated because the formation of a carbocation is an important step during a S_N1 reaction.

7. B In a propagation step of a radical mechanism, there is no net change in the number of radicals in the reaction, as shown in this example. An initiation step results in a net increase in the number of radicals in the reaction (eliminate A). A termination results in a net decrease in the number of radicals in the reaction (eliminate C). Elimination and substitution reactions are not part of a typical radical reaction. Lastly, eliminate D since in this reaction a pi bond is broken.

8. C S_N1 and E1 reactions both involve the initial formation of a carbocation and therefore may involve carbocation rearrangements. Type 2 reactions cannot form carbocations as their mechanism involves 1 concerted step.

9. C When an alkyne is treated with two equivalents of hydrogen in the presence of platinum, it is reduced to an alkane. This results in the loss of both pi bonds from the triple bond, so eliminate A. The two pi bonds are converted to four C—H sigma bonds, so B and D can be eliminated.

10. B Although a minor product, given enough catalyst, heat, and time, the disubstituted products can form. In this reaction, two atoms of bromine will replace two hydrogens previously attached to the benzene ring. The bromine atoms can have either an *ortho* or *para* relationship to each other. This makes two possible isomers.

11. B Addition of water to 1-butene will only add one OH group, so cannot form a diol (eliminate D). Since there are no tertiary carbons on the starting material, a tertiary alcohol cannot be formed (eliminate C). Markovnikov addition results in the addition of the hydroxyl group to the most substituted carbon of a double bond. A can be eliminated because it represents addition of the hydroxyl group to the least substituted carbon. E may be eliminated because does not represent an addition reaction.

12. D Of the answers, only the nitro substituent is meta-directing and therefore, D is the best answer.

14. C Because H_a is bound to a carbon that is adjacent to two carbonyl groups, it is the easiest proton for a base to abstract since the conjugate base has the most resonance structures. Therefore, you can eliminate A. Because this molecule has a mirror plane, H_b and H_d are equivalent, so you can eliminates B and D, which leaves C as the correct answer. H_c is on a carbon that is not adjacent to any electron withdrawing groups or pi electrons, so it is the least acidic.

15. A A symmetrical aldol condensation is the same thing as a self-condensation reaction; it is an aldol condensation between two of the same molecule. In order for an aldol condensation to occur, at least one of the carbonyl compounds must be able to form an enolate through deprotonation of an a-carbon. Since 2,2,4,4-tetramethylpentan-3-one contains no a-hydrogens, it cannot form an enolate, and therefore cannot undergo a self-condensation reaction. All of the other molecules listed to have at least one a-hydrogen, and therefore can undergo self-condensation reactions.

16. A One signal on the ^{13}C NMR spectrum implies that either the molecule has only one carbon, or that all carbons in the molecule are equivalent. Since the empirical formula of Compound X is CH and the molecule contains no electronegative elements to shift the signal downfield, the single peak, located in the region common for alkenes and aromatic carbons (128 ppm), must represent some sort of sp^2-hybridized carbon(s). Any compound with only sp^2 hybridized carbons will have no stereoisomers, and in this case, the compound is benzene (C_6H_6).

17. C TLC separates compounds based on their polarities. The more polar a compound is, the more it adheres to the silica gel plate, giving it a smaller R_f value. A and D are inconsistent with this type of interaction. The product for this reaction is bromocyclohexane, which is more polar than the reactant due to the presence of the halogen.

18. C The structure of isobutane is shown below. All three terminal CH_3 groups are chemically identical, and will show up as one resonance. More specifically, they will correspond to a doublet as they are split by the sole proton on the central carbon. The proton on the central carbon will show up as a multiplet, as it is split by 9 equivalent H atoms. Thus, one 9H doublet and one 1H multiplet is the correct answer, A, which corresponds to *n*-butane.

Clockwise = R
Counter = S

NOTES

Chiral → non superimposable
centre: has 4 diff groups.

Constitutional: same formula, diff. order
Sterioisomers: same formula, diff spacial arrangement
① - enantiomer - mirror images
② - diasteriomers - more than one chiral centres.

Substitution = nucleophilic attack Ove w extra electrons to share

leaving group + attack.
SN_2 → all one step, rate = K[substrate][nuc]
SN_1 → multiple steps rate = K[substrate]

OH not a good leaving group
E → opposite   Z → same   based on priority

Elimination occurs @ Beta position

Saponification = Esters to carboxylic acids